D0886655

Explorers of the Body

Explorers
of the Body

STEVEN LEHRER

Doubleday & Company, Inc., Garden City, New York
1979

Library of Congress Catalog Card Number 78-14685
ISBN: 0-385-13497-5
Copyright © 1979 by Steven Lehrer

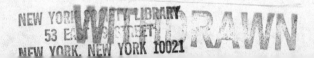

For Pamela

I wish to acknowledge my gratitude to the following:

Pamela Dunn Lehrer for her help with the research
Dr. Bernard Roswit for his support
Dr. Herbert Rosenthal for his assistance
Mr. Hugh O'Neill of Doubleday, "accoucheur par excellence"

Steven Lehrer
New York City

CONTENTS

---

ance of Chemotherapy; Antagonisms; The Fight Over
Streptomycin

"Write the things which thou hast seen, and the things which are, and the things which shall be hereafter."

Revelation 1:19

Explorers of the Body

INTRODUCTION

The art of healing is an old one. It antedates even the evolution of modern man more than one hundred thousand years ago and is also practiced by other primates. Chimpanzees, for example, have been observed to perform certain medical maneuvers on each other. They extract splinters from hands and feet by a method humans use: levering the splinter upward with two fingernails, to be caught and removed by the teeth. In Louisiana's Delta Regional Primate Center one chimp was photographed using a red cedar twig to pull a deciduous tooth from the mouth of another.

The science of healing is somewhat newer than the art. The decisive turn from supernaturalism to naturalistic, rational explanations of disease appears to have been made in Greece, sometime between 500 B.C. and A.D. 500. Hippocrates, a Greek physician, is generally credited with this innovation in medical thought.

Very little is known about Hippocrates. He was born on the small island of Cos, in the Aegean Sea, about 460 B.C. Evidently he traveled widely, and the writings of Plato and Aristotle indicate that he achieved great renown during his long life. While his existence cannot be doubted, most of the manuscripts attributed to him are of questionable authenticity.

Numerous contributions to the science of healing have been made since Hippocrates' time. A few, because of their revolutionary nature, stand out from the rest. This book tells the story of these great discoveries—and of the men and women responsible for them.

CHAPTER ONE

Muscle and Blood

How does the body work?

This question about the general nature of the life process is as old as human thought. Both philosophers and physicians have speculated and written about the mechanism of life and the special functions of body organs. Ancient man believed that the heart was the home of the soul. Fortunetellers used the livers of animals to try to predict the future. From these crude beginnings arose the science of physiology.

At first physiology appeared a gruesome and reprehensible business—certainly not a gentleman's pursuit. A first-century Roman scholar, Celsus, wrote a horrifying description of the activities of Alexandrian scientists: "They laid open men whilst alive—criminals received out of prison from the kings—and whilst these were still breathing, observed parts which beforehand nature had concealed, their position, colour, shape, size, arrangement, hardness, softness, smoothness, relation, processes, and depressions of each, and whether any part is inserted into or is received into another." Celsus deplored these experiments. "I believe that medicine should be rational. . . . But to open the bodies of men still alive is as cruel as it is needless." Further advances in physiology came from the dissection of dead animals and live ones.

The busiest dissector and vivisector in Rome was the second-century physician Galen. Though he never cut up ants, gnats, fleas, "and other minuscule creatures," Galen did manage to dissect the remainder of the animal kingdom: apes, horses, asses, mules, cows, camels, sheep, lions, wolves, dogs, lynxes, stags, bears, weasels, mice, snakes, a variety of fish and birds, and several elephants.

Galen limited dissection of live animals to pigs or goats, which he strapped to a board. Although he obtained much anatomical information from the barbary ape, he usually would not vivisect this little tailless creature, and recommended to other scientists that they "leave live apes alone." Perhaps the ape's facial expressions and cries while being cut up were human enough to be disturbing.

From his animal studies Galen managed to learn a few fundamental facts about how the body works. In one experiment, he cut the recurrent laryngeal nerve of a live pig and found that the animal could no longer squeal, thus identifying the origin of the voice and part of its control mechanism. Even more elegant was his identification of the optic nerve as being responsible for vision:

"When you have divided the frontal bone . . . you will be met by two nerves that go to the eye. If you divide the larger of the two, then the visual sense of the animal will be impaired. . . . But that the animal can no longer see . . . you can only appraise by deduction, from the fact that you find that it does not blink with its eye at anything which you bring near it, pretending to be about to stab home with it."

Galen also made the first correct observations of the functions of the spinal cord and the kidney. He noted that if the cord is cut "behind the first thoracic rib, then that damages the hand of the ape. And should the cut follow a line behind the second thoracic rib, then that does not damage the arm, except that the skin of the axillary cavity and upper arm become deprived of sensibility." In another experiment, the ureter of a living animal was tied, proving that urine is produced in the kidney.

Galen should have stopped here, but unfortunately he didn't. Instead, he tried to use what he had found and what he could contrive to explain one of the oldest of all mysteries: what the heart does, and why it is necessary to breathe. He failed, and fifteen centuries elapsed before this interaction of muscle and blood was understood—the first great triumph of the science of healing.

Of Pumps and Valves

The discovery of the circulation of the blood was made by a single scientist—William Harvey. Even today, more than three hundred years later, Harvey's finding is considered the most important advance in all of physiology, on a par with Newton's discovery of universal gravitation in physics. Our knowledge of the spread of infections and of the cause of many diseases depends on comprehension of blood circulation; without this comprehension, most of medicine as we know it today would not exist and doctors would be little more than witch doctors.

The recognition that the heart and blood are necessary for life is a primitive one. An association between cold, pallor, bloodlessness, and death has been common knowledge since antiquity. Vampires were believed to kill a victim by sucking out his blood, and the bloodiest of all wounds—a heart wound—was known to be invariably fatal.

The first detailed anatomic study of the heart was made around 400 B.C. and is included in a collection of ancient Greek medical treatises known as the Hippocratic corpus. The author, perhaps a Greek from Sicily, dissected the mammalian heart with exceptional skill, and though he saw it as having only two chambers rather than the four we know today, he discovered within it two interesting sets of membranes. There are two great vessels, he wrote, and "at the entrance of each are arranged three membranes, rounded at their extremities, in the shape of a half circle; and when they come together, it is marvelous to see how they close their orifices. . . . And if someone . . . takes the heart after death, and the membranes are spread out and made to lean against each other, water poured in will not penetrate into the heart, nor will air blown in; and this especially on the left; for that side has been constructed more precisely, as it should be, since the intelligence of man lies in the left cavity."

The marvelous membranes this unknown anatomist describes are the aortic and pulmonary valves. He obviously interprets them as static safety devices to prevent a messy mixing of blood and intelligence, testing his conclusion by pouring water into the stumps of the aorta and pulmonary artery to check whether the valves close properly; this is now routine in modern pathology. But he goes further by blowing into the severed vessels, a procedure fortunately not taught in pathology residencies today.

About 270 B.C., an Alexandrian physician, Erasistratos, made the next great contribution to cardiac physiology. Erasistratos discovered that the heart is not a static reservoir. It is a pump, with the right and left portions subdivided into upper and lower chambers (atrium and ventricle) separated by the bicuspid and tricuspid valves. These valves are made respectively of two and three roughly triangular flaps, anchored to the inner surface of the heart by cords. When the heart contracts, the valve flaps are pressed together to prevent blood from returning to the upper chambers. Erasistratos concluded correctly from his observations that the heart must receive blood from the veins and pump it out through the arteries.

Where the blood came from and went, however, remained a mystery. Veins and arteries were seen as sets of independent, dead-end canals. Blood and air were supposed to seep slowly toward the periphery, where they were used up. The lungs were considered to be chiefly for the purpose of cooling the blood. Galen recognized that the arteries contained blood, and not air as had been believed, but he still managed to explain the nature of the pulse beat incorrectly, and his faulty explanation was perpetuated by his writings for nearly fifteen hundred years.

A correct description of the anatomy of the heart was finally published in 1543 by Andreas Vesalius, a professor of surgery and anatomy at the University of Padua. In his book *De Humani Corporis Fabrica,* Vesalius showed that Galen had made two serious mistakes. The ascending vena cava, which Galen had originating in the liver, was demonstrated to be one of the two great veins which bring blood from the body back to the right side of the heart. Perhaps Galen had confused the vena cava with the hepatic vein, which does arise from the liver.

Galen's description of the septum dividing the right side of the heart from the left was also incorrect, for he somehow believed that it had openings connecting the two ventricles. How Galen could have arrived at this conclusion remains uncertain. Some abnormal hearts do have a septal opening, and surgeons today correct this problem by sewing a dacron patch over it. Galen might have noted such an orifice in one or two animal hearts and regarded it as the norm.

Vesalius, however, was able to show conclusively that the cardiac septum contains no openings.

For rectifying these and other mistakes Galen had made, Vesalius was showered with a torrent of abuse by his contemporaries. Sylvius, a former teacher, turned against his pupil angrily, calling Vesalius a madman. A former assistant, Colombo, sought to discredit and deride his teacher. Vesalius was not insensitive to such criticism; out of rage and disappointment he was reported to have burned notes being prepared for another publication.

Within a few years, however, the findings of Vesalius had been verified. And when combined with the work of two other men—Servetus and Colombo—they formed the anatomic basis for understanding blood circulation.

Miguel Servetus was a fellow student with Vesalius in Paris. At some period during his life as a physician he began to study the lungs and realized that blood filtered through them, mixed with air, changed color, and entered the left side of the heart. Unfortunately, Servetus turned his attention to religion and wrote a book critical of the holy Trinity. Persecuted, he fled to Geneva, hoping to find protection with another fellow student from Paris, the reformer John Calvin. But Calvin was not sympathetic and had him tried and condemned for heresy. Servetus was burned at the stake in 1553, supposedly with all copies of his works. Three did escape the flames, though we are uncertain as to whether his anatomical ideas were immediately appreciated.

Another anatomist working at the same time as Servetus, Realdus Colombo, also observed the circulation of blood through the lungs and the mixing there with air, and in addition noted the simultaneous beat of the two ventricles of the heart. Colombo published his findings in a book that appeared in the year of his death, 1559.

Now the anatomical information necessary for understanding the circulation of the blood was available, and the parallels with Newton's accomplishment, which occurred in the same century as William Harvey's, can be seen. Newton was able to take Kepler's laws of planetary motion, combine them with Galileo's laws of the motion of a falling body, and from these derive the notion of universal gravitation. Harvey was able to take the isolated facts known about the cardiovascular system and use them to explain just how this system works. In doing so, he laid the scientific basis for all of modern medicine.

William Harvey was born at Folkestone, in England, April 1, 1578. He was the eldest child in the large family of Thomas Harvey, a prosperous merchant and civic official. Several brothers became successful merchants, but William's scholarly nature destined him early in life for one of the professions. The scholarliness was still in evidence years later: While accompanying King Charles I and taking care of the princes during the battle of Edgehill, Harvey is described as sitting at the outskirts of the fight under a hedge reading a book.

Harvey was sent to King's School at Canterbury and then to Caius College at Cambridge, where he received the Bachelor of Arts degree in 1597. Shortly afterward, he enrolled at the medical school of the University of Padua. Here, where Vesalius had written his famous book, another great anatomist, Fabricius of Aquapendente, was at the peak of a distinguished career, lecturing in the windowless, six-tiered, oval amphitheater he had had specially designed for teaching anatomy. By candlelight, Harvey and several hundred other students stood and watched as the master dissected, disposing quickly of the unpreserved corpses to prevent their reek from overpowering everyone in the closed room. Years later, Harvey was to credit Fabricius with the discovery that first inspired the young anatomy student to consider the circulation of the blood. This was the identification of the venous valves.

Actually, the little venous valves had been observed long before Fabricius by Johannes Baptista Cannanus, a contemporary of Vesalius. But the first meticulous descriptions were not made until Fabricius published his book devoted to the subject, *De Venarum Ostiolis*. In this work, the structure, position, and distribution of the little valves are carefully noted and illustrated by fairly good drawings. Fabricius also clearly recognized that the valves offer opposition to the flow of blood from the heart towards the periphery, but failed to comprehend their true function of preventing retrograde flow, believing instead that they merely prevented too much blood from being heaped in one place. Harvey did not make this mistake.

After receiving the Doctor of Medicine degree from the University of Padua in 1602, Harvey returned to England, and in the same year was awarded another doctoral degree in medicine from Cambridge. He then settled in London to practice medicine, and was admitted as a candidate to the College of Physicians in 1604. In November of that year he married Elizabeth Browne, daughter of Lancelot Browne, former first physician to Queen Elizabeth.

What sort of man was this rising young doctor? Like Shakespeare, his contemporary, Harvey left us his works but not very much about himself. Most of our knowledge about his character derives from a librarian and biographer, John Aubrey. Harvey, wrote Aubrey, was a very short man with a "little eie, round, very black, full of spirit." He was temperamental and somewhat eccentric. As a young man he wore a dagger, in the fashion of the day, but was prone to draw it upon the slightest provocation. In his later years he liked to be in the dark because, he said, he could think better, and had underground caves constructed at his house in Surrey for meditation.

We do not know when Harvey began to form his notion of the circulation of the blood. His first musings on the subject appeared in a series of anatomical lectures that he delivered in 1616. His ninety-eight page set of notes still exists, and besides his genius these demonstrate that Harvey was a copious scribbler. He wrote hastily and almost illegibly in a mixture of Latin and English, and was a careless speller. In one place in his notes the word "piggg" appears, with a rather large number of g's even for seventeenth-century English.

His writings tell us that Harvey was initially quite overwhelmed by the enormous complexity of the cardiovascular system:

"When I first gave my mind to vivisections, as a means of discovering the motions and uses of the heart, and sought to discover these from actual inspection, and not from the writings of others, I found the task so truly arduous, so full of difficulties, that I was almost tempted to think . . . that the motion of the heart was only to be comprehended by God. For I could neither rightly perceive at first when the systole [contraction] and when the diastole [relaxation] took place, nor when and where dilatation and contraction occurred, by reason of the rapidity of the motion, which in many animals is accomplished in the twinkling of an eye, coming and going like a flash of lightning; so that the systole presented itself to me now from this point, now from that; the diastole the same; and then everything was reversed, the motions occurring, as it seemed, variously and confusedly together. My mind was therefore greatly unsettled, nor did I know what I should myself conclude, nor what to believe from others. . . ."

He solved the problem with a set of ingenious experiments. Though in some his calculations were incorrect, he managed to come to the right conclusions. There can be no doubt that Harvey had realized what he was going to find even before he formally began to look for it.

The first step was to prove that the amount of blood transmitted from the veins to the arteries is so great that all the blood in the body must pass through the heart in a short time. Physicians since Galen had erroneously believed that blood was constantly being produced from food consumed. To accomplish his proof, Harvey attempted to measure the amount of blood that the heart ejects with each beat and to establish the pulse rate.

Even today, the measurement of cardiac output is a complex and difficult procedure, and there are wide variations in results obtained by various methods. It is not surprising, then, that Harvey's measurements were not correct; but he came out with such a ridiculous figure —far below the lowest estimate used today—as to suggest that he lacked the ability of a skilled experimenter. He derived his results by measuring the volume of the left ventricle in one cadaver, then multiplying this figure by the pulse rate. But, in the first place, he measured the volume incorrectly, and then he made an enormous error by using a pulse rate of thirty-three beats per minute, about half the actual average rate. The final figure he obtained for cardiac output is less than one thirty-sixth of the lowest value accepted today. Nonetheless, Harvey had proved his point, because even by his calculations the output of the heart in thirty minutes far exceeded the total weight of blood in the body. Obviously Galen had been quite wrong in believing that the amount of food a man eats could produce blood continuously in any such volume.

The second step of Harvey's proof was to demonstrate that the amount of blood going to the extremities is much greater than is needed for the nutrition of the body. Here he used no specific measurements and argued instead largely by inference. In doing so, he made the important point that the blood must pass from the arteries to the veins in the extremities. This was ingeniously demonstrated by employing a bandage in such a way as to stop the flow in the veins of a man's arm while leaving the arteries open. As a result, the veins swelled but not the arteries. When the pressure was increased sufficiently to cut off arterial circulation as well, the veins did not swell. From his observations, Harvey reasoned correctly that the blood entered the extremities through the arteries and passed somehow to the veins. He looked for the channels of connection but, lacking a microscope, failed to find them. In 1661, four years after Harvey's death, Marcello Malpighi, using a crude microscope, located these tiny channels we now call capillaries in the lung of a frog.

The third step was to prove that blood in the veins flows toward the heart and not away from it, as Galen had believed. Harvey demonstrated this in an elegantly simple manner: He pressed one finger on a vein in a man's arm and moved the finger along the vein from below one valve to above the next. The blood thus pushed up the vein did not return to the emptied section. This established beyond doubt that the valves were one-way devices, thus destroying Galen's old theory that blood moved back and forth in the venous system like the ebb and flow of the tide.

In 1628 Harvey published his experiments in a little book entitled *Exercitatio Anatomica de Motu Cordis et Sanguinis in Animalibus*— "An Anatomical Treatise on the Movement of the Heart and Blood in Animals"—or *De Motu Cordis*. Here are his famous conclusions, soon destined to change the course of all medical thought:

"Since all things, both argument and ocular demonstration, show that the blood passes through the lungs and heart by force of the ventricles, and is sent for distribution to all parts of the body, where it makes its way into the veins and pores of the flesh, and then flows by the veins from the circumference on every side to the centre from the lesser to the greater veins, and is by them finally discharged into the vena cava and right auricle of the heart, and this in such quantity or in such afflux and reflux, thither by the arteries, hither by the veins, as cannot possibly be supplied by the ingesta, and is much greater than can be required for mere purposes of nutrition; it is absolutely necessary to conclude that the blood in the animal body is impelled in a circle, and is in a state of ceaseless movement; that this is the act or function which the heart performs by means of its pulse, and that it is the sole and only end of the movement and contraction of the heart."

Harvey probably never had any notion of the far-reaching consequences his discovery would have. Nothing else can explain the lack of care devoted to *De Motu Cordis*. The manuscript was sent to an obscure German printer, Wilhelm Fitzer of Frankfort-on-Main, and was produced on thin, cheap paper that quickly deteriorated. The finished work literally teemed with typographical errors, suggesting that Harvey did not even take the trouble to read proof. Except for the title page and two plates borrowed from Fabricius, there were no illustrations. But there was no lack of controversy.

The loudest critics were Jean Riolan, an anatomist on the faculty of the University of Paris, and his English student James Primrose. Riolan managed to induce his university to prohibit the teaching of Harvey's doctrine. Primrose, who had just been certified to practice medicine in England the year before with Harvey as one of his examiners, locked himself in a room for two weeks and produced quite a large book that refuted *De Motu Cordis* by rehashing all the old ideas. Harvey began to be referred to in some circles as "Circulator" —in the Latin sense of the word, which means quack. He preserved a stoic silence and in the end lived to see his work vindicated. In the meantime, his professional standing was quite unaffected because of his royal patrons.

This patronage began in 1609, when his brother John Harvey, who had obtained employment in the king's household, influenced James I to recommend William for an appointment at St. Bartholomew's Hospital as assistant physician. When the physician died in the summer of that year, Harvey succeeded him. The hospital at that time had about two hundred beds for patients in twelve wards, and the new physician's duties consisted of attending in the hall of the hospital for at least one day a week throughout the year and prescribing for treatment at any other time when specially needed. The physician was usually expected to live within the hospital grounds, but the rule was waived for Harvey since he lived not far away. He received an annual salary of twenty-five pounds, with two pounds extra for livery and a further eight pounds since he did not use the official residence. Three surgeons and an apothecary in charge of the dispensary formed the remainder of the staff.

In his free time, Harvey developed a large private practice, attending many of the most distinguished citizens, including Sir Francis Bacon and, after about 1618, King James himself as physician extraordinary. Though advanced in his physiologic views, Harvey was quite conservative in the remedies he prescribed for his patients; considering the wealth of worthless drugs and primitive state of medical therapeutics, such conservatism was probably best.

In 1625 King James fell ill for the last time, and Harvey led the team of doctors in attendance. After the king's death, a rumor quickly spread that his favorite, the Duke of Buckingham, had hastened the fatal outcome by applying remedies not approved by the doctors. As suspicion grew, the duke was actually accused of having poisoned the king, and in 1626 an inquiry was ordered by Parliament. Harvey was the most important witness of several who contributed to saving the duke's neck.

What may be called the best years of Harvey's life began with the ascent of the new king, Charles I. The appointment as physician extraordinary was continued, and Harvey received a special award for the care he had given the previous monarch. The new king and his physician quickly became the closest of friends, with the king always ready to help in furthering the biologic research. Harvey, in return, delighted in showing Charles anything of scientific interest. On one occasion a courtier received a severe chest injury that exposed his heart. Harvey was called to attend and he summoned the king, who was permitted to stick his fingers into the wound to feel the beating heart. If infection subsequently developed, at least the organisms were royal.

Harvey might have lived the rest of his days as a close confidant of the king with an excellent position but for the Civil War in England. Like many great scientists before and since, Harvey had little interest in politics, but he was soon to learn how a changed political climate could so sour his life as to make it barely tolerable.

Parliament had become quite restive under Elizabeth, though deferring to her as an aging woman and a national symbol. Neither James I nor his son Charles was to have this good fortune. Parliament would not grant either of these rulers adequate revenue, because it distrusted them both. Many members were Puritans, dissatisfied with the organization and doctrine of the Church of England. And Parliament was organized so that it could make resistance effective.

In 1629 the king and Parliament came to a deadlock. Charles attempted to rule without Parliament, which could legally meet only at the royal summons. The Scots were the first to rebel, rioting in Edinburgh in 1637 against attempts to impose the Anglican religion in Scotland. To raise funds to put down the Scottish rebellion, Charles convoked the English Parliament in 1640, for the first time in eleven years. When it proved hostile to him, he dissolved it and called for new elections. The same men were returned. The resulting body, since it sat theoretically for the next twenty years without new elections, is known historically as the Long Parliament.

The Long Parliament, far from assisting the king against the Scots, used the Scottish rebellion as a means of pressing its own demands. These were revolutionary from the outset. Parliament insisted that the chief royal advisers—Harvey was one—be not merely removed but impeached and put to death. In 1642 Parliament and king came to open war.

At the start of this civil war, Harvey was with the king. When Charles later established his headquarters at Oxford, Harvey remained with him, and in 1645 was made warden of Merton College. Here he resumed the work on embryology that he had begun years earlier with deer embryos, which was to result in the publication of his second book, *De Generatione Animalium; or, Anatomical Excitations, Concerning the Generation of Living Creatures*. But while he puttered with eggs and yolks, a powerful leader was coming to the fore.

This was a hitherto unknown gentleman named Oliver Cromwell, a devout Puritan and member of the parliamentary forces called Roundheads from the close haircuts they wore. Cromwell was able to organize a new and more effective military force, the Ironsides, in which extreme Protestant exaltation provided the basis for morale, discipline, and the will to fight. Gradually these men were able to crush the Royalist opposition.

Cromwell concluded that the defeated King Charles could not be trusted, that "ungodly" persons of all kinds put their hopes in him (what later ages would call counterrevolution), and that he must be put to death. Since Parliament resisted, Cromwell, with the support of the army, broke Parliament up.

When the defeated Charles fled from Oxford to surrender himself to the Scots, Harvey joined him for a time at Newcastle but was forced to leave the king when he was handed over to the parliamentary army, and was not allowed to go to him when he was imprisoned in the Isle of Wight. Charles' execution in 1649 left Harvey a broken and unhappy man, though even before this he had begun to suffer the consequences of having supported the wrong faction.

In 1643 he had been stripped of the post at St. Bartholomew's Hospital, one he had occupied for thirty-four years. His professional reputation was gradually eroded, and in his last years under Cromwell's Protectorate he was regarded as a political "delinquent," being forced to spend much of his time lodging in one or another of his brothers' houses outside London. During the Civil War his house was sacked and most of his papers were destroyed by parliamentary soldiers. The once-prominent physician was reduced at the end almost to incompetence in the eyes of his patients, as one, the Lady Anne Conway, describes in a letter to a friend:

"I heare that you have a great good opinion of Dr. Harvey. I thinke you do well . . . : he is a most excellent anatomist, and I conceive that to be his Masterpiece, which knowledge is many times of great use in consultations, but in the practicke parte of Physicke I conceive him to be too mutch, many times governed by his Phantasy, the excellency and strength whereof did produce his two workes to the world. . . .

"I grieve much Dearest that you are not yet out of Dr. Harvey's hands. . . .

"When once I have ended my tryalles of Dr. Harvey which I thinke will be very shortly. He is very ill himselfe of the gowte almost continually, and that must needs indispose him to the mindings of such things as relates not to his owne perticuler (yet he pretends very much to study and lay my case to heart)."

Another colleague put the matter more succinctly: "I know several practitioners that would not have given threepence for one of his bills."

Deeply despondent, racked with pain by gout and kidney stones, Harvey at age eighty was forced to move once again, this time to his brother Eliab Harvey's house at Roehampton. There he awoke one morning, partially paralyzed and unable to speak, and shortly after, on June 3, 1657, he died.

The Flower of English Medicine

At the time of Harvey's death his great discovery was still only of theoretical interest. What, after all, could a physician offer a patient whose heart was not contracting properly? This question probably never even occurred to Harvey, because no one at the time recognized the relationship between heart disease and dropsy, a condition in which the tissues and cavities of the body fill up with water, frequently on account of a weak heart.

The greatest discovery in the field of cardiology was made by a man who identified digitalis, a drug so effective for treating a weakened heart muscle that no better substitute has been found for two hundred years. This man was an English physician, William Withering.

For centuries the common form of dropsy—now called cardiac edema—was one of the most frequent causes of death, and an unpleasant death it was. Dr. Samuel Johnson, the great eighteenth-century lexicographer, died of dropsy after suffering intensely, his legs becoming so painfully bloated that his physicians vainly tried to let the fluid out by making large knife incisions.

Yet since antiquity a few rather bizarre and unreliable concoctions sometimes helped a patient with dropsy. The dried bulb of the squill, a plant of the lily family native to the Mediterranean area, was known as a medicine to the ancient Egyptians and is mentioned in the Ebers Papyrus, written around 1500 B.C. The Romans used squill to treat dropsy, to strengthen the heart, to induce vomiting, and— ominously—to poison rats, for the effective ingredient in squill, called a cardiac glycoside, will accomplish all these functions as the dose is increased. Strophanthus, the seeds of a genus of African shrubs and woody vines used to make arrow poison, contains another cardiac glycoside and was also introduced into medicine. The dried skin of the common toad has been used for centuries as a drug by the Chinese. Called *ch'an su,* it was highly recommended for toothache and bleeding of the gums, as well as dropsy. We now know that *ch'an su* contains epinephrine, an arterial constrictor, combined with a cardiac glycoside. The beneficial effects were also known to the peasants of Western Europe, who had used powdered toad skins medicinally for centuries.

One folk remedy, however, was favored by these same peasants above all others. This medicine came from a tall plant with long pointed leaves and lovely, delicate purple flowers shaped like bells. For centuries it had grown wild through most of Europe, and its dried, powdered leaves were known to bring relief for many dropsy-sufferers. This plant was *Digitalis purpurea,* the purple foxglove.

We know that digitalis had been used since at least the thirteenth century by Welsh physicians, for they mentioned it in their writings as *menygellydon,* which means "elves gloves." The word foxglove is of uncertain origin, but some etymologists believe it is derived from the name of an ancient musical instrument that consisted of bells hung from an arched support; very likely the little purple bell-shaped flowers hanging from the foxglove stalk looked similar. Even the Norwegian word for foxglove means "fox music."

In 1542 the first accurate scientific description of foxglove was given by a German botanist, Leonhard Fuchs. He named the plant genus *Digitalis,* from the Latin *digitus,* meaning "finger"; but why he chose this word is uncertain. Perhaps the German name for the plant, *Fingerhut,* meaning "thimble," was the origin. More likely, the tall, fingerlike vertical stalk from which the foxglove flowers hang suggested the word.

Fuchs did more than name *Digitalis purpurea.* In his 1542 history of plants, he categorized digitalis as being of value in inducing vomiting and "in its action to thin, to dry up, to purge, and to free of obstructions." John Gerard confirmed one of these observations in 1597, noting that he had used foxglove to induce vomiting. More important, the plant's value in treating dropsy was noted a few years after Fuchs's account by the Dutch medical biologist Rembert Dodoens, who wrote that "for those who have water in the belly . . . it draws off the watery fluid, purifies the choleric fluid, and opens the obstruction."

Digitalis had been included in the London Pharmacopoeia by 1661, though recommended for the wrong purposes—for epilepsy and as a sedative. And a few years later an English physician, William Salmon, became convinced that digitalis was the long-sought treatment for tuberculosis.

Salmon's error was a logical one at the time, since there was still a great deal of confusion between pulmonary tuberculosis, where digitalis is of no value, and pulmonary edema or fluid in the lungs due to heart failure, which can be dramatically helped by digitalis. When an eighteenth-century physician administered digitalis to a patient with pulmonary edema thinking the patient had tuberculosis, and the patient's condition improved, no conclusion could be more obvious than that here was a remedy for tuberculosis. This mixup between pulmonary tuberculosis and pulmonary edema persisted well into the nineteenth century.

No confusion, however, existed in Salmon's mind about the side effects and toxicity of digitalis when given in excessive amounts. For this reason he recommended that the drug be given only in very small doses. When doctors ignored this advice and subsequently killed patients with digitalis, the Dutch physician Hermann Boerhaave, one of the most respected men in eighteenth-century Europe, declared that digitalis was a poison and cautioned against its use.

The most crushing indictment of digitalis came with the experiments of a Dr. Salerne of Orleans in 1748. Hearing that a turkey had died after eating foxglove, Salerne proceeded to stuff foxglove powder down the throats of two healthy turkeys in the vigorous manner that Frenchmen usually reserve for geese in the making of pâté de foie gras. The two turkeys did not survive these ministrations, and an autopsy revealed that their intestines had been squeezed as dry as grapes in a wine press.

Salerne should have concluded that digitalis was indeed a good drug for ridding the body of excess fluid, but instead he reported to the French Academy of Sciences that the compound was a powerful poison. The Academy, at that time the final authority in European medicine, condemned the use of digitalis in medical practice, and here matters stood for a quarter century until William Withering decided to reinvestigate the subject.

Withering was born in 1741 into a family of distinguished physicians. His maternal grandfather had delivered Samuel Johnson, and his father was a successful physician at Wellington in Shropshire. William was afforded the impeccable education of the English upper class, which included mathematics, the classical languages, geography, and history. He was an average student and showed no sign in school of the remarkable insight that was to result in his great discovery.

At the age of twenty-one Withering decided to study medicine, and entered the University of Edinburgh, a school which had great appeal for English students in the eighteenth and nineteenth centuries. Oxford and Cambridge had degenerated into shadows of their former selves, becoming chiefly schools for the training of clergymen. The great historian Edward Gibbon had left Oxford in disgust after one year because he found his tutors "plunged deep in port and prejudice." But the Edinburgh faculty was superb, numbering among its members some of the greatest scientists of the day.

Withering made many warm friends at Edinburgh, and throughout his life continued to correspond with teachers and classmates of his student days. He learned to play golf on the famous Scottish greens, and also became an accomplished musician with an incredible mastery of the German flute, the harpsichord, and the bagpipes. He took his degree of doctor of physic on July 31, 1766, after a successful defense of an inaugural dissertation on malignant putrid sore throat, later published under the title *De Angina Gangrenosa.*

In the eighteenth century no fashionable young English gentleman could consider his formal education complete until he had made the *de rigueur* trip to the Continent. Withering made such a journey during the summer and autumn of 1766 with a companion, a Mr. Townsend, described as "a gentleman of independent fortune familiar with the manners and language of the French." Midway through the trip Mr. Townsend had a bit of bad luck, described by Withering in a note to his parents: "I have been so much taken up for some days past that it was impossible to find time to write; I have lost my Fellow traveller Mr. Townsend; an abscess formed upon his shoulder, a Fever came on, the wound gangren'd and yesterday he died." This was the not infrequent result of an infection before the days of antibiotics.

After arriving home at Christmas, Withering began to consider the matter of setting himself up in a general practice. Flattering offers came from Chester and Coventry, but he finally selected the small town of Stafford, county seat of Staffordshire. This was a spot fairly near home, where the medical reputation both of his father and his uncles was well known. He became physician to the newly built infirmary, and though he was well liked, the people of the community were slow to accept a newcomer, leaving a great deal of free time for the new doctor to fill.

Withering chose to occupy this time engaged in the study of botany, and for a rather romantic reason. As a student he had detested the subject, speaking of "the disagreeable ideas I have formed of the study of botany." But one of his first Stafford patients was a charming young woman, Helena Cooke, whom it was necessary to visit almost daily. Miss Cooke passed the hours of her long convalescence by painting flowers, and Withering fell into the habit of searching the countryside for new specimens. Her style was so greatly admired that on September 17, 1772, Miss Cooke became Mrs. Withering.

Along with a new wife, Withering had managed to acquire a first-rate knowledge of plants, and he soon published *A Botannical Arrangement of All the Vegetables Naturally Grown in Great Britain According to the System of the Celebrated Linnaeus,* still considered a classic text. One particular section is of great interest today, because it contains the first cautious comments on the medicinal properties of the foxglove: "A dram of it taken inwardly excites violent vomiting. It is certainly a very active medicine and merits more attention than modern practice bestows on it."

The study of foxglove that was to make Withering famous was prompted by a medical consultation: "In the year 1775, my opinion was asked concerning a family receipt for the cure of the dropsy. I was told that it had long been kept a secret by an old woman in Shropshire, who had sometimes made cures after the more regular practitioners had failed. I was informed also, that the effects produced were violent vomiting and purging; for the diuretic effects seemed to have been overlooked. The medicine was composed of twenty or more different herbs; but it was not very difficult for one conversant in these subjects, to perceive, that the active herb could be no other than the Foxglove."

The diuretic effect referred to is the one so valuable in the treatment of dropsy, for when it occurs, the body rids itself of copious quantities of unwanted fluid through the kidneys. Withering noted this beneficial action in a few patients he treated in Stafford, but presently an even greater opportunity to use digitalis arose. An offer came from Erasmus Darwin, grandfather of Charles Darwin, to sponsor a practice in Birmingham, and Withering was soon busier than ever before with dropsy cases. Here is a record of the remarkable results in one, a Miss Hill of Aston, who was in the last stages of heart failure with extreme shortness of breath when a liquid digitalis preparation was administered by mouth:

"The patient took five . . . draughts, which made her very sick, and acted very powerfully on the kidneys, for within the first twenty-four hours she made upwards of eight quarts of water. The sense of fulness and oppression across her stomach was greatly diminished, her breath was eased, her pulse became more full and regular, and the swellings of her legs subsided.

"26th. Our patient being thus snatched from impending destruction, Dr. Darwin proposed to give her a decoction of pareira brava and guiacum shavings, with pills of myrrh and white vitriol; and if costive, a pill with calomel and aloes. To these propositions I gave a ready assent.

"30th. This day Dr. Darwin saw her, and directed a continuation of the medicines last prescribed."

This case is quite a notorious one in the history of digitalis. Withering, writing the report nine years later, stated that when he suggested the drug, "Dr. Darwin very politely acceded immediately to my proposition and, as he had never seen it given, left the preparation and dose to my direction." Yet Darwin jumped into print almost immediately after with a paper that did not mention Withering, and forgot him again in another article, "An Account of the Successful Use of Foxglove in Some Dropsies and in the Pulmonary Consumption," published in the *Medical Transactions of the College of Physicians*. The two men then became bitter enemies, though Withering was to retain priority for his great discovery.

Darwin was not able to convince the medical profession with his two unscrupulously published works that he had found anything worthwhile. Withering, however, managed to inaugurate the systematic use of digitalis. He kept full records of his extensive case experience, and after ten years' careful observation published in 1785 a detailed and systematic treatise, *An Account of the Foxglove, and Some of its Medical Uses: with Practical Remarks on Dropsy and Other Diseases*.

In this book, the fundamentals of digitalis treatment were correctly established for the first time. A dose of one or two grains twice daily was advised for patients beginning therapy—the amount still prescribed today. Withering also recognized that slow digitalization required several days to achieve. Equally important, he appreciated digitalis toxicity and cautioned against overdosage. He found that the drug was effective until evidence of its action upon "the kidneys, the stomach, the pulse, or the bowels" was apparent; then it was to be stopped. The description of an overdosed patient is most striking.

"I have lately been told that a person in the neighborhood of Warwick possesses a famous family recipe for the dropsy, in which the Foxglove is the active medicine, and a lady from the western part of Yorkshire assures me that the people in her country often cure themselves of dropsical complaints by taking Foxglove tea. In confirmation of this I recollect about two years ago being desired to visit a travelling Yorkshire tradesman. I found him incessantly vomiting, his vision indistinct, his pulse 40 in a minute. On enquiry it came out that his wife had stewed a large handful of green foxglove leaves in half a pint of water and given him the liquor which he drank at a draught in order to cure him of an asthmatic affection. This good woman knew the medicine of her county, but not the dose of it, for her husband narrowly escaped with his life."

Especially important in the *Account* was Withering's brilliant recognition of the action of digitalis, "a power over the motion of the heart, to a degree yet unobserved in any other medicine." Thus did Harvey's discovery of the circulation first become applicable to a pathologic condition.

By the time the *Account* was published, Withering had become highly successful. His practice had grown to bring him an annual income of two thousand pounds per year—an immense sum at that time —despite the fact that he held a daily free clinic for the poor and is said to have treated three thousand cases annually without charge. He had also become a member of the Lunar Society, a select scientific organization which numbered among its members James Watt, inventor of the steam engine, Josiah Wedgewood, the pottery manufacturer, and Joseph Priestley, the discoverer of oxygen. Benjamin Franklin was a guest at one meeting, and he consulted Withering by letter regarding the treatment of his kidney stones.

But just as he reached the peak of his career, Withering was struck by consumption. Two serious attacks in 1783 and 1786 forced him to give up work entirely and go to the country to regain his health. In 1790 he had a serious attack of pleurisy, and until his death he was plagued by shortness of breath and frequent coughing up of blood. To escape the damp English winters, he spent two seasons in Portugal, somehow finding strength to study the tropical and semi-tropical plants not seen in England.

The 1793 trip to Portugal proved to be his last. He bought a beautiful country estate in September 1799, but on the date he was to move in, Mrs. Withering was taken ill and could not accompany him; this, in addition to the fatigue of the journey, sent him to bed, and he died October 6, 1799. During the last days, a friend who came to see him produced the most distasteful pun in the whole history of medicine: "The flower of English medicine is indeed withering."

The Flame of Life

In 1794, five years before William Withering's quiet death in bed, another scientist had died much more violently—on the guillotine. This man, Antoine Lavoisier, made the final great contribution to our understanding of the circulation by demonstrating conclusively why breathing is necessary. Lavoisier, a chemist and not a physician, was able to show that breathing allows the flame of life to burn in essentially the same way as the flame of a candle—by combustion of carbon.

Though respiration is one of the oldest physiologic functions man has observed, for thousands of years it remained the most mysterious. The eyes were necessary to see, the ears to hear, the kidneys to make urine, the heart to pump; but what did the lungs do?

The ancient Greeks thought they had the answer: The lungs somehow sucked the blood from one part of the body to another. Aristotle was sure he had a better idea. Noting that the lungs were well supplied with blood, he postulated that their function must be to cool the blood and produce mucus. A few years later, Erasistratos, who had brilliantly recognized the pumping function of the heart, stated that the arteries were empty pipes filled with air by the lungs. Galen rectified this error by demonstrating that the arteries contained blood and not air, but was unable to explain breathing.

So matters stood for seventeen centuries until an Englishman, Robert Boyle, began to experiment. Today every high school chemistry student recognizes the name of this scientist in Boyle's law: The volume of a gas is inversely proportional to the pressure on it, provided temperature is kept constant. But Boyle was responsible for much more, including investigation of the physics of colors, the chemistry of acids and bases, and the specific gravity of body fluids.

Boyle's work on respiration was stimulated by news of a novel invention. In 1650 a German, Otto von Guericke, had used a suction pump to empty a wine barrel filled with water and produce what all philosophers had believed to be impossible—a vacuum. Going further, Guericke pumped the air from two metal hemispheres and then amazed a large group of spectators by connecting a team of horses to each hemisphere. Straining in opposite directions, the two teams could not pull the hemispheres apart. Guericke was obviously something of a showman, since he probably knew that one of the teams of horses could have been eliminated simply by anchoring one of the hemispheres to a wall.

When in 1657 Boyle read the first accounts of these experiments, he set out to construct a similar device. The resulting pump designed by his assistant, Robert Hooke, was easily operated by one man and moderately airtight—the first deliberately designed air pump. Its receiver, seven to eight gallons in volume, was made of glass and fitted so that objects could be readily put into it before pumping and then could be manipulated in the vacuum.

With his new air pump, Boyle was able to carry out a large number of experiments. He demonstrated how a deflated bladder swelled in the vacuum, how the mercury in a barometer fell, and how the ticking of a watch suspended by a thread grew fainter and stopped as air was removed. Most dramatic was the way a bird or kitten without air languished and eventually died in an environment that would not allow a candle to burn. Throughout the next century this fascination with the effect on animals was so great that Boyle's experiment was widely repeated by amateur scientists and is now represented by a famous painting in the Tate Gallery in London, "The Air Pump," by Joseph Wright of Derby. In a charming genre scene, Wright depicted an experimenter using the pump to suffocate a bird in a bell jar, while a small child looks on in horror.

Robert Hooke, working on his own, went a bit further than Boyle had. Opening widely the thorax of a dog, he demonstrated that the animal could be kept alive by artificial respiration in absence of all movements of the chest wall. This experiment had been done before, and is described in the writings of Vesalius. But Hooke ingeniously demonstrated that the animal could also be kept alive without any movement of the lung at all. To do this, the lung was kept motionless but thoroughly distended by maintaining a powerful blast with a bellows, the air driven in escaping continually through minute holes pricked in the lung. Thus the mere movement of the lungs in breathing, previously believed to be the essential factor, was shown to be unimportant. The purpose of breathing was to keep a supply of fresh air in constant contact with the lung tissue.

Hooke is perhaps the most eccentric figure in the history of science. One of the greatest of all experimenters, he left his imprint in chemistry and physics as well as physiology. By physics students he is remembered for Hooke's law: The displacement of an elastic body is directly proportional to the force applied to it. He was also the foremost English microscopist. But during his lifetime visitors attracted by his fame must have been surprised when meeting him.

No artist or rock musician of today has a shaggier or more unkempt appearance than did Hooke. His great uncombed mane almost covered an ashen face, while his crooked figure and shrunken limbs grew smaller and more deformed with the years. His parsimony and his crabbed, sour, jealous, vain, and morbid character made him one of the most well-known misers in England.

Not being satisfied to make many of the great discoveries of his age, Hooke also demanded the rest. When Newton's *Principia* was in the process of publication, Hooke so insistently claimed part of the work was stolen from him that Newton determined to suppress a third of the volume, and would have done so except for the intervention of Edmund Halley. Later, when Newton completed *Optics,* he ascertained that Hooke had claims upon it, and steadfastly refused to publish until after Hooke's death. When this occurred, several thousand pounds were found in an old iron chest in Hooke's dingy lodgings; the rusty key was said to have been unused for thirty years, though his physiologic experiments had provided another key that was employed almost immediately.

In 1669 Richard Lower, an English physician, used Hooke's method of artificial respiration to observe the blood in the pulmonary veins—the vessels that go from the lungs to the heart. Lower noted that when an animal was suffocated, the blood in the pulmonary veins and the left side of the heart became dark and venous. Taking this dark blood and injecting it into the lungs, he found that it became bright red only if fresh air was driven through the lungs simultaneously. He then concluded correctly that the change in color was due simply to the exposure of the blood to air in the lungs. This was confirmed by the fact that a clot of dark venous blood soon became bright red on the upper surface where it had been exposed to air, and if it was turned upside down, the dark undersurface also turned bright red.

Following Lower's work, the final important seventeenth-century observation of respiration was made by another Englishman, John Mayow. Mayow used a bell jar inverted over water in which he placed small animals, lighted candles, and combustible materials, noting that the extinction of life and flame were associated with a reduction in volume of the contained air. Though thereby proving that only a portion of the air is necessary to support life and flame, Mayow failed to identify this portion as oxygen. Here knowledge of respiration might have remained indefinitely fixed but for the revolution that was taking place in chemistry.

Chemistry had evolved from the alchemy of the Middle Ages and its preoccupation with converting metals such as lead into gold. To the alchemists, all matter was supposed to be made up of a "prima materia" modified by four elements—earth, air, fire, and water. By the eighteenth century, these had been differentiated into three varieties—mercurial, vitreous, and combustible. In addition to the elements, there were four spirits—sulfur, mercury, arsenic, and sal ammoniac. There were also six bodies—gold, silver, copper, lead, tin, and iron. And the "soul" of all matter was believed to be a hypothetical substance—phlogiston—by virtue of which all combustible bodies burned.

The first large cracks in this imposing alchemical structure were made by Joseph Priestley, the son of a weaver in the small English town of Leeds. Orphaned at an early age, he had been adopted by an aunt, a strong-minded woman of independent temper, whose influence led to his ordination as a Calvinist minister who eventually adopted Unitarian views.

On a trip to London shortly after his marriage, Priestley met the famous philosopher from the American colonies Benjamin Franklin, and the encounter was a turning point. Up to this time, the young minister had taken only a casual interest in science, but when he suggested to Franklin that someone ought to write a popular book on electricity, Franklin urged him to do so. The result was Priestley's brilliant work *The History and Present State of Electricity*. In writing, he was led to investigate for himself certain disputed points of electrical theory, and, through his natural flair for research, he made some original discoveries, one of which was the fact that carbon is an excellent conductor of electricity. So successful was the book that a year after its publication Priestley was elected to the Royal Society.

Priestley's great blow to the old alchemical theories came with his discovery that air is not an elementary substance. Instead, it is composed of several gases, one of which, oxygen—which he called "dephlogisticated air"—is the one essential to the life of animals. On August 1, 1774, he made some oxygen and was astonished at how brightly a candle burned in it. On March 8, 1775, he put a mouse into oxygen and noted how well the animal breathed in it. Shortly thereafter he wrote to Franklin, "Hitherto only two mice and myself have had the privilege of breathing it." His further experiments revealed that green plants breathe out oxygen in sunlight, thus providing for the animals that need it.

Though extremely conservative scientifically, Priestley was quite radical in his theological and political beliefs, and was as well a rather difficult, cold, cantankerous, precise, prim, puritanical individual. Naturally, a great scientist does not achieve immortality for his pleasing personality, but in Priestley's case, a more acceptable disposition and set of political convictions might have made life much smoother.

Priestley finally got into trouble with his support of the French Revolution, a very unpopular issue in some parts of England. In 1791, on the second anniversary of the fall of the Bastille, he had joined a group of friends to celebrate the event when a hysterical mob that had set fire to two dissident churches set out to burn down Priestley's house, hoping to be able to lynch him and his family as well. Priestley tried to bribe the leaders and, failing, took refuge with friends while the howling crowd looted his house, scattered his papers, battered down the walls, and made a bonfire of the debris.

Several hours later the mob went in search of Priestley. He and his family escaped in a coach with only a few minutes to spare, emigrating to the United States not long afterward. In America he continued to be hounded by tragedy. First his favorite son died and, shortly afterward, his wife, who had never recovered from the shock of the riots. Yet the great scientist did become a close friend of President Thomas Jefferson, who once told him, "Yours is one of the few lives precious to mankind."

More fortunate than Priestley was his contemporary at the University of Edinburgh, Joseph Black, a man able to engage in research unhindered by violent mobs. Studying the decomposition by heat of caustic lime, Black identified a by-product, the gas carbon dioxide, then known as "fixed air." This substance had been produced a hundred years before by Jean Baptiste van Helmont, but Black went further by demonstrating that it was present in the expired air of man and would not support life.

Now most of the information needed to understand the process of respiration was at hand. The man who finally provided this understanding—with theory supported by experiment—was Antoine Laurent Lavoisier.

Some scientists are great theoreticians but poor experimenters. William Harvey, who recognized the circulation of the blood though he could not even measure the pulse rate accurately, was one such, and Gregor Mendel, who perceived that individual hereditary characteristics are determined by two particles, though he very probably falsified his experimental results to prove this, was another. Two further examples are James Watson and Francis Crick, who determined the DNA structure using only chemical theory and the facts about the molecule already known. Other scientists are skilled experimenters without being great theoreticians. Rosalind Franklin, who identified and made elegant X-ray crystallographic studies of the A and B forms of DNA, is an example. But Lavoisier was both a superb experimentalist and a brilliant theoretician, and his contribution to the science of healing is universally regarded as the most important of all those made in the eighteenth century.

Lavoisier was born in Paris on August 26, 1743, the only son of well-to-do parents. His mother died when he was quite young, and he was brought up with loving care by his father and a maiden aunt. His father wanted him to become a lawyer, and Antoine dutifully complied, studying law at Mazarin College, qualifying as Bachelor of Law in 1763 and as Licentiate in 1764.

A taste for science, however, had developed in the young man. In college he had taken courses in astronomy, botany, chemistry, and geology, and upon finishing law school he quickly turned to science again. In 1765 Lavoisier published his first paper on chemistry, using the careful quantitative approach that was later to make him famous. He also won a medal from the king in a prize essay contest on metropolitan street lighting. In 1768, when he was but twenty-five years old, he was admitted to membership in the Academy of Sciences. Soon Lavoisier was being assigned to commissions upon the recommendation of the greatest scientists in France, usually also writing the reports of the commissions' findings for presentation to the Academy. But at just this time he made the mistake which was to cost him his head.

Because of his resolve to pursue a career in science, Lavoisier arranged to assure himself of sufficient financial means by buying a part share in the Ferme Générale, a widely hated, privately owned organization to which the French monarchy farmed out a profitable tax-gathering monopoly. Throughout his life, Lavoisier profited by his association with this organization and he seems to have been quite fair with those from whom the taxes were collected.

At age twenty-eight, Lavoisier married Marie Anne Pierrette Paulze, the fourteen-year-old daughter of a prominent member of the Ferme. Though it was a marriage of convenience arranged by the father to save his daughter from marrying an elderly, disreputable nobleman, Lavoisier and his young bride proved to be a happy pair. Marie was both a gifted linguist and a skilled artist, who translated scientific works for her husband and prepared excellent illustrations of his experiments. As a hostess she made the Lavoisier home a popular meeting place for French and foreign scientists. And after her husband's execution she edited and printed privately his last work, compiled in prison, *Mémoires de Chimie*. Her life was ultimately embittered by an unhappy, short second marriage to Count Rumford. Rumford was a renowned scientist and inventor, but also an adventurer possessing no patience with his wife's domestic inclinations. During one party, to show his disdain for Marie, he publicly threw a pot of boiling water over her prized bed of flowers. During such times, the former Mme. Lavoisier no doubt longed for the period during which she assisted her first husband in his experiments.

Of these, the greatest are the ones Lavoisier performed at age twenty-nine, one year after his marriage. While they were in part a repetition of Priestley's work, both men were actually performing almost a caricature of one of the classic experiments of alchemy.

First, red oxide of mercury was heated using a burning glass, in a vessel in which the gas produced—oxygen—could be observed and collected. This was the qualitative part of the experiment, but to Lavoisier's mind a revolutionary new idea was suggested: Run the experiment in both directions and measure exactly the quantities that are exchanged. Initially, mercury was burned so that it absorbed oxygen, and the exact amount of oxygen taken up from a closed vessel was determined from the difference in weight between the beginning of the burning and the end. Then the process was reversed by vigorously heating the mercuric oxide formed so that it would again expel the oxygen. When elemental mercury was left behind and the oxygen had flowed into the vessel, Lavoisier once more measured the proportions and found exactly the same amount of oxygen was given off as had been taken up before.

Quite suddenly, the process of chemical combination had been revealed for what it is, the coupling and uncoupling occurring between fixed quantities of two substances. Lavoisier had brilliantly dispatched the old notions of phlogiston, essences, and principles by showing that two elements, mercury and oxygen, had been demonstrably put together and taken apart. As he said, "This discovery, which I have established by experiments that I regard as decisive, has led me to think that what is observed . . . may well take place in the case of all substances that gain weight by combustion. . . ."

These new principles were slowly accepted by most scientists, though a few continued to cling to the old theory. A whole new nomenclature had to be devised, for "earth," "air," "fire," and "water" were no longer sufficient. Lavoisier, with other leading French chemists, composed this terminology, and with minor revision it is still in use today.

Early during his studies of combustion Lavoisier guessed that what had occurred in his glass beakers might also occur in the animal body. Working with the French mathematician Pierre Laplace, he designed a set of elegant experiments to verify this theory. By accurately measuring a guinea pig's intake of oxygen and output of carbon dioxide and heat—the latter with an ice calorimeter they invented—the two men were able to demonstrate that the animal produced the same amount of heat during consumption of a predetermined amount of oxygen as was produced by burning charcoal consuming the same amount of oxygen. From their studies, Lavoisier and Laplace concluded: "Respiration is therefore a combustion, admittedly very slow, but otherwise exactly similar to that of charcoal; it takes place in the interior of the lungs, without the evolution of light, since the matter of fire set free is immediately absorbed by the moisture of those organs. . . ."

Lavoisier erred in believing that combustion took place in the lungs rather than in the tissues, but this mistake may certainly be said to have been made up for by the breadth and depth of his other investigations. He was the first scientist to show that water is made of hydrogen and oxygen and is, therefore, a compound rather than an element—another blow to alchemy. He also made valuable contributions to the study of political economy, the science of agriculture, and public education. There is no way to guess what else this brilliant man might have achieved had he lived longer, for the most violent segment of the French Revolution tragically coincided with the peak of his scientific career.

In 1793, to repress all counterrevolution, the revolutionary government of France, called the Convention, created a kind of supreme political police and set up what we now call "the Terror." Designed to protect the new republic from its internal enemies, the Terror struck at those who were in league against the republic, and at those who were merely suspected of hostile activities. The number of persons who lost their lives in the Terror, from the late summer of 1793 to July 1794, is small by twentieth-century standards. Yet about forty thousand persons died in it, most on the guillotine, though some by other methods. At Nantes, for example, two thousand people were loaded on barges and deliberately drowned. Victims of the Terror included Marie Antoinette and other royalists, former revolutionaries, and Lavoisier.

The tax-collecting Ferme Générale was, after the royal family, one of the first targets. No one then had any more love for revenue agents than we do today. On November 14, 1793, Lavoisier, his father-in-law, and their colleagues on the Ferme were ordered arrested. Since he had been scrupulously honest in his dealings, Lavoisier was finally accused of such crimes as trying to poison the Paris air by erecting a large wall in the city. When his attorney asked that consideration be given to Lavoisier's scientific achievements and their benefit to the nation, the judge, one Jean Baptiste Coffinhal, snapped back that the republic had no need for scientists.

Lavoisier, dignified and aristocratic until the end, was executed on May 8, 1794, for "plotting against the people of France." Shortly before he went to the guillotine, he calmly remarked, "This probably saves me from the inconveniences of old age."

His body was dumped, along with dozens of others, into an unmarked mass grave.

CHAPTER TWO

The Spiral Threads of Life

The newspaper headlines were frightening.

MAN-MADE BACTERIA COULD RAVAGE EARTH

SCIENCE THAT FRIGHTENS SCIENTISTS

NEW STRAINS OF LIFE—OR DEATH

The organism that caused this outcry is *Escherichia coli,* a rod-shaped structure less than one ten-thousandth of an inch long. Named for its German pediatrician discoverer, Theodor Escherich, who isolated it from feces, *E. coli* is a normal—and usually harmless —resident of the colon.

Yet this tiny parcel of protoplasm has now become the center of a stormy controversy that has divided the scientific community and reached the highest levels of government. Congress has been asked to impose federal restrictions on recombinant DNA research, a new form of genetic inquiry involving *E. coli.* And though this research is bound to continue, questions about the ultimate outcome and the need for regulation will surely reverberate for many years to come. Robert Sinsheimer, chairman of the biology department at the California Institute of Technology, has defined the problem best: "Biologists have become, without wanting it, the custodians of great and terrible power. It is idle to pretend otherwise."

This great and terrible power evolved suddenly from the fusion of two scientific disciplines which had been quite content to ignore one another in years gone by. One is genetics, a formerly sleepy branch of biology. The other is chemistry. For better or worse, they have now placed control of DNA—the spiral threads of life—within the grasp of man.

The Biologic Legacy

Not just for centuries but for thousands of years ordinary observation has suggested that some characteristics are literally handed down from parent to offspring. A Babylonian tablet more than six thousand years old, for example, shows pedigrees of horses and indicates possible inherited characteristics; other old carvings show cross-pollination of date palm trees. In the Bible, Adam's fall was passed on in the moment of conception. The Habsburg jaw could be objectively recognized and was taken as a guarantee of the legitimacy of the heir.

Observers also took note of oddities. For example, not all off-spring strongly resemble either mother or father. And sometimes "throwbacks" to earlier ancestors occur, a phenomenon known as atavism. Observation, however, effectively stopped here, though incorrect explanations did not.

The earliest theory of heredity was offered by the great Greek mathematician Pythagoras around 500 B.C. and shows nothing except that he should have stuck to analyzing triangles. A better guess, though still a shot in the dark, was made by Aristotle, who postulated that life begins with a blending of male and female blood. Though he had the details wrong, Aristotle had come close to the truth in recognizing that the biologic legacy of inheritance implies, somehow, the transmission of what might be called a plan for development, passed on by some means or other from parent to offspring.

About 1651 William Harvey managed to disprove the old Greek concept. As physician to Charles I, Harvey had so impressed the king that the royal deer were put at his disposal for scientific purposes. The discovery that deer embryos have the appearance of a tiny ball during early developmental stages and resemble a deer only later in development led Harvey to conclude that the origin of the tiny ball was not blood, as Aristotle had surmised, but a small egg. Before the end of the seventeenth century, some scientists had recognized that the female structures called ovaries are the source of eggs, and that sperm might carry the hereditary material of the male. These simple facts suggested to the mind of Gregor Mendel, an obscure Augustinian monk, a remarkable set of experiments that revolutionized man's knowledge of the mechanism of biologic inheritance.

The Curious Mendel

Mendel was a riddle in his own lifetime and still puzzles us today. The conventional idyllic image of a simple, uncomplicated, gentle priest and amateur naturalist, totally unaware of the supreme importance of his work, simply does not fit. This man who founded the science of genetics—and probably falsified his experimental results to do so—left us no revealing autobiography, unlike his contemporary Charles Darwin. Fortunately, some letters, documents, and personal belongings have survived. From these, an unusual image emerges.

As a boy, Mendel seems to have been healthy and happy, deeply attached to his mother and two sisters. Though we know little of his relations with his father, a poor Silesian farmer, there is nothing to suggest that Mendel was subject to domestic psychological stresses through domineering parents and sisters, as was Darwin. But he did show early on the personal instability that became quite evident later in his life.

Mendel's first recorded breakdown occurred after he had left his home for a grammar school in a nearby provincial town. Of course, the physical deprivations of a poor scholar in a strange environment may have triggered the illness. Yet how many students are subjected to the same or worse stresses without ill effect? The symptoms—excessive fatigue, lack of concentration, and headaches—were slow to subside. Only after several months' rest in the shelter of his home was he able to complete his studies successfully and to proceed to the

Philosophical Institute attached to the University of Olmütz (or Olomouc), in the small Moravian fortress town of that name.

At Olmütz, Mendel read mathematics, Latin, natural sciences, and religious subjects. His school record testifies to the young man's diligence in his studies, but it also contains an ominous comment that foreshadowed the increasing difficulties to come: "Withdrew from the final examinations because of illness." The symptoms of this inconvenient malady just at the critical examination period are apparently the same as those he demonstrated at grammar school a few years before.

Because of this second breakdown, Mendel was required to repeat one year of university studies. His decision to become a priest was made at this time. What was the reason for this step? Mendel's biographers are still hotly disputing this point, the argument centering on part of a *curriculum vitae* submitted ten years later to the University of Vienna. Note the strange, self-effacing style: ". . . the humbly undersigned felt that he was unable to bear further strain and deprivations; after completing his philosophical studies he felt compelled to enter a station of life which would free him from the bitter struggle for material existence. In 1843, at the age of twenty-one, he requested and received permission to enter the Augustine monastery of St. Thomas in Brünn (modern Brno). This step radically changed the material situation of the undersigned. The physical security, which is so conducive to the pursuit of studies, gave him new courage and strength. . . ."

Mendel had obviously joined the order of St. Augustine first and foremost to acquire an education and a sheltered life. Within the quiet cloisters, the natural sciences could be studied and taught with few interruptions. There is, however, no reason to doubt a sincere religious belief. Unfortunately, after acting for a few days as pastor to the infirmary at Brünn, Mendel was again bedeviled by the old emotional problem. As the abbot, Father Napp, reported, "Mendel is quite unsuited to become a parish priest; he is incapable of witnessing suffering and disease. As the result of such confrontations he had a dangerous breakdown, and I had to relieve him from all duties. . . ."

Mendel's breakdown when faced with the stress of confronting severe illness is quite reminiscent of Darwin's experience at Edinburgh Medical School: "I also attended on two occasions the operating theatres in the hospital, and saw two very bad operations, one on a child, but I rushed away before they were completed. Nor did I ever attend again for hardly any inducement would have been strong enough to make me do so. . . ."

As an alternative to being a pastor, Mendel was sent by his abbot to a small Moravian town to teach Latin and mathematics temporarily. In addition, he was to prepare himself for an examination at the University of Vienna, which would confer the rank of fully established grammar school teacher. Again the old emotional problems surfaced, and Mendel suffered what was to prove the worst setback of his life.

In the summer of 1850 the young priest presented himself for his first examination. The university records of this painful ordeal have been preserved and portray a vivid picture. Mendel must have tried to cover his nervousness and perhaps some lack of preparation with a few tongue-in-cheek answers. This is how he replied to a written question, "Give an account of the classification of mammals with regard to their usefulness to man":

"I.   Handed animals
 II.   Pawed animals
       1. The kangaroo, which provides the natives with excellent meat
       2. The hare
       3. The beaver
III.   Flatfooted animals
 IV.   Clawed animals
       1. The dog
       2. The wolf
       3. The cat (she is useful for catching mice)
       4. The civet (secretes an aromatic substance which is useful for trade)
  V.   Hoofed animals
       The horse
       The donkey
       The ox
       The sheep
       The goat, the roebuck, and the chamois."

Then, as an afterthought he added, "the llama, the musk, and the reindeer, which is for the North what the camel is for the hot desert. The elephant is excellent for carrying loads."

The examiners, needless to say, were not at all amused. In reply to a question obviously meant to test for a knowledge of correct taxonomic terms, Mendel had provided such a list as a totally untutored grammar school child might scribble on a slate. Years later, biographers tried to explain the failure as being the result of unsupervised preparation. But the report issued at the time was hardly so charitable: "[These] answers were regarded as a sign of a mental defect." The angry examiners, who had had to postpone their summer holidays in order to arrange this session, gave their luckless subject twelve months to prepare himself more thoroughly.

Anyone who compares the superbly clear and logical style of Mendel's scientific papers with the answers produced under the stress of an examination can see at once that there is no question of mental defect; certainly Mendel never could have believed that he possessed an inferior intellect. As at Olmütz ten years earlier, he had simply broken down under stress.

Mendel stretched the one-year period before re-examination into five years. And for two years during this time he read physics, chemistry, zoology, botany, and paleontology at the University of Vienna. Two of his teachers, the physicist Christian Doppler and the botanist Franz Unger, were world-famous scientists. Yet again all this effort was wasted. A letter by a close friend, Matheus Klacel, describes the second failure:

"Father Gregor was unlucky again. His examination questions were easy, but after the first session he broke down and became unable to write. He seems to suffer from nervous troubles, and it is known that he had previous similar attacks, even that he suffered from fits. We are all terribly sorry for him especially as the written papers he had submitted from here were considered to be excellent. However, rules are rules, and nothing further could be done for him. In fear of further attacks he has now returned home, without having achieved anything at all. I am very sorry for him; he is despondent and is eating his heart out. . . ."

Mendel returned for the second and last time to his cloister, never to become a fully established teacher. His head was swathed in bandages, and his family had to be quickly summoned to Brünn in order to comfort their hapless son. Today, the presence of this possible head injury suggests one serious disorder.

Father Klacel's mention of fits in his letter reinforces other impressions that Mendel was not only hysteric but epileptic as well. There is, however, no objective evidence for seizures, and at autopsy, no gross brain changes were found. Perhaps the bandage-swathed head after the return from the second disaster at Vienna was merely a plea for sympathy and attention. We only know for certain that in the following year, 1856, Mendel began his important experiments with *Pisum sativum,* the garden pea.

When Mendel started his work on the operation of heredity, little was known to explain the puzzling patterns observed. As early as 1669, Johann Joachim Becher had written, "When a black cock pigeon and a white hen pigeon unite, the young birds of the first generation are usually some of them entirely black and others entirely white; and it is only when we allow some of these blacks and some of these whites to unite that we get young birds which are spotted black and white. In arboriculture nature achieves similar results, for when there occurs a union between trees bearing white and red fruits respectively, spotted fruits appear only after the second crossing."

Around the time of Mendel's birth, some of the first experiments with garden peas were performed. In 1822 an Englishman named John Goss, living in a Devonshire village, reported to the London Horticultural Society some of the odd results he had obtained. Goss crossed plants yielding green peas with others yielding yellowish-white peas and in the first generation obtained only yellowish-white peas. Breeding from these hybrids, he was surprised to get three types of plants: One had only green peas, one only yellowish white, and the third kind had both green and yellowish-white in the same pod. Goss could offer no explanation; and a few years later, one of the world's greatest scientists fared little better when faced with similar results.

Charles Darwin made a careful study of what happened when various types of garden peas are crossed. He also crossed antirrhinums, or snapdragons, using two varieties known as normal and peloric—the latter having symmetrical blossoms instead of the common asymmetric ones. In the first generation only normal plants were obtained; but when these were bred, the result was about one peloric plant to every three normal plants. Try as he might, the first man to recognize the evolution of species was unable to frame a satisfactory explanation for the outcome of his own plant-breeding experiments or the observations made by others. It was Mendel's genius, when confronted by the same information, to realize what was actually happening.

When Mendel began his pea-breeding experiments, he carefully picked out seven characters for comparison: shape of seed, color of seed, and so forth, the last on the list being tall stem versus short stem. To ensure control of the crossings, he would open the pea flower before it was fully developed, remove its anthers (the pollen producers) by means of forceps, and dust its stigma or female part with preselected pollen carried on a camel's hair brush. Once this was done, he tied a little paper bag around the flower to protect it from visits by any insects such as bees or pea weevils which might bring different pollen to it. The other monks who knew that Mendel was making studies involving the sexuality of plants were probably not pleased; neither was the bishop, but fortunately he did not interfere.

Mendel's results were similar to Darwin's. In the first generation all the plants had long stems, which we now call the dominant trait. In the second generation there were three long-stemmed plants to each short-stemmed one. Botanists had long held the view that the characters of hybrids fall between those of their parents. This was now disproved, and to explain what he had found, Mendel postulated a radically different theory, one that he had probably thought out even before he started his study.

Mendel had guessed that a simple character is regulated by two particles that we now call genes. Each parent contributes one of the two particles. If one of these particles is different from the other, then one will be dominant and the other recessive. All the first-generation hybrids will show the dominant trait but will have one dominant and one recessive gene. When these are crossed, one plant in four will have two recessive genes and show the recessive trait. This is the famous ratio of one out of four or one to three that everyone associates with Mendel's name. Unfortunately, however, it seems that Mendel was so strongly convinced of the correctness of his assumptions that he probably falsified his experimental data to fit the expected results—one of the most serious breaches of ethics a scientist can commit.

In 1936 a statistician, Dr. R. A. Fisher, made a meticulous analysis of Mendel's experiments as carried out year by year, knowing the garden space available and the number of years involved. Fisher found that Mendel's reported numbers and ratios were much closer to expectation than sampling theory would lead one to expect. For example, if a coin were tossed a thousand times, a statistician might raise his eyebrows if he were told that the outcome was 500 heads and 500 tails, even though that is the most probable specified result. On the other hand, if he were told that 481 heads and 519 tails resulted, he would say that that is about what one would expect— even though the particular result is less probable than the 500:500 one.

In all of Mendel's data, Fisher found the outcomes extremely close to perfect ratios. Taking the whole series of experiments, Fisher calculated that Mendel stood only one chance in fourteen thousand of getting the close results he reported. If this were all, however, it might not be too disturbing: Maybe Mendel was just lucky. But there is more. It appears that in one series of experiments Mendel got an equally close fit to a wrong expectation because of a genetic peculiarity known today but not in the nineteenth century. The outcome Mendel reported is so near to the one he would, mistakenly, have expected but so far from the ratio now known to be correct that the odds are only one in two thousand that it could have happened by chance. But no one at the time seems to have noticed; in fact, the entire theory initially had very little effect at all.

One evening in February 1865, Mendel and some friends set out for the Brünn Society for the Study of the Natural Sciences, where the results were to be announced. Wearing his teacher's garb of tall hat, long black coat, and trousers tucked into top boots, he strode through the streets with his precious manuscript under his arm, full of excitement and apprehension.

About forty persons heard Mendel that evening describe the ratios he had obtained. The same forty stalwart listeners duly turned up again at the next month's meeting to hear the ratios explained. Surprisingly, the significance of the work was totally unappreciated. Both presentations made so little impact that there was not even any discussion—a rare phenomenon indeed at a scientific meeting. There is no record of the degree of Mendel's disappointment, but it must have been intense.

Nonetheless, the lectures were printed in the official proceedings of the society and were sent, as was customary, to more than 120 other learned societies, universities, and academies throughout the world, all to no avail. If Mendel had been a professional scientist, he would have pushed to get his results known and, at the least, would have published his paper more widely in France or Britain in a journal that botanists and biologists read. He did none of these things, though he did attempt to reach scientists abroad by sending them reprints of his paper. And at least one showed an interest.

This was the German botanist Karl Wilhelm von Nägeli at Munich, considered at the time the world's foremost expert on plant hybridization. Nägeli's pet experimental subject was the *Hieracium* or hawkweed, and Mendel was persuaded to repeat with that plant the experiments already conducted with the garden pea. All this work, unfortunately, was doomed to fail, for the hawkweed is a more complex genetic puzzle than the pea.

Nägeli not only set Mendel on a sort of wild-weed chase, but did so in a haughty manner. The correspondence between the two is almost embarrassing to read because of the sterile, condescending, and patronizing attitude of a German university professor of the nineteenth century toward a man he considered a lowly, self-taught amateur. After Mendel had concluded several thousand experiments, Nägeli advised him, "I believe your experiments cannot yet be considered concluded; they have hardly started. . . ." This must have been quite difficult to stomach, and the assurance, "Your intention of extending your experiments to further plants is excellent, and I am convinced that with other varied forms you will obtain substantially different results," must have come close to causing another fit. Yet Mendel followed Nägeli's advice, though the terribly discouraging results with the hawkweed led eventually to his discontinuing his botanical studies and concentrating on sunspots, tornadoes, and the behavior of bees.

Actually, Mendel had always wanted to push his work from plants to animals. But the choice was unlucky. He bred a strain of hybrid bees which gave excellent honey. Alas, they were so ferocious that they stung everyone for miles around and soon had to be destroyed. And when the bees met their end, so did his scientific career.

In 1868, at the early age of forty-six, only two years after the publication of his pea genetics papers, Mendel was elected abbot and handed the heavy responsibility of administering one of the richest cloisters in the whole Habsburg empire. He had had no forewarning of this appointment to high office, and the reason for his election was not only the respect and love of his fellow monks. Austrian law subjected monasteries to a heavy tax when abbots changed, and sensibly enough the church tended to choose young men with a reasonable life expectancy for the top job.

Mendel accepted the new position with a typically odd, self-effacing remark: "From a humble teacher I find myself transferred into a position where everything is strange to me. It will require a great effort to get used to it."

The effort was certainly greater than it might otherwise have been because of some inflammatory political sentiments quite unsuited to a pillar of Catholicism. Though he never took an active role in national or local politics, there is abundant evidence that he supported the Austro-German Liberal Party and was regarded as unreliable by the emperor's secret police. It was this party which caused the Vatican to renounce unilaterally a previous agreement with the Habsburg monarchy; as a result, in 1874 the Viennese Parliament abolished the tax exemption of the Catholic Church.

When the time came for a valuation of the monastery property, Mendel showed his distaste for the government by turning in an absurdly low estimate. Surprisingly, this was cheerfully accepted by the secular authorities, who then set the annual tax at 7,000 Austrian guilders. On receiving the bill, Mendel forwarded a check for 2,000 guilders and enclosed a contemptuous note suggesting that the tax authorities had no right to the money anyway and would probably never see another pfennig from him. All other Austrian church officials might choose grudgingly to take advantage of the compromise which a lenient government offered, but not Gregor Mendel. Such intransigence, needless to say, produced an awful brouhaha.

The "affair Mendel" was front-page news in the Vienna papers, especially when the recalcitrant abbot received the sheriff in full regalia at the monastery gates and dared him to extract the keys from the holy pocket. Ironically, Mendel's only fame during his lifetime was achieved on account of this incident. With considerable psychological insight, the county lieutenant of Moravia wrote in one of his reports to Vienna, "Abbot Mendel's attitude seems to be based on regrettable mental stress."

The eccentric "Fight for the Right," as Mendel called it, dragged on until his death in January 1884, at the age of sixty-two. The other monasteries had long before come to terms with the tax authorities. Years of fighting were accompanied by a rapid deterioration of Mendel's health. With severe heart and kidney disease he developed a marked paranoia manifested by fear of assassination or confinement to an asylum. So great was his terror of being buried alive that strict instructions were left that an autopsy be performed.

The funeral was carried on with all the pomp and ceremony due the abbot of a large monastery. The requiem mass was conducted by the great Czech composer Leoš Janáček, at that time a little-known organist and musician. The new abbot elected by the monks burned all of Mendel's papers at the monastery.

Two years earlier Charles Darwin had been buried among England's greatest scientists in Westminster Abbey. Probably no one in the funeral cortege at Brünn could have foreseen that the temperamental, unstable, yet good-hearted man they had come to mourn would one day achieve a fame almost as great as Darwin's, or that Mendel had provided the answers so long sought to validate the theory of natural selection. But sixteen years after his death, Mendel's work was suddenly and dramatically rediscovered by three investigators working independently.

Hugo de Vries, a Dutch botanist, published a paper in 1900 of very extensive research he had done with plant hybrids. He proposed two laws which he said "were, in essentials, formulated long ago by Mendel for a special case. . . . They fell into oblivion, however, and were misunderstood. According to my own experiments they are generally valid for true hybrids." De Vries had not seen Mendel's papers until after he had reached the same conclusions on his own.

A month later, a German scientist at Tübingen, Karl Correns, reported that he had independently worked out the ideas of dominant and recessive traits, and of the separation of the factors for these in pairs in the sex cells. Like de Vries, Correns soon discovered that Mendel had anticipated him, though he did go further than Mendel, noting that "in the case of a great many pairs of characters, we do not find that either is dominant."

In June of 1900 a Viennese botanist, Erich Tschermak, published the results of his own genetic study of peas that followed upon Darwin's observations of snapdragons. Tschermak, also, had arrived independently at the same conclusions as Mendel, and in a postscript to the paper he added, "The simultaneous discovery of Mendel by Correns, de Vries, and myself seems to me peculiarly gratifying. I, too, as late as the second year of my experiments, believed that I had happened upon something new."

Dividends from Pus

In 1869, just four years after Mendel's publication of his now-famous papers, a young Swiss chemist, Friedrich Miescher, found a strange substance within white blood cells that he called *nuclein*. The intersection of the discoveries by these two men has brought science to the verge of controlling life.

Miescher was the son of a Swiss physician who practiced in Basel and taught at the university there, and he followed his father into medicine. As a medical student he came under the influence of his uncle, Wilhelm His, a professor of anatomy whose son became famous for his descriptions of the electrical conducting fibers of the heart—the bundles of His.

Uncel Wilhelm had a profound, lifelong influence on his nephew, and urged him almost immediately to devote himself to histochemistry, the study of the chemical composition of tissues. In his own investigations, His later said, "I was constantly reminded that the ultimate problems of tissue development would be solved on the basis of chemistry."

Miescher took his uncle's advice, and, after receiving his degree in 1868, he went to the University of Tübingen, first to learn organic chemistry and then to work in the laboratory of the biochemist Felix Hoppe-Seyler. In an ancient castle overlooking the Neckar River, with narrow, deep-set windows and dark vaults, in a room that might have belonged to a medieval alchemist, Miescher began his studies on pus. Within a few months, he had isolated nuclein, known today as deoxyribonucleic acid or DNA.

To most of us, pus seems a lowly and repulsive substance—certainly not a subject for serious study. But Miescher considered the white blood cells present in pus to be among the simplest of animal cells, and there was a fresh supply of pus every day in the Tübingen surgical clinic. He was given the bandages removed from postoperative wounds, and from these the white cells were washed for experiments. If the bandages were soaked in ordinary saline solution, the cells swelled to form a useless gelatinous mass. In a dilute sodium sulfate solution, however, the cells were well preserved and sedimented rapidly, facilitating their separation from the blood serum and other material in pus. The obtaining and processing of the pus was not a job that anyone else might envy, and Miescher himself once confessed, "I feel as if I am mired in a swamp."

Miescher's method of extracting DNA was much more indirect than that used today. After treatment with dilute alkali, a substance was obtained which could be precipitated from the solution by addition of acid and redissolved with a trace of alkali. Miescher made this observation about what he had accomplished: "According to recognized histochemical data I had to ascribe such material to the nuclei, and I therefore tried to isolate the nuclei."

The isolation of the nucleus—or any other cell part, for that matter —had not been attempted before, though the nucleus had been identified in 1831. Miescher's primary observation, and one upon which isolation of nuclei still depends, was that dilute hydrochloric acid dissolves most of the materials of a cell while leaving the nucleus behind.

When Miescher examined the isolated nuclei under his microscope, he could still see contamination that he suspected was cell protein. So, to obtain clear nuclei, he made a hydrochloric acid extract of pig stomach, which contains the protein-digesting enzyme pepsin, and applied it to the pus cells. Though the isolated nuclei so prepared were shrunken like raisins, they were clean enough for chemical study.

Miescher proceeded to analyze this material into its elements, and found it to contain both nitrogen and phosphorus. Since the newly extracted compound did not fit into any known group of substances, it was obviously *sui generis* and so was given a new name—nuclein. A modern study of the analytical data reveals that 30 per cent of the preparation consisted of pure DNA.

The year at Tübingen had now ended. Hoppe-Seyler, who agreed that a new substance had been discovered, was sufficiently interested to repeat the preparation of nuclein after Miescher's departure but sufficiently cautious to delay the publication of the results until the work was proved sound. The paper was published in 1871.

During his vacation in the fall of 1869, Miescher decided he would broaden his study of nuclein by looking for it in various cells. Unfortunately, the first material he chose was the hen's egg, because his uncle Wilhelm had recently claimed that the microscopic particles called yolk platelets were genuine cells of connective tissue origin. This was a controversial assertion, and Miescher believed that attempting to extract the nuclein from platelets would help to establish its validity.

Following the procedure already worked out for pus cells, Miescher soon isolated from yolk platelets what he took to be nuclein. Though the phosphorous content and some of the other properties of platelet nuclein did differ somewhat from those of pus nuclein, Miescher, like many another investigator, was determined to find what he was looking for, and he was convinced this was nuclein. In spite of the curious appearance of the platelets, he wrote, "Nobody would any longer deny that they have genuine nuclei, because it is not in the optical properties but in the chemical nature of a structure that its role in the molecular events of a cell's life is rooted."

Miescher was wrong, as he was soon to find out. After the new work was written up and sent off to Hoppe-Seyler, it was published along with the Tübingen research. The paper on pus cells remains a classic, but the one on yolk platelets is almost forgotten. The microscopists, considering what Miescher called the "optical properties" of platelets, never did accept the idea that they were cells. In time, detailed chemical analysis showed, and Miescher had to agree, that what had been taken for platelet nuclein in fact had a very different composition. Only recently, careful microscopic observation has demonstrated that yolk platelets are derived from tiny intracellular particles called mitochondria, and they do indeed contain a small trace of DNA, but not nearly so much as Miescher originally believed.

When he returned to Basel in 1870, Miescher began the investigation which was to result in his finest piece of work: an analysis of nuclein and other components in salmon spermatazoa. Uncle Wilhelm was again instrumental in this decision, having introduced his nephew to the salmon fishery then flourishing on the banks of the Rhine at Basel, though today wiped out by pollution.

The salmon, having made the considerable exertion of swimming upstream all the way from the North Sea to spawn, were sexually mature and full of huge quantities of ripe sperm. In any sperm cell, the nucleus is extremely large, but in the salmon sperm exceptionally so, accounting for more than 90 per cent of the mass. To a young scientist who had recently discovered nuclein in pus cells washed out of bandages, the investigation of Rhine salmon sperm must have seemed, at the least, a definitely more aesthetic opportunity. Yet much hard work under uncomfortable conditions was required.

To prepare the nucleic acid, the sperm heads had to be dissolved in strong salt solution; the fibers of nucleic acid were then precipitated by adding water. The preparations had to be kept as cold as possible, and in those pre-refrigerator days Miescher was forced to work through the winter in an unheated room. In a letter to a friend he described his methods: "When nucleic acid is to be prepared, I go at five o'clock in the morning to the laboratory. . . . No solution can stand for more than five minutes, no precipitate more than an hour being placed under absolute alcohol. Often it goes on until late in the night. . . ."

Using these methods, Miescher extracted an organic base with a high content of nitrogen. This material accounted for 27 per cent of the mass of the sperm, and was named *protamine* by its discoverer. Today, protamine is of vital importance to diabetics, because when mixed with regular insulin the glucose-lowering effect is prolonged. Thus one injection of protamine insulin in the morning can be used instead of many injections of regular insulin throughout the day.

Miescher recognized that nuclein was an acid containing a number of acid groups, and that it combined with protamine, a base, to form an insoluble salt in the nucleus. He experimented with modifying the chemical equilibrium of the nuclein-protamine combination, finding that if sperm washed with acetic acid and alcohol were treated with sodium chloride solution, then much of the protamine was released from combination and passed into solution. If, however, fresh sperm were treated with the same salt solution, the material became a lumpy gel that could almost be cut with a pair of scissors; today we know that the DNA in this preparation is present as an extremely long, linear molecule called a polymer.

Miescher's work—unlike Mendel's—was immediately recognized as a significant contribution to science, and led to his appointment at age twenty-eight as professor of physiology at Basel. The young professor became a leading figure at his university and in time built a new physiological institute and stocked it with the precision instruments becoming available.

From time to time Miescher undertook public-service projects. The canton of Basel asked his advice on the nutrition of inmates in prisons, and he also gave a series of public lectures on nutrition and home economics. Living in a country that produced milk but did not consume much of it, he was aware of milk's food value and in one lecture heaped scorn on the "sordid avarice" of peasants who withheld milk from their children in order to make the last drop into salable cheese. "If you ask these pale and feeble people what they eat," he said, "they reply: potatoes, coffee, more potatoes, and schnapps to keep down hunger." This social concern led one colleague to comment that Professor Miescher would surely have been active in politics had he not been so deaf.

Did Friedrich Miescher finally come to understand the significance of DNA, the substance which he studied almost his entire professional career? Probably not. "The riddle of fertilization is not hidden in a particular substance," he wrote. "The sperm acts as a whole through the co-operation of all its parts, and fertilization is a physical procedure in which a certain movement of the sperm is transmitted to the egg." In other words, an energetic sperm with the right shimmy could be expected to produce a different organism than a lethargic one, much in the way an energetically stimulated nerve would produce a different movement than a mildly stimulated one.

Miescher held these quaint beliefs until the end of his life. After a long day of many hours spent in a freezing cold laboratory analyzing nuclein, he developed pneumonia and died. But not many years were to pass before Miescher's nuclein and Mendel's units of heredity were seen to be the same substance—DNA—situated within the nucleus of the cells.

The Last Parts of the Puzzle

Cells were receiving a good bit of attention in the nineteenth century. Though first described in 1665 by Robert Hooke, their interiors remained formless blobs to scientists until the mid-eighteen-hundreds, when improved microscopes allowed the first glimpses of the inner parts. By 1839 the German zoologist Theodor Schwann recognized that plants and animals were "aggregates of cells which are arranged according to definite laws." Meanwhile, a German cytologist, Walther Flemming, studying animal cells, found that scattered within the nucleus were spots of material that strongly absorbed certain dyes. These spots stood out brightly against the colorless background and so were called *chromatin,* from the Greek word for color.

When Flemming dyed a section of growing tissue, the cells were killed, of course, but each was caught at some stage of division. After much painstaking observation, the changes in chromatin that accompanied division could be recognized, and here a remarkable discovery was made. As division began, the chromatin material was seen to coalesce into short, threadlike objects: chromosomes. A few years later, a Belgian cytologist, Eduard van Beneden, demonstrated that the number of chromosomes was constant in the various cells of an organism, and that each species has a characteristic number.

There was good evidence by 1900 that Mendel's units of heredity, now called genes, resided on the chromosomes, and the definitive proof was not long in coming. Thomas Hunt Morgan, an American biologist studying the genetics of the fruit fly *Drosophila,* showed that the behavior of *Drosophila*'s chromosomes so closely paralleled the requirements of Mendel's theory that the association between gene and chromosome could be positively made. Since there were obviously an enormous number of genes and a small number of chromosomes, the genes must be contained within the chromosomes. Morgan was even able to localize specific genes to particular chromosomes, allowing various genetic characteristics of the fly to be mapped along the chromosomes like towns on a country highway.

While Morgan was doing his genetic studies, knowledge of the chemistry of DNA was becoming more complete. A German chemist, Albrecht Kossel, proceeded to take Friedrich Miescher's nuclein and identify within it four nitrogenous compounds called bases, a five-carbon sugar, and phosphoric acid. Two of the bases, called purines, which Kossel called adenine and guanine, were made up of two carbon rings each. Three other bases, pyrimidines, made of single carbon rings, were named cytosine, thymine, and uracil.

By 1950 an enormous amount of further study had made it apparent that the DNA molecule carried encoded within itself the message of heredity. How? Four of the bases—adenine, guanine, cytosine, and thymine—were arranged in very long molecular lines, like the dots and dashes of the Morse code on a ticker tape, and these dots and dashes signaled the genetic information to a reading mechanism.

The stage was now set for what might be called the final solution of the DNA problem: the determining of the structure of the DNA molecule. This feat is considered the crowning achievement of twentieth-century biology and one of the greatest scientific advances of all time. But because information obtained by one of the four scientists involved was appropriated in a deplorable manner by another, an aura of impropriety still lingers even decades later.

The Path to the Double Helix

The approach to the final solution began early in 1951 with the arrival of a young physical chemist, Rosalind Franklin, at King's College in London. She had come to study DNA.

Rosalind Franklin was born July 25, 1920, the second child and first daughter of a wealthy and distinguished family of English merchant bankers. When she was very young, Franklin suffered a severe infection that first resolved itself and then recurred. For some time afterward she was quite frail and subject to fatigue. Her concerned parents at first sent her away from home to seek a cure at a coastal boarding school which specialized in the care of frail children, but a case of homesickness worse than the original illness soon developed. She was brought home and sent to St. Paul's Girls' School, where she quickly developed an interest in science—especially physics and chemistry. By the age of fifteen her mind was made up to become a scientist.

Her father, Ellis Franklin, was at first quite skeptical about this career choice. His daughter was under no compulsion to earn a living, since her family could provide for her quite adequately. Very few women were working seriously and professionally at science in the 1930s, he pointed out, so why then not take up some type of voluntary social work.

Rosalind would have none of this, however, and in 1938 entered Cambridge to study chemistry. She worked hard and did quite well until her last term, when, somewhat like Mendel, she entered her final examinations in a terrible state of weariness and nervous tension. As a result, she failed to receive a first-class degree, ending up with a high second, and her disappointment was bitter.

Nonetheless, Franklin received a good research fellowship, and after a year joined the British Coal Utilization Research Association, called CURA. Here she did excellent fundamental work on the microstructures of various coals, writing five papers still considered classics in the field. After finishing her doctoral thesis on the structure of coal, she went to Paris in 1947 with an appointment as researcher in the Central State Chemical Services Laboratory. Here she learned the technique of X-ray crystallography, which was to prove so important in finally elucidating the structure of DNA.

When Franklin began to study X-ray crystallography, the methods used were scarcely more than thirty years old. A German physicist, Max von Laue, and his students had done the pioneering work in 1912, showing simply that when a beam of X rays is passed through a crystal, the beam is scattered in such a way as to record upon film a visible pattern—the X-ray diffraction pattern—which varies from substance to substance, but which is always identical for identical substances.

Very shortly afterward, in England, Dr. W. L. Bragg, employing a trial and error method, was able to use an X-ray diffraction pattern to determine the structure of zinc blende. This was done by constructing atomic models until one with just the right arrangement precisely fitted the film image obtained. In the process, a fundamental theorem, Bragg's law, was formulated. Bragg, a modest man, later remarked about the naming of the law after him, "It is, I have always felt, a cheaply earned honor, because the principle had been well known for some time in the optics of visible light."

Unfortunately, the trial and error method was suited to finding the structures of only the simplest molecules. But in 1915 W. H. Bragg, father of W.L., made the next important advance. Applying a mathematical method called the Fourier transform to the spotted X-ray diffraction pictures, which often don't look like very much, W.H. was able to determine molecular structures by direct calculation. And with this striking innovation, X-ray crystallography expanded from an adjunct of metallurgy to a tool for the study of more complex organic molecules; it continued to grow steadily more sophisticated until scientists began to think that even complex biologic molecules might be profitably investigated.

By the 1930s, biologists had begun to suspect that an understanding of the structure of biologic molecules might prove of crucial importance to finding their function. X-ray diffraction methods were plainly one of the most promising approaches, although nothing was then so simple, since the diffraction patterns become increasingly complex as the size of a molecule increases. Because of the enormous size of most biologically important molecules, there was hardly time enough in a single human life to calculate their structure mathematically.

An example of these difficulties may be seen in the Nobel Prize–winning experiments of Max Perutz. In 1937 Perutz began work as a young man on the structure of hemoglobin, the vital oxygen-carrying protein within the red blood cells. Twenty-five years later, he had successfully elucidated the exact configuration of the molecule. By the time he made the trip to Stockholm to collect his award, he was certainly much older and wiser than when he started his studies. Perutz managed to live long enough to win his prize because of the development of helpful tricks and short cuts that came with improvements in crystallographic methods.

In 1951 these improvements lured Rosalind Franklin, now an expert crystallographer, away from Paris to a laboratory at King's College in London in order to set up the X-ray diffraction equipment for studying DNA. Here was a chance to solve one of the oldest of questions—how heredity works. Yet there was great risk involved because previous attempts had not gotten very far beyond indicating that DNA was a poor subject for X-ray photography, producing too little data to permit any significant analysis.

Unfortunately for Franklin, the excitement and promise of the project was quickly soured by a bad interpersonal situation that arose shortly after she arrived at King's College. For she quickly grew to hate Maurice Wilkins, a colleague in the same laboratory working on the biochemical and biophysical aspects of DNA.

This was not her first difficulty with a scientific associate. While she was a graduate student at Cambridge, her preceptor, R. W. Norrish, described Franklin as "stubborn and difficult to supervise" as well as "not easy to collaborate with." For her part, she later referred to Norrish—unkindly and not at all accurately—as an "ogre." But the problems with Wilkins were to prove much more serious, and in the end were partially responsible for her not obtaining proper credit in the DNA work.

Wilkins, a shy and sensitive man, had moved into biophysics from physics, after some years spent working first on the Manhattan Project, then later at the University of California on the separation of uranium isotopes by mass spectrography. He should have gotten on well with Franklin from the beginning since they had many characteristics in common. Yet even their first recorded contact was a clash.

The exact nature of what happened is difficult to know, but Wilkins' version is probably the most accurate. When Franklin arrived at the laboratory, the group working under Wilkins' direction had been for some time attempting to hydrate fibers of DNA, as many compounds show very different characteristics and possibly informative ones in a hydrated form. There had been little success, however, since DNA is one of the least thirsty of all molecules.

Franklin quickly solved the annoying hydration problem by suggesting that appropriate gases be bubbled through the water bath; this, in fact, worked very well, though nothing very innovative was involved. Such a method of hydration is well known and described in most textbooks. Wilkins describes Franklin as taking "a very superior attitude" after this event, and very likely she had offered her advice mixed with an equal part of disdain. As Raymond Gosling, her graduate student, once commented, "She didn't suffer fools gladly at all. You either had to be on the ball, or you were lost in any discussion about anything, and that was constant."

Wilkins portrays the same characteristic even more pointedly. She was, he remembered, "very fierce, you know. She denounced, and this made it quite impossible as far as I was concerned to have a civil conversation. I simply had to walk away."

This trait that Wilkins relates was worse for Franklin than she could know. Because while she labored to perform meticulous crystallographic studies, quite isolated from Wilkins, two other scientists doing no DNA experiments at all watched and waited, hoping to be able to obtain enough information to work out the DNA structure without ever lighting a Bunsen burner or filling a beaker. These two were James D. Watson and Francis Crick.

Watson, a brilliant, unpredictable man, had been a child prodigy and was a college student at the University of Chicago by the age of fifteen. After obtaining his doctorate in genetics at Indiana University, he had come to the Cavendish Laboratory at Cambridge on a fellowship. By his own admission he had no experimental skill. As he writes in his book *The Double Helix,* "Briefly the Indiana biochemists encouraged me to learn organic chemistry, but after I used a Bunsen burner to warm up some benzene, I was relieved from further true chemistry. It was safer to turn out an uneducated Ph.D. than to risk another explosion."

Francis Crick was trained in physics and had spent the war years designing mines for the British Admiralty. Then, like many another physicist after the war, he had turned to molecular biology, first working on X-ray diffraction pictures at the Polytechnic Institute of Brooklyn before coming to the Cavendish Laboratory. But Crick had very little ability as an experimentalist; as Watson relates: "On two occasions the corridor . . . was flooded with water pouring out of a laboratory in which Crick was working. Francis, with his interest in theory, had neglected to fasten securely the rubber tubing around his suction pump."

In later years, after they had become famous, these two men would have teams of graduate students and skilled technicians to do their experiments for them. In 1951, however, they had no one and so were dependent on the work of others, obtaining such information in whatever way they could. Yet even in this uncertain milieu, Watson was able to achieve a stunning success because he was possessed of an attribute which separates a great scientist from a merely intelligent one—a certain kind of instinct that guides the scientist to the right problem at the right moment before the rightness can be demonstrated. For Watson had grasped how important it was to understand the structure of DNA at a time when very few other people agreed with him.

To solve the DNA structure, Watson again showed an uncanny instinct by settling on the technique of model-building as opposed to Fourier analysis. In this method, molecular models are employed which have the same relative dimensions as real molecules and atoms. Though to a layman such models may look like nothing more than a child's Tinkertoys, the method is an extremely powerful one because if no rules of chemistry are violated and distances between atoms are correct, exact molecular configurations may be deduced by using only isolated bits of information about the substance in question.

Watson had quite a few bits of data about DNA when he started to think about building models. First, the exact chemical composition was known, and it was also apparent that the four bases—adenine, guanine, thymine, and cytosine—must be arranged in some type of linear manner in order to form a code for genetic information. In addition, an American biochemist, Erwin Chargaff, had recently made an important discovery regarding the proportions of the bases.

Chargaff and his students had analyzed various DNA samples for the relative amounts of their bases. They had found that in all the DNA preparations the number of adenine molecules was very similar to the number of thymine molecules, while the number of guanine molecules was correspondingly close to the number of cytosine molecules. This was true although the proportions of adenine and thymine groups varied with the biologic origin of the material. Chargaff offered no explanation for his results, nor did anyone else at the time.

Another valuable piece of information came to Watson from Jerry Donohue, an American crystallographer visiting the Cavendish Laboratory. Watson had originally believed that the bases must lie within the molecule in a chemical configuration known as the enol form. Donohue, however, told him that after years of work with related compounds he was very certain that the bases were in another form, called the keto form.

Both Watson and Linus Pauling, a Nobel Prize–winning American chemist, suspected that the DNA molecule must consist of multiple strands in the form of a helix or spiral. Pauling had already suggested one configuration, an alpha helix, quickly shown to be incorrect. Watson and Crick also had built one helical model that would not conform to the known chemistry of the molecule. And the truth was that an infinite number of wrong models could still have been built had Watson not been able to obtain one further piece of evidence.

Watson had initially seen X-ray diffraction films of only one form of DNA, the unhydrated or A form. But after a great deal of experimental work, Rosalind Franklin had managed to produce and film a second form of the DNA molecule, the hydrated or B form. Examination of her notes and laboratory records now reveals that, very likely, before her data had been published Franklin would have worked out the correct DNA structure for herself; however, sometime in February 1953, Wilkins showed Watson an unpublished X-ray diffraction picture of the B form.

Watson reacted intensely, with a dropped jaw and racing pulse. The simple pattern with its prominent black cross gave irrefutable evidence of the helical structure. And the picture itself provided several vital parameters of the molecule which could be derived after a little calculation.

Now all of the pieces had fallen into place. With a brilliant flash of insight Watson guessed that the DNA helix must consist of two chains, since most important biologic entities come in pairs.

Chargaff's work also suggested that adenine was somehow paired with thymine and guanine with cytosine. "This pairing is likely to be so fundamental for biology," Crick wrote later, "that I cannot help wondering whether some day an enthusiastic scientist will christen his newborn twins Adenine and Thymine."

Within a few days the correct model had been built, and this was published by Watson and Crick in the April 25, 1953, issue of *Nature*. Besides the remarkable achievement of determining the correct structure, one other important question, the method of DNA replication, had been answered. As the authors succinctly stated, "It has not escaped our notice that the specific pairing we have postulated immediately suggests a possible copying mechanism for the genetic material." The chains, they surmised, separated, and each chain then served as the template for a new DNA strand.

Rosalind Franklin died of cancer in 1958 without ever realizing she had not been treated quite fairly by Watson. In 1962 the Nobel Prize was awarded to Watson, Crick, and Wilkins, without the slightest mention of her. But probably still gnawed at by some rudimentary conscience, Watson wrote *The Double Helix* in 1968 in order to explain his side of the story.

In the book, Rosalind Franklin is presented as "Rosy," an ardent, angry, violent feminist. Anne Sayre, who knew Franklin well and later wrote an excellent biography of her, demonstrates quite plausibly that Watson's portrait of Rosy hardly bears even the mildest resemblance to the actual Rosalind Franklin. As Sayre points out, the shabby treatment in Watson's memoir was quite obviously the result of guilt, "it being easier to indulge happily in breaches of faith with those we can convince ourselves we despise." Watson also overemphasized the threat posed by Linus Pauling's incorrect models in order to minimize Franklin's importance as a competitor.

Recombinant DNA and Beyond

The understanding of DNA brought about by the Watson-Crick model and the subsequent cracking of the genetic code has ushered us suddenly into a new era of genetic engineering. Such engineering is most commonly performed today on the bacterium *Escherichia coli*. In the process, DNA containing genes of a plant, animal, or virus may be inserted within the bacteria. Thus these organisms become forms of life potentially different from what they had been before—imbued with characteristics dictated not only by their own *E. coli* genes but also by genes of an entirely different species.

This dramatic technique of DNA recombination holds both promise and peril. On the one hand, the bacteria could be made to churn out great quantities of human insulin for diabetics. Insulin is now obtained from pigs and other animals, and because of its nonhuman nature is not as effective as human insulin would be. Other useful substances could also be made in this way: clotting factor for hemophiliacs, which is now both scarce and expensive, as well as vitamins and antibiotics.

But peril is involved. What could happen if *E. coli* containing a cancer virus such as the SV 40 monkey virus escaped from the laboratory? Would these bacteria be capable of infecting a large human population and causing a cancer epidemic?

Only the years to come will tell.

CHAPTER THREE

The White Light

Consciousness can be altered to relieve severe pain. Artie Ross knew how.

Artie Ross, born of a wealthy New York family, went to the University of California at Berkeley in 1963. There he majored in drama, became a campus hotshot, and let his hair grow, sometimes decorating it with roses. Soon he was smoking marihuana, taking LSD, and going to rock concerts. "He had a knack for pinpointing other people's states of mind," said a former girlfriend. "You felt he was constantly searching you. And he projected a very romantic image of himself as a kind of a rake or a scoundrel. He was incredibly perceptive and articulate."

Through family connections, Artie Ross met Bert Schneider, another former New Yorker with a similar background, though vastly more successful. Schneider, one of the better-known Hollywood producers, is said to have revolutionized the industry with his second motion picture, *Easy Rider.* He followed this with two more hits— *Five Easy Pieces* and *The Last Picture Show*—and in 1975 won an Academy Award for *Hearts and Minds,* a documentary about U.S. involvement in Vietnam. Schneider used the ceremony to achieve some notoriety, reading a message to the American people from the Provisional Revolutionary Government of South Vietnam. Because it came on the eve of the Communist victory in Indochina, the action caused a commotion among the stars. But Schneider, a long-time member of the counterculture movement, was not upset; in fact, he thrived on needling the establishment.

Artie Ross formed a strong relationship with Schneider during the early seventies. Schneider often visited Big Sur with actress Candice Bergen; Artie, a charter member of the local counterculture, delighted in serving as host and guide. He arranged accommodations for the couple and took them to points of interest, notably the famous communal warm sulfur baths. There they would sit for hours, naked and sweaty, absorbing the good vibrations.

In 1973 Artie struck out for Los Angeles, and was hired by Schneider as associate producer of a Charlie Chaplin film biography, *The Gentleman Tramp*. Later, Artie completed an unsuccessful screenplay, but did manage to save money, with which he planned to set up his own movie production company. Unfortunately, he used some of the money to acquire a dangerous new toy.

This was a tank of nitrous oxide or laughing gas and an inhalation mask. Most nitrous oxide freaks use a balloon or beach ball filled with the gas so that when they black out, the balloon or ball will slip away. Artie, however, always inventive, thought he could prolong or maybe amplify the high by strapping the inhalation mask on his face to prevent it from dropping away as he lapsed into unconsciousness.

One afternoon, Artie put the tank in a closet that opened onto a staircase. Then he strapped on the mask, seated himself on the steps, and turned on the gas. Later he told friends he had never had such an experience. He had felt himself getting higher and higher. He had seen the "white light," an almost mystical phenomenon. When he woke up, he was lying at the bottom of the stairs. He had fallen and ripped off the mask.

Artie's friends were shocked. Don't do this, they said. It's too dangerous. You'll get killed. He ignored their warnings.

On June 20, 1975, Bert Schneider was planning to have dinner with his ex-wife and his daughter. They invited Artie; he accepted. At five that afternoon a friend telephoned Artie and they talked for several minutes. At six-fifteen another friend knocked on his door. There was no answer. On entering the apartment, the visitor heard a hissing sound, shouted Artie's name, then looked toward the staircase. There he lay, slumped on the steps, with the mask clamped to his face, the tank in the closet, the gas turned on.

The friend telephoned Schneider, saying, "You better get over here. I think Artie is dead."

Schneider had scheduled a trip to Havana to visit Huey Newton, the Black Panther leader. But the producer postponed his departure a few days to help arrange a small funeral. He himself delivered a eulogy: "Artie lived on the edge. There are many ways to measure the fullness of life besides quantity. Artie packed several lifetimes into his thirty years."

Other friends continued to wonder about the loose ends of Artie's life. Had he committed suicide? He left no suicide note and had not been depressed. When asked, one acquaintance shrugged, then said, "Well, we know this much: Artie Ross died laughing."

Almost two centuries before Artie Ross's death, men had begun to play with nitrous oxide for much the same reason as Artie did—they wanted a kick. Undoubtedly some also died laughing. But a few more perceptive—and lucky—than the rest made the remarkable observation that nitrous oxide, as well as chloroform and ether, were capable of allaying even the most agonizing forms of pain when inhaled. Surgical anesthesia, one of the greatest advances in the science of healing, was introduced by these men who had first seen the white light.

The Painful Knife

"Now a surgeon should be youthful or at any rate nearer youth than age; with a strong and steady hand which never trembles, and ready to use the left hand as well as the right; with vision sharp and clear, and spirit undaunted; filled with pity, so that he wishes to cure his patient, yet is not moved by his cries, to go too fast, or cut less than is necessary; but he does everything just as if the cries of pain cause him no emotion."

Thus Celsus, the first-century Roman encyclopedist, characterized the ideal attributes of a surgeon. The vigorous appearance, the strong and steady hand, the sharp and clear vision, the undaunted spirit—who can turn on a television set or peruse the pages of *Time* without noticing most of these qualities in such supersurgeons as Dr. Christiaan Barnard, Dr. Michael De Bakey, or Dr. Denton Cooley?

But the ability to be unmoved by cries of pain is no longer sought after, and one wonders how today's supersurgeon would react to the unease in this early-nineteenth-century female patient: "At the first clear crisp cut of the scalpel, agonizing screams burst from her and with convulsive struggles she endeavours to leap from the table. But the force is nigh. Strong men throw themselves upon her and pinion her limbs. Shrieks upon shrieks make their horrible way into the stillness of the room. . . . At length it is finished, and, prostrated with pain, weak from her exertions, and bruised by the violence used, she is borne from the amphitheatre to her bed in the wards, to recover from the shock by slow degrees."

No doubt a modern surgeon suddenly confronted by a life filled with such disagreeable cases would immediately chuck his medical diploma in the nearest garbage can and enroll in law school. Yet until the mid-nineteenth century, a surgeon's working day was filled routinely with screams of agony not even to be heard in the most modern, well-equipped torture chamber.

Naturally, only the simplest operations could be performed under such conditions or the patient would die on the operating table from pain and shock. Any prolonged operation usually resulted in death of the patient from heart failure, and the best surgeons were those who worked most quickly. William Cheselden, a friend of Alexander Pope, could cut out a bladder stone in fifty-four seconds. The chief surgeon of the Hanoverian army, a Dr. Langenbeck, could amputate an arm at the shoulder joint in the time needed to take a pinch of snuff. Robert Liston, a Scottish surgeon famed for his operating speed, could complete an amputation, including ligature of the bleeding vessels, in twenty-nine seconds; he accomplished this by holding instruments in both hands, and in his teeth as well.

Even an apparently simple orthopedic procedure, resetting a dislocated hip, was rendered almost impossible by the pain and muscle spasm involved, although the method used had been considerably refined since being first described in the Hippocratic corpus in 400 B.C. Here is a mid-nineteenth-century account: "A pulley is attached to the affected limb, while the body, trussed up by appropriate bands, is fastened to another; now several powerful muscular assistants seize the ropes, and with a careful steady drawing, tighten the cords. Soon the tension makes itself felt, and as the stubborn muscles stretch and yield to the strain, one can almost imagine that he hears the crack of parting sinews. Big drops of perspiration, started by the excess of agony, bestrew the patient's forehead, sharp screams burst from him in peal after peal—all his struggles to free himself and escape from the horrid torture are valueless, for he is in the powerful hands of men then as inexorable as death. . . . Stronger comes the pull, more force is added to the ropes, the tugs, cruel and unyielding, seem as if they would burst the tendons where they stand out like whipcords. At last the agony becomes too great for human endurance, and with a wild, despairing yell, the suffering patient relapses into unconsciousness. The surgeon avails himself of this opportunity and . . . seizing the limb by a dexterous twist snaps the head of the bone into its socket. The operation is done, and the poor prostrated, bruised sufferer can be removed to his pallet to recover from the fearful results of the operation as best he can."

A brave patient usually scorned ropes or straps as effeminate, and would not permit himself to be tied down. The biographer Plutarch described a second-century B.C. operation on the Roman general Marius: "There is testimony both to the temperance of Marius, and also to his fortitude, of which his behavior under a surgical operation is proof. He was afflicted in both legs, as it would appear, with varicose veins, and as he disliked the deformity, he resolved to put himself into the physician's hands. Refusing to be bound, he presented to him one leg, and then, without a motion or a groan, but with steadfast countenance and in silence, endured incredible pain under the knife. When, however, the physician was proceeding to treat the other leg, Marius would suffer him no further, declaring the cure to be not worth the pain."

The frightening and formidable nature of operative pain prodded surgeons from antiquity onward to search for an effective anesthetic. The Egyptians, who practiced surgery widely, knew of the effects of the opium poppy. There is strong evidence that opium reached Egypt sometime during the Eighteenth Dynasty (c. 1590–1340 B.C.). Even earlier, in 1650 B.C., the Edwin Smith Surgical Papyrus recommended the "red shepenn," probably opium, as a pain-relieving wound salve.

Less effective and reliable analgesics were also tried. Alcohol was freely given before some operations. Pliny, Dioscorides, and Apuleius recommended the mandrake plant, which we now know to contain the belladonna alkaloids. Assyrian surgeons asphyxiated children by strangulation before circumcision, a practice used in Italy as late as the seventeenth century. Cerebral concussion, produced by striking a wooden bowl placed on the head, was also employed.

The relatively ineffective or dangerous nature of all these agents was finally accepted with sad resignation by the medical profession. By the nineteenth century, operative pain came to be regarded as absolutely inevitable; all the greatest scientific authorities agreed that no good preventive measure existed. But just as the situation began to look most bleak, a series of discoveries provided an answer to the problem.

Laughing Pain Away

In 1772 Joseph Priestley, the discoverer of oxygen, produced the gas nitrous oxide by heating iron filings dampened with nitric acid. A short time later, after administering oxygen to mice, Priestley also determined to observe the physiologic effects of nitrous oxide. Unfortunately, he was driven from his home by the screaming mob before he could attempt this, and dropped the idea after his arrival in America.

In 1795 an English chemist, Humphry Davy, using Priestley's technique, prepared a flaskful of nitrous oxide and then proceeded to inhale it, a whiff at a time. He noted a feeling of lightness in his body, a relaxation of the muscles, and a sense of pleasure so intense that he actually burst out laughing. Seizing a pen, he quickly wrote the following poem to describe his experience:

> Not in the ideal dreams of wild desire
> Have I beheld a rapture-wakening form:
> My bosom burns with no unhallow'd fire,
> Yet is my cheek with rosy blushes warm;
> Yet are my eyes with sparkling lustre fill'd;
> Yet is my mouth replete with murmuring sound;
> Yet are my limbs with inward transport fill'd;
> And clad with new-born mightiness around.

Not without reason, it would seem, do textbooks refer to this period of English history as the Romantic Age.

Davy soon began giving nitrous oxide to some of his very prominent friends: the poets Southey and Coleridge, Peter Mark Roget, compiler of the well-known *Thesaurus,* and Dr. Robert Kinglake, then a leading authority on gout. Their reactions were quite similar to his.

To observe further the action of the gas, Davy undertook and described the following animal experiment: "A stout and healthy young cat, of four or five months old, was introduced into a large jar of nitrous oxide. For ten or twelve moments he remained perfectly quiet, and then began to make violent motions, throwing himself round the jar in every direction. In two minutes he appeared quite exhausted, and sunk quietly to the bottom of the jar. On applying my hand to the thorax, I found that the heart beat with extreme violence; on feeling about the neck, I could distinctly perceive a strong and quick pulsation of the carotids. In about three minutes the animal revived, and panted very much; but still continued to lie on his side."

On another occasion, Davy inhaled nitrous oxide while suffering the pain of erupting wisdom teeth and recorded the following remarkable result: "The power of the immediate operation of the gas in removing intense physical pain, I had a very good opportunity of ascertaining. . . . In cutting the unlucky teeth called dentes sapientiae, I experienced an extensive inflammation of the gums, accompanied with great pain. . . . On the day when the inflammation was most troublesome, I breathed three large doses of nitrous oxide. The pain always diminished after the first three or four inspirations; the thrilling came on as usual. . . ."

With these experiments, Davy became the first man to describe what we now call the planes of anesthesia. The first plane, or stage of analgesia, occurs just after administration of anesthetic, and was noted by Davy during his dental pain. The second plane, the stage of delirium, begins at the loss of consciousness, and was observed in the cat experiment as the perfectly quiet animal suddenly began to thrash wildly around the jar. The third plane, the stage of surgical anesthesia, commenced as the exhausted animal sank quietly to the bottom of the jar. The fourth plane, the stage of respiratory paralysis, was reached in other experimental animals, and on those that died Davy performed careful post-mortem studies.

In 1800 Davy wrote a book on his work with nitrous oxide, *Researches, Chemical and Philosophical; Chiefly Concerning Nitrous Oxide, or Dephlogisticated Nitrous Air, and Its Respiration.* Though this work is now considered one of the classics of chemistry, it contains a few important oversights. Davy did not realize that the reactions to nitrous oxide he recorded are almost identical to those produced by other general anesthetic agents such as ether and chloroform. He also probably did not appreciate that the third plane of anesthesia, occurring after delirium, was the surgical stage. But the most important observation of all did not escape him, and toward the end of his book, on page 556, he wrote: "As nitrous oxide in its extensive operation appears capable of destroying physical pain, it may probably be used with advantage during surgical operations in which no great effusion of blood takes place."

No surgeon of the time appears to have taken note of this recommendation, but Davy probably didn't care. In his later work he made numerous other important discoveries: the elements sodium and potassium, electrochemistry, and the miner's safety lamp. After being knighted, he actually began to look back with disdain on his nitrous oxide research, expressing some embarrassment that this youthful work had ever been published and regarding the time spent on it as "misemployed."

In the light of the age in which he lived, Davy's contempt for nitrous oxide was not entirely unjustified. After the first elemental gases had been discovered late in the eighteenth century, a new medical specialty called pneumatology developed. The pneumatologist used all types of gases, including nitrous oxide, to treat all types of illness. One of the most famous pneumatologists was Dr. Thomas Beddoes, with whom Davy had worked.

But at length, doubts about the efficacy and safety of pneumatology began to arise. Dr. Latham Mitchell, after nearly killing a few animals with nitrous oxide, concluded that this gas was the cause of all contagious disease. Other physicians, recognizing the potential hazards and seeing no ultimate benefits, also became concerned. Finally, inhalation of laughing gas was made illegal in England. Beddoes was discredited, and in 1808, on his death bed, he wrote to Davy, "Greetings from Dr. Beddoes, one who has scattered abroad the Avena Fatua [wild oats] of knowledge, from which neither branch nor blossom nor fruit has resulted." The situation was almost a repetition of history, for fifty years earlier Boerhaave and Salerne had destroyed confidence in digitalis by much the same method.

Anesthesia by Suffocation

The difficulties involved in resurrecting pneumatic medicine after it had fallen into disrepute are well illustrated by the experience of Henry Hill Hickman. Hickman was an English country doctor who heard of Beddoes and came to believe that maybe therapeutic gases did have some value. The young physician looked up the work of Priestley, Davy, and others, going on to make some fresh inquiries of his own. On March 20, 1824, he recorded the following: "I took a puppy a month old and placed it on a piece of wood, surrounded by water, over which I put a glass cover so as to prevent the access of atmospheric air; in ten minutes he showed great marks of uneasiness, in twelve minutes respiration became difficult, and in seventeen minutes ceased altogether; at eighteen minutes I took off one of the ears, which was not followed by hemorrhage; respiration soon returned and the animal did not appear to be the least sensible of pain; in three days the ear was perfectly healed."

A few days later, these more gruesome variations were tried: "A mouse was confined under a glass, surrounded by water; by means of a small tube a foot long, I passed carbonic acid gas very slowly into the glass; respiration ceased in the minute. I cut all its legs off and plunged it into a basin of cold water. The animal immediately recovered . . . apparently without pain. . . . Later I took a fully grown dog and plunged him into an atmosphere of the same gas. Within twelve seconds he was completely insensible. He remained so for seventeen minutes. Meanwhile I amputated a leg without his giving any sign of pain. . . . Next day, I filled a glass globe with the gas exhaled from my own lungs, into it I put a kitten. In twenty seconds I took off its ears and tail, there was very little hemorrhage and no appearance of pain to the animal."

Convinced he had found a method to relieve surgical pain, Hickman attempted to have his work recognized. But in doing so he made a careless error that eliminated any small chance for success he may have had. Having become acquainted with a Fellow of the Royal Society, Thomas Andrew Knight, Hickman somehow took Knight to be "one of the presidents of the Royal Society." Knight was president of the horticultural society, but never of the Royal Society. On February 21, 1824, Hickman sent the following letter to Knight:

"There is not an individual who does not shudder at the idea of an operation, however skillful the surgeon or urgent the case, knowing the great pain that the patient must endure, and I have frequently lamented, when performing my own duties as a surgeon that something has not been thought of whereby the fears may be tranquilised and suffering relieved. . . . Having made experiments on various animals, I feel perfectly satisfied that any surgical operation might be performed with quite as much safety in an insensible state, for the performance of the most tedious operation. . . . I believe there are few if any Surgeons who could not operate more skillfully, when they were conscious they were not inflicting pain. . . . I certainly should not hesitate a moment to become the subject of such an experiment, if I were under the necessity of suffering any long or severe operation."

Hickman then added, in an affectingly modest touch, "If by my labours I could add a grain of knowledge to what has been ascertained about the means for dulling pain, I should be amply rewarded."

In the summer of 1824 Hickman enlarged on his four-page letter by writing a pamphlet entitled "A letter on suspended animation, containing experiments showing that it may be safely employed during operations of animals, with the view of ascertaining its probable utility in surgical operations on the human subject, addressed to T. A. Knight, Esq., of Downton Castle, Herefordshire, one of the presidents of the Royal Society." The pamphlet was printed at Ironbridge in Shropshire and was then distributed, a copy eventually coming into the hands of the actual president of the Royal Society, Sir Humphry Davy.

Davy, by then quite disillusioned with pneumatology, would probably have been little inclined to pay much attention to gas studies in any case. But probably because the report was sent in by someone so unbelievably ignorant that he did not even know the name of the president of the Royal Society, Davy completely ignored the pamphlet and Hickman, too. Still undaunted, Hickman managed to wangle a chance for a public reading of his work before the Medical Society of London. The eminent audience listened politely, but with obvious disinterest, and at the end responded to the presentation with bone-chilling silence that suddenly erupted into laughter.

Hickman did not give up. In April 1828 he sent a letter to Charles X of France that was similar in content to the one he had previously sent to Knight. The letter was passed to the minister of the royal palace, who forwarded it to the Academy of Medicine.

Hickman traveled to Paris and there awaited permission to present his experiments to the French medical community. But again he was ignored. Two years later he died at the age of thirty.

Surprisingly, pneumatology and carbon dioxide inhalation did not die with Hickman. In 1928, nearly a hundred years after his death, a study entitled "The Anesthetic Value of Carbon Dioxide" appeared in the *Journal of Pharmacology and Experimental Therapeutics* and confirmed his results. Further investigation by researchers in 1929 showed that catatonic schizophrenics could be made momentarily normal with a carbon dioxide flush. Dr. L. J. Meduna, the originator of psychiatric electroshock therapy, in 1950 stunned the medical community by announcing that after several years of experimentation he had determined that carbon dioxide inhalation had the capacity to cure neurosis. Proponents of the technique were soon publishing studies in respected medical journals announcing carbon dioxide cures of asthma, exfoliative dermatitis, rheumatoid arthritis, alcoholism, stuttering, and hives. "You could see the hives disappear before your eyes as you administered the treatment," commented a prominent New York physician. A speech therapist declared that all other treatments for stuttering should be abandoned. Old Dr. Beddoes would have been pleased.

Perhaps the most bizarre pneumatologist of recent times is New York's Dr. Albert A. LaVerne. Long after most doctors had abandoned carbon dioxide in the early 1950s, LaVerne continued to advocate gas inhalation therapy as a cure for a multitude of ills: alcoholism, mental retardation, and drug addiction. He also gained notoriety by developing the LaVerne Diet Bread, for which he toiled into the early morning hours behind locked kitchen doors, mixing, molding, and baking according to his own secret recipe. One full-page ad placed to promote the bread in the New York Sunday *News* made extravagant claims for its therapeutic value.

As might be expected, the diet bread did not have the powerful impact of the carbon dioxide drug addiction cure. In 1971 Dr. Wharton Shober, president of Hahnemann Medical College and Hospital

in Philadelphia, invited LaVerne to Hahnemann to set up a pilot
program for drug addicts despite the strenuous objections of the
medical faculty. Within three months the experiment was dismantled
in disgrace. But by this time the procedure had caught the eye of State
Supreme Court Judge Vito Titone of Staten Island, who urged New
York City to adopt carbon dioxide therapy as an alternative to meth-
adone.

The city never did, principally because of the unsavory reputation
LaVerne had managed to acquire. The doctor was extracting four-
thousand-dollar fees from alcoholics and addicts desperate to kick
their habits and making glowing reports of his therapeutic triumphs
to the *Star* and the *National Enquirer*. In June 1977 the New York
Post devoted most of a two-page spread to the story of a woman desperately appealing for five thousand dollars so that Dr. LaVerne
could treat her mentally retarded son. Yet despite such sensational
publicity, respected Manhattan psychiatrists continued referring patients to LaVerne, though Dr. Robert Campbell, the head of the
American Psychiatric Association's New York chapter, expressed the
opinion that LaVerne "is skirting right on the edge all the time."

Men skirting right on the edge of professional ethics are not new
to the science of healing. And the story of one, Franz Anton
Mesmer, forms an interesting sidelight to the history of surgical anesthesia.

Anesthesia by Suggestion

Mesmer was born May 23, 1734, in Iznang, a small German village
on Lake Constance, very near the Swiss border. His father, Anton
Mesmer was a forester employed by the archbishop of Constance; his
mother was the daughter of a locksmith. Franz Anton was the third
of nine children.

When he was nine, Mesmer was sent by his parents to a monastery
school, where the monks were principally concerned with Latin and
music. His work was looked on with favor, and at the age of fifteen
he was awarded a scholarship for a well-known Jesuit college at
Dillingen in Bavaria. From Dillingen he went to the University of In-

golstadt to study theology but soon switched to law and finally to medicine at the University of Vienna. On November 20, 1765, at the age of thirty-one, he passed his medical examinations with honors.

In his doctoral thesis, *Disputatio de Planetarum Influxu* ("Concerning the Influence of the Planets"), Mesmer first set forth the notions which were to make him famous. He asserted that the sun, the moon, and other heavenly bodies might have a direct influence on human beings by way of a subtle "fluid"; this, he said, followed logically from the fact that the moon controls the earth's ocean tides. "Animal magnetism" was the name he gave to that property of the animal body that renders it sensitive to the motion of the planets, and he further suggested that human bodies themselves might carry a magnetic, curative fluid.

These theories may now seem bizarre, but they were much less so two hundred years ago. Even today, the nature of the magnetic force remains obscure though elegant mathematical and physical descriptions of this force have made possible all electrical and electronic devices. In the eighteenth century, the puzzling nature of the compass and the strange attraction of the lodestone for iron filings fascinated many and no doubt suggested to Mesmer that magnets might influence human maladies.

The physician's doctoral thesis is still a quaint tradition in European universities, but it has never received serious attention and is regarded by most medical students as nothing more than another piece of busy work. Thus Mesmer's startling essay received little notice by the medical faculty at Vienna. And for five years its author appeared to be nothing more than an increasingly prosperous and cultured Viennese physician.

On January 10, 1768, Mesmer married Marie Anna von Bosh, a wealthy and well-connected woman ten years his senior. Frau von Bosh was the daughter of an army apothecary at court by the name of Georg Friedrich von Eulenschenk and the widow of a high government official. Her former husband, a lieutenant colonel in army supply, had been an influential court and social figure. No doubt Mesmer believed that he had acquired a spouse who would be a great social asset.

The marriage proved to be an unhappy one, though it did have some redeeming features. The wife was a spoiled woman, lavish in her spending. In a letter to a friend, Mesmer mentioned her "stupidity" and "extravagance." The doctor was frequently accused of having affairs with his patients. But the father of the bride had given the couple a big house with a large garden in the Landstrasse, the Park Avenue of Vienna. The garden, with its marble fountain, shady paths, and statues, soon became a center of attraction. Prominent guests could sit in the gazebo and enjoy a lovely river view. Always a lover of music, Mesmer constructed an outdoor theater in his garden for concerts and recitals.

Gluck, Haydn, and Mozart, who was then only twelve, came to this theater to perform some of their greatest compositions, often before publication. Mozart had a high admiration for Mesmer's musical sensibility, and the relationship that developed between the two was an especially enduring one. The Empress Maria Theresa had commissioned the young Mozart's first opera, *La Finta Semplice,* to be performed at the palace, but the plans fell through due to jealousy on the part of the impresario Giuseppe Affligio. Upon learning this, Mesmer offered his garden theater for the performance. When the opera turned out to be too big a production for the space available, Mozart composed an operetta, *Bastien et Bastienne,* which was performed in the garden in 1768. Some years later, Mozart wrote the "magnetizer" into his opera *Così Fan Tutte:*

> This magnetic stone
> Should give the traveler pause.
> Once it was used by Mesmer,
> Who was born
> In Germany's green fields,
> And who won great fame
> In France.

As this verse suggests, Mesmer quickly became famous using his hands and his magnets to cure a wide variety of human ailments that would now be labeled psychosomatic. Cures effected by suggestion alone were not new, of course, and formed the basis of spiritualism and faith healing. But the eighteenth century had been shaped by the impact of Newton's theory of universal gravitation and the search for other natural laws. Into this framework Mesmer's explanation for the successes he achieved seemed to dovetail nicely—at least to the general public. In a 1776 report, the Augsburg Academy wrote, "What Dr. Mesmer has achieved in the way of curing the most diverse maladies leads us to suppose that he has discovered one of nature's mysterious motive energies."

The Viennese physicians, however, showed themselves to be as conservative and cautious as any group of bankers. Their skepticism about the phenomenal cures and the magnetic doctrine was intense. Finally, the notorious case of Maria Theresa von Paradis allowed them to rid themselves of their annoyingly successful magnetic colleague.

Fräulein von Paradis was an infant prodigy, an extremely talented pianist, and a protégée of the Empress Maria Theresa. The girl had been blind since the age of four, supposedly because of a shock or fright. Her mother was a hysteric, who was unable to control her daughter; her father was private secretary to the empress.

The young girl had many talents besides musical ones. She could knit and make lace. An amazing memory allowed her to play cards by remembering moves made by the other players. She even took part in amateur theatricals. The entranced empress conferred a generous allowance for the education of her namesake; she later arranged for the girl's first public appearance in Austria and first continental concert tour. By the time she had reached her teens, the young Fräulein von Paradis was famous throughout Europe. She had played in Paris and London to such acclaim that Mozart became interested in her career, composing a concerto especially for her.

For years, physicians had tried to relieve the girl's blindness without success. After she had become the idol of musical Vienna, these efforts were redoubled. The doctors noted especially a terrible twitching of Maria Theresa's eyes, and believed this to be the cause of her blindness. Today this twitching would be recognized as *nystagmus,* a rhythmic horizontal oscillation of the eyes seen in longstanding blindness that is organic but never seen in hysteric blindness. Nystagmus, however, does not cause blindness; some people, especially albinos, with severe congenital nystagmus still have reasonably good vision.

Mesmer knew Fräulein von Paradis and convinced her parents that he should be allowed to treat her. Though he must have recognized early that his methods were of no value in organic disease, he obviously mistook the case as hysterical blindness—a serious error. The father and mother were eager to try anything and placed their daughter in Mesmer's hands.

Maria Theresa first visited Mesmer's clinic regularly for a few

weeks. In the beginning of 1777 she moved into the small private
nursing home he had established in one wing of his house. On January 20, continuous treatments were begun. Her eyes were bandaged
and unbandaged. She was placed before a mirror while a magnetized
wand was moved back and forth over her reflection.

As a result, the girl is said to have become more sensitive to light
and to have been able eventually to follow the movements of the
magnetized wand with her head. Also she is said to have been able to
discern through three thicknesses of bandage whether she was in a
darkened room. In light of the probable organic nature of her
blindness, this improvement is hard to believe today, especially when
one other fact is taken into account.

There is some evidence that soon after she moved into his house,
Mesmer began having sexual relations with young Maria Theresa,
and she fell in love with him. Then, to oblige her lover, she agreed to
participate in fake demonstrations of the "cure," though soon the
love affair and the deception she was involved in produced terrible
anxiety and guilt. Noting the increased emotional disturbance with
alarm, her father wrote, "Now that her senses are more diffused, she
requires greater concentration when she plays the piano, whereas formerly she played long concertos with great accuracy and was able to
carry on a conversation at the same time. Now, with open eyes, it is
difficult for her even to play one piece. She watches her fingers moving over the keyboard, and misses most of the chords."

The parents grew concerned that their daughter's future as a concert pianist was being ruined. The family's principal source of income, including the allowance from the empress, was in jeopardy.
Their distress was no doubt aggravated by the fact that Professor
Barth, an expert on the anatomy and diseases of the eye, had avowed
that the girl "must still be considered blind, because she did not
know what the objects shown her were called." In other words, environmental cues let her know an object was being held up, but she
could not see the object to identify it.

Frau and Herr von Paradis went to Mesmer's clinic to demand the
release of Maria Theresa. By this time, the furious father must have
suspected the affair between Mesmer and his daughter. When
Mesmer refused to give the girl up, the father drew a sword and
threatened him.

Meanwhile, Frau von Paradis had pulled Maria Theresa from her
room and dragged her along the corridor to confront Mesmer and

her husband. The poor girl shrank between her fuming parents, shaking and vomiting. Mesmer urged her to leave with her father and mother, but she refused to go. Though her mother struck her in the face, she continued to cling to Mesmer, and managed to remain in his house for five weeks longer.

On May 2 a Commission of Investigation ordered Mesmer to end his "fraudulent practice," and he was expelled from the medical faculty. Not disappointed when his wife decided to remain in Vienna, he traveled in Switzerland and Bavaria for a few months. In early 1778 he settled in Paris.

Again Mesmer managed to build up a highly successful practice, treating such luminaries as Marie Antoinette, Lafayette, and the entire Parisian court. When his home in Montmartre became too flooded with patients for him to be able to treat the sufferers individually, he began charging and distributing various objects—trees, bowls, mirrors, tubs—in order to obtain remote cures. The direct descendants of this method are today's electronic faith healers who can cure a distant sufferer via a television set.

At first, the French believed that Mesmer was a natural resource. The State offered to build him an institute to work in and to give him a pension of forty thousand livres. Mesmer was prepared to accept this provided he was given some official form of scientific recognition.

At this point, Louis XVI convinced the Academy of Sciences to investigate Mesmer's methods. Among its members were Lavoisier, Dr. Joseph Guillotin, and Benjamin Franklin. In their report, they tactfully stated that they were unable to sanction such techniques, though some inexplicable natural phenomenon did seem to be involved.

Yet the immense popularity of animal magnetism remained undiminished. "It is impossible to conceive the sensation which Mesmer's experiments created in Paris," wrote Baron Dupotet. "No theological controversy in the earlier ages of the church was ever conducted with greater bitterness." When Mesmer, mortified by the results of the investigating commission, threatened to leave Paris, the queen sank into despair. Maurepas, the minister of state, was authorized to offer every conceivable honor and a large sum of money in compensation to keep the famous healer in France. A public subscription was held in order to organize another academy—in opposition to the Academy of Sciences—that would be pro-Mesmer. The subscription was a huge success, in spite of the fact that many believed Mesmer's fees were outrageous. Madame Du Barry, the king's mistress, had a private Mesmer apparatus by her bed, but complained, "The fee demanded by this doctor for explaining the use of his magnetic apparatus was no less than one hundred louis. I was surprised, and my faith was shaken, because this man who declared his sole object was to serve humanity should have expected so vast a sum from his supporters."

The French Revolution soon cut short the controversy. In 1792 Mesmer was forced to flee Paris, leaving his money and manuscripts behind. He went first to Germany, to Karlsruhe in Baden. Then in 1793 he decided to return to Vienna, for the first time in fifteen years.

The Viennese government and the police were very fearful lest the revolution should spread to Austria and therefore were suspicious of all émigrés from France. When Mesmer was questioned, he did little to allay their fears, commenting that in the France of Louis there had been great inequalities, and though as a victim he had lost everything, he still felt constrained to see both sides of the situation. As a consequence of this incredible naïveté, he was arrested as a possible revolutionary plotting to overthrow the Austrian government and kept in prison for two months, being discharged on December 18, 1793.

He traveled to Switzerland and became a Swiss citizen. In 1798, at the age of sixty-four, he returned to Paris. Eventually the French government awarded him a pension of three thousand francs. Now financially secure, he moved back to Switzerland, where he died at the age of eighty.

In the 1820s a general revival of interest in mesmerism occurred, and sometime during this period the observation was made that pain could be obliterated in a mesmerized state. On April 12, 1829, Jules Cloquet, a French surgeon, removed the breast of a patient in mesmeric sleep. The method was promulgated by Richard Chenevix, a Parisian practitioner, who visited London and gave several demonstrations of mesmeric phenomena.

At St. Thomas' Hospital in London, Chenevix mesmerized patients before John Elliotson, an English physician. Elliotson was keenly interested, but did not become thoroughly convinced of the technique's efficacy until 1837, when the French mesmerist Baron Dupotet visited London to show the results he had obtained in Paris.

By this time, Elliotson was considered one of the ablest physicians in London and had risen to the rank of first professor of the practice of medicine at the new University of London, as well as senior physician at the newly founded college hospital attached to the university. Great public interest was aroused by his own demonstrations of mesmerism, and they were attended by many celebrities, including Charles Dickens and members of the nobility. But opposition within the medical community soon became so intense that the council of University College passed a resolution forbidding further practice of mesmerism within the hospital. In protest, Elliotson promptly resigned.

Now the former professor of the practice of medicine became a man with a mission—to demonstrate the truth of mesmerism. To do this, he and his supporters started *The Zoist: A Journal of Cerebral Physiology and Mesmerism, and their Application to Human Welfare.* In its first issue *The Zoist* announced that "the science of Mesmerism is a new physiological truth of incalculable value and importance. . . . Already it has established its claim to be considered a most potent remedy in the cure of disease; already enabled the knife of the operator to traverse and divide the living fibre unfelt by the patient. If such are the results of its infancy, what may not its maturity bring forth?"

Ultimately, very little, though in the beginning there was great promise, which is shown by the articles Elliotson reprinted to strengthen his argument. "A Case of Excision of a Wen without pain, in the Mesmeric State," was taken from the *Illinois Telegraph and Review* of August 19, 1843. A report of the removal of a tumor from the shoulder was reproduced from the *Missouri Republican,* February 21, 1843.

Meanwhile, surgical mesmerism was becoming more widely practiced, especially in America, where the medical establishment seemed to be less hostile to new ideas. Dr. A. Sidney Doane painlessly removed a neck tumor in New York. Another neck tumor was removed at the Cleveland Medical College. Dr. L. A. Dugas, of the Medical College of Georgia, amputated a breast. The excision of a nasal polyp was reported in the *Boston Medical and Surgical Journal.*

In India, too, surgical mesmerism was being used by James Esdaille, a follower of John Elliotson. While in charge of the Native Hospital at Hooghly, Esdaille reported performing seventy-three "painless surgical operations." These included amputations of the arm and breast, removal of tumors, hydroceles, cataracts, and tooth extractions. After publishing his results in *The Zoist,* Esdaille continued to use mesmerism, executing a total of several thousand operations, about three hundred of which were major.

But by 1851 Esdaille and others had come to recognize the basic weakness and inefficiency of mesmerism. Anesthesia could not be produced in every case, since not everyone needing surgery could be mesmerized. An especially serious defect was the failure of mesmerism in surgical emergencies; there simply was not enough time to induce the trance. Fortunately, all of these deficiencies could be circumvented by the chemical agents then coming into widespread use.

Chemical Anesthesia

The introduction of chemical anesthetic agents to abolish surgical pain occurred in an epoch-making five-year period between 1842 and 1847, though the first of these agents—diethyl ether—had been known for hundreds of years. In 1540 an alchemist, Valerius Cordus, gave the earliest account of the synthesis of this fluid, which he called *oleum dulci vitrioli* or "sweet oil of vitriol." To "very biting wine" (ethyl alcohol) "sour oil of vitriol" (sulfuric acid) was added. The mixture was then heated and the sweet oil of vitriol distilled from it. Or in modern chemical terms

$$2 \ CH_3CH_2OH \xrightarrow{\ H_2SO_4\ } CH_3CH_2OCH_2CH_3 + H_2O$$

Two molecules of ethyl alcohol (CH_3CH_2OH) heated in the presence of sulfuric acid (H_2SO_4) combine to form one molecule of ether ($CH_3CH_2OCH_2CH_3$) and one molecule of water.

Cordus found that sweet vitriol was an excellent solvent for many substances, and noted that it "may be used in pleurisy, peripneumonia, and hacking cough to draw from the lungs pus and mucus." F. G. Frobenius, a German chemist, gave sweet vitriol the name "ether" in 1730.

At the same time that Cordus was experimenting, another alchemist-physician Theophrastus Bombastus von Hohenheim, called Paracelsus, prepared ether independently. After administering the fluid to chickens, he made the following remarkable observation: "Of all the things extracted from vitriol it is most remarkable because it is stable. And besides, it has associated with it such a sweetness that it is taken even by chickens, and they fall asleep from it for a while but awaken later without harm. . . . In diseases which need to be treated with anodynes it quiets all suffering without any harm, and relieves all pain, and quenches all fevers, and prevents complications in all illnesses."

Paracelsus is one of the most controversial figures in the science of healing. Though he was first to recognize the analgesic effect of ether and advocate the use of chemicals in medicine, he was attacked by colleagues as a charlatan and a quack. A violent iconoclast, a prodigious drinker and fighter, he never went anywhere without a large sword buckled to his waist, and he died following a tavern brawl in Salzburg at the age of forty-eight. During his years of wandering from town to town throughout Europe, he lectured and wrote extensively, but infuriated other physicians by doing so in his native Swiss dialect rather than the customary Latin. Yet his discoveries survived him. Maupassant, the great French writer, used ether to relieve his headaches, remarking in *Sur l'Eau:* "Migraine is atrocious torment, one of the worst in the world, weakening the nerves, driving one mad, scattering one's thoughts to the winds and impairing the memory. So terrible are these headaches that I can do nothing but lie on a couch and try to dull the pain by sniffing ether."

Early in the nineteenth century, another use for ether was found: the ether party or ether frolic. This use is possible because inhalation of small amounts of ether has a similar effect to that of nitrous oxide. After observing one ether frolic, an American doctor, Crawford Williamson Long, became the first to use ether as a surgical anesthetic.

Long was a young doctor fresh from the medical school of the University of Pennsylvania when he hung out a shingle in the little village of Jefferson, Georgia. At that time, Jefferson was a crossroads far from a railroad. The nearest hospital, in New Orleans, was four hundred miles away.

The traveling showman with his laughing gas demonstrations was a familiar figure of the period, and such a showman passed through Jefferson in the winter of 1841. Having been called out to attend a patient, Long had missed the performance, but many of his friends had not. They waited for him at his house and gave him an uproarious welcome, telling him everything that had happened and remarking, "You're supposed to be a doctor and know something about chemistry. Make us some gas and we'll go on a fine tear."

Long did not have the means to prepare nitrous oxide. He did, however, have a bottle of ether in his surgery, and suggested that inhalation of this might produce the same effect. No sooner had he shoved an ether-saturated handkerchief under the nose of a friend than the man began to talk nonsense, dance, and sing. After the others had also enjoyed the effects of the ether, Long told them, "You see, your doctor here in Jefferson can give as good measure as any stranger."

Next day the friends came again and begged to be given more ether. Thereafter, there would be ether frolics at the young doctor's house two or three nights a week. The girls from the neighborhood soon also begged to join in. Because the tall, handsome doctor did not want to refuse them, he was forced to continue ordering ether from Robert Goodman's drug store in Athens, Georgia, and with one order sent this letter:

> Dear Bob,
>
> I am under the necessity of troubling you a little. I am entirely out of ether and wish some by tomorrow night if it is possible to receive it by that time. We have some girls in Jefferson who are anxious to see it taken, and you know nothing would afford me more pleasure than to take it in their presence and to get a few sweet kisses (?) . . . if you can meet with the opportunity to send the medicines to me tomorrow you will confer a great favour by doing so. If you cannot send them tomorrow, get Dr. Reese to send them by the stage on Wednesday, I can persuade the girls to remain until Wednesday night, but would prefer receiving the ether sooner.
>
> > Your friend,
> > Crawford Long

On the day of the party, Long told the girls that he would not inhale the ether himself, because there was no telling what he might do while intoxicated. Of course, the women insisted that he do so.

"All right," said Long, "I'll inhale some if y'all promise not to hold me responsible for anything I may do."

Because he boarded with two strait-laced elderly sisters who were strict Quakers, Long was careful to lock the door to his room. Then, with great solemnity, he poured the ether onto a cloth, put it to his face, and pretended to sleepwalk gravely around the room as he kissed every girl in turn. As an old man, he would slap his thigh with glee and roar with laughter as he recounted this prank, recalling that "the girls must have liked it for they were so anxious to try the drug themselves."

Long later married one of these beautiful young girls, and here is her recollection of him at that period: "I yet see him, dressed in a light blue summer suit, collars and cuffs black, tan coloured silk gloves, wide-brimmed white hat, sitting superbly on his dapple grey charger, firm dignified—he rides like one to command."

Though Long may have looked like a dandified version of Robert E. Lee, he proved himself to be an extremely astute and perceptive observer. For he noticed after several of the ether parties that he had bruised himself, though he had absolutely no recollection of doing so. Convinced that ether might be of value as the long-sought surgical analgesic, he resolved to use it on the next patient requiring an operation. This historic first case of ether anesthesia was a man who suffered from what now appear to be sebacious cysts. Seven years afterward, Long described the procedure as follows:

"The first patient to whom I administered ether in a surgical operation was Mr. James M. Venable, who then resided within two miles of Jefferson, and at present lives in Cobb County, Georgia. Mr. Venable consulted me on several occasions in regard to the propriety of removing two small tumors situated on the back part of his neck, but would postpone from time to time having the operations performed, from dread of pain. At length I mentioned to him the fact of my receiving bruises while under the vapour of ether, without suffering, and as I knew him to be fond of, and accustomed to inhale ether, I suggested to him the probability that the operation might be performed without pain, and proposed operating on him while under its influence. He consented to have one tumor removed, and the operation was performed the same evening. The ether was given to Mr. Venable on a towel; and when fully under its influence I extirpated the tumor. It was encysted, and about half an inch in diameter. The patient continued to inhale ether during the time of the operation; and when informed it was over seemed incredulous, until the tumor was shown to him. He gave no evidence of suffering during the operation, and assured me, after it was over, that he did not experience the slightest degree of pain from its performance. This operation was performed on the 20th March, 1842."

Within the next three years, Long used ether to perform several more operations, two of these being amputation of toes and fingers. Unfortunately, other doctors in the neighborhood began to complain that their colleague was recklessly using a new poison that was bound to kill someone sooner or later. As word got around, Long's practice began to dwindle; finally the village elders threatened to lynch him if he used ether any longer.

Not inclined to be a revolutionary or martyr, Long gave up. He didn't even publish the results of his first case until 1849, three years after the general acceptance of ether by the medical profession. The only record he made at the time of surgery was this simple ledger entry: "James Venable, 1842. Ether and excising tumor, $2.00."

When he realized the significance of the discovery he had allowed to slip through his grasp, Long struggled the rest of his life for recognition. During his flight before the oncoming forces of General Sherman in 1864 he carried with him a glass jar containing a roll of papers, "my proofs of the discovery of ether anesthesia." But by hesitating to publish until well after the fact, he had lost for all time the credit for influencing the development of anesthesia. This credit belongs to another man—William Thomas Green Morton, a dentist.

Today it may seem odd to some people that a dentist should be involved with the discovery of surgical anesthesia. After all, can a patient suffer so intensely in a dental chair that such a powerful agent as ether is necessary?

Indeed he can. The terrible pain associated with dental procedures has long been known as one of the most effective forms of torture. At Alexandria during a persecution, St. Apollonia and Blasius the Blessed were tied to pillars while their teeth were extracted to persuade them to renounce Christianity. A thousand years later, King John of England extorted money by yanking teeth. When a wealthy citizen of Bristol would not pay ten thousand ducats, John had the man brought to his palace and with his own royal hands extracted a tooth a day for a week until finally resistance was broken.

Dentists had long agonized over the killing pain they inflicted during oral surgery and extractions, yet it seemed insurmountable. Then in 1844 one dentist, Horace Wells, observed the analgesic effect of nitrous oxide, just as Sir Humphry Davy had almost half a century before.

On December 10 an itinerant laughing-gas showman named Gardner Colton gave a frock-coated exhibition of chemical wonders before a large audience in Hartford, Connecticut. As "Professor" Colton, he invited a few members of the audience to come on stage and inhale. Among those who came forward was Wells.

Wells was a well-educated, inquisitive, restless man. At nineteen, he had begun the study of dentistry in Boston by reading under preceptors and working in dental offices. Soon he had established a large practice in Hartford while finding time to invent and construct novel dental instruments. But though several of these were subsequently patented, he quickly lost interest in them, impulsively jumping from one new project to the next. Colton's laughing gas demonstration was to bring an unfortunate repetition of this erratic behavior.

Wells watched as a young man named Cooley inhaled the gas and, while under its influence, ran against some wooden settees on the stage and bruised his legs badly.

"You must have hurt yourself," said Wells to Cooley.

"No," Cooley replied, but then, after beginning to feel some pain, was astonished to find his legs bloody. When Wells inquired about this, Cooley said he felt no pain until the effects of the gas had worn off.

Now quite excited, Wells approached Colton after the performance and asked, "Why cannot a man have a tooth extracted under the gas, and not feel it?"

When Colton said that he did not know, Wells insisted that a painless extraction could be so performed. Furthermore, he would try it on himself if the "Professor" would bring a bag of gas to his office. The reluctant Colton was induced to participate in the experiment only after Wells described in glowing terms the huge fortune that the two could make as painless dentists.

The next day, December 11, 1844, Wells summoned a colleague, John Mankey Riggs, to perform the extraction of a wisdom tooth that had troubled Wells for some time. Riggs, who later became known as the discoverer of alveolar pyorrhea, or Riggs' disease, was quite skeptical and hesitant; only after Wells' bubbling enthusiasm had thoroughly infected him did he agree to help.

After Wells sat down in his dental chair, Colton put the mouthpiece of the gasbag to the patient's lips and turned the tap to release the gas. Wells inhaled deeply, coughed, and then continued to breathe the gas slowly and regularly. Suddenly, his usually pale face went ashen and his lips turned blue. Riggs immediately picked up the dental forceps, reached in for the tooth, and extracted it. Wells' eyes were glazed over. His head fell forward on his chest. His breathing stopped. But then his hands fluttered, he began to breathe naturally, and his eyes opened.

"A new era in tooth pulling!" shouted the startled Wells when he awoke to find Riggs holding the tooth. "I did not feel it so much as the prick of a pin!"

Not wasting a minute, Wells assembled all the materials needed to produce nitrous oxide. Convinced by Riggs that some scientific authority should endorse the method in order to reassure potential patients, he then hurried to Boston to consult Charles T. Jackson, a chemist, who had a few years earlier given a similar endorsement to a new dental solder concocted by his student William Morton and Wells. But this time Jackson was unconvinced and scornfully ordered Wells to go no further with his crazy idea. Pain, the chemist said, was an integral part of life; all scientists knew this fact, and it was certainly not to be questioned by a mere dentist.

Wells left Jackson's house in a fury, but still certain that laughing gas was an effective surgical anesthetic. To prove this, he decided to arrange a public demonstration by approaching Dr. John Collins Warren, an eminent Boston surgeon. Warren was accustomed to evaluating such remedies as Wells claimed to possess and agreed to allow the dentist to demonstrate a painless extraction before a class of students at the Massachusetts General Hospital.

On the appointed day, Wells appeared before the assembled group with the gas apparatus. William Morton, who was boarding in Boston with Jackson, accompanied his former dental preceptor and brought along his own instruments to assist. Dr. Warren's voice was full of scorn as he introduced Wells to the students: "There is a gentleman here who purports to have something which will destroy pain in surgical operations. He wants to address you. If any of you would like to hear him, you are at liberty to do so."

A Harvard student with a troublesome tooth volunteered to be the guinea pig. Wells tried to adopt a calm and confident air, but just could not control his nervousness. He kept fumbling and dropping the instruments. Finally he managed to give what he thought was an adequate dose of laughing gas. He gripped the tooth firmly with the dental forceps, but as he began to pull, the patient emitted an awful shriek.

The whole room erupted. "The spectators laughed and hissed when the patient screamed from pain," said Morton. Actually, the student had felt no pain, and later admitted this. But there was no consolation for Wells at the moment of his humiliation as he rushed out of the room to escape the insults and jeers. He returned to Hartford the following morning to arrange another demonstration, determined to give a larger dose of gas. But this time the patient almost died.

Wells could stand no more and gave up. He turned his dental practice over to his friend Riggs and tried to make a living as a salesman. First he traveled through Connecticut peddling singing canaries, then patented shower baths, then coal-sifters. When these products were not snapped up as expected, he went to Europe to buy paintings and engravings cheaply, hoping to receive high prices for them in America.

In the meantime William Morton had made the first successful public demonstration of ether anesthesia. Upon learning this, Wells published a letter, dated February 17, 1847, in *Galignani's Messenger,* stating his claims to priority and asserting that he had used ether as well as nitrous oxide. An American dentist, C. Starr Brewster, met Wells in Paris, believed his story, and brought his claims before several French learned societies, though the Paris Medical Institute had already made an award for the discovery of ether.

By this time Wells had become deeply depressed. He returned to America to try to promote the use of nitrous oxide in surgery, but shortly afterward became psychotic. He was arrested in the streets of New York while attempting to hurl concentrated acid at passers-by and was incarcerated in the notorious Tombs Prison to await sentence. On January 24, 1848, he managed to get hold of some chloroform and a razor. After writing a suicide note begging forgiveness for the act he was about to commit, he anesthetized himself with chloroform and in his last conscious second slashed the femoral artery in his thigh. He was thirty-five years old.

Twelve days before this gruesome event, Dr. Brewster had sent a letter that its addressee did not survive to receive:

My Dear Wells:

   I have just returned from a meeting of the Paris Medical Society, where they have voted that to Horace Wells, of Hartford, Connecticut, United States of America, is due all the honor of having successfully discovered and successfully applied the use of vapors or gases whereby surgical operations could be performed without pain. They have done even more, for they have elected you honorary member of their Society. This was the third meeting that the Society had deliberated on the subject. On the two previous occasions, Mr. Warren, the agent of Dr. Morton, was present and endeavored to show that to his client was due the honor but he, having completely failed, did not attend the last meeting. The use of ether took the place of nitrous oxide gas, but chloroform has supplanted both, yet the first person, who first discovered and performed surgical operations without pain, was Horace Wells, and to the last day of time must suffering humanity bless his name.

Your diploma and the vote of the Paris Medical Society shall be forwarded to you. In the interim, you may use this letter as you please.

> Believe me ever truly yours,
> Brewster

Wells died with the belief that the ultimate credit for anesthesia would go to Morton. Even Brewster's letter might not have been sufficiently reassuring. But had he lived, he would have seen that Morton was also to suffer embitterment over priority for the discovery.

William Morton was born in 1814 at Charlton, Massachusetts, the son of a farmer. After a spotty elementary education, he went to Boston at the age of seventeen, where he held various jobs as a clerk and a salesman. Then he moved to Baltimore to study dentistry at the College of Dental Surgery. Two years later he returned to Boston, where he first met and worked with Wells.

In March 1844 Morton decided to study medicine and enrolled at the Harvard Medical School. Though eventually completing two terms at Harvard, he did not receive a medical degree. While a student, he was assigned the chemist Charles T. Jackson as preceptor and lived in his house.

Morton had meanwhile continued to practice dentistry, and one day at home with Jackson the subject of deadening dental pain was brought up. A few years later, at the peak of their subsequent bitter feud, Morton recalled the conversation: "I spoke of the operation of destroying the nerve of a tooth. . . . Dr. Jackson said, in a humorous manner, that I must try some of his tooth ache drops." As the drops had ether as their active ingredient, "Dr. Jackson then added, that as this ether might be applied with advantage to sensitive teeth, he would send me some. The conversation then turned upon the effect of ether upon the system, and he told me how the students at Cambridge used to inhale sulphuric ether from their handkerchiefs, and that it intoxicated them, making them reel and stagger."

In July 1844 Morton tried the ether Jackson had given him on the aching tooth of a Miss Parrot from Gloucester. The treatment worked, and Miss Parrot returned several times for a reapplication. One day, after using more ether than before, Morton was astonished to notice how the surrounding tissues had also been numbed. It was at this moment that the idea of systemic administration of ether to relieve intense pain occurred to him, as he later recounted: "The successful application I had made of the ether in destroying the sensibility of a tooth, together with what Dr. Jackson told me of its effects when inhaled by students at college, awakened my attention, and having free access to Dr. Jackson's books, I began to read on the subject of its effects upon the animal system. I became satisfied there was nothing new or particularly dangerous in the inhaling of ether, that it had long been the toy of professors and students, known as a powerful anti-spasmodic, anodyne, and narcotic, capable of intoxicating and stupefying, when taken in sufficient quantity. I found that even the apparatus for inhaling it was described in some treatises, but in most cases it was described as inhaled from a saturated sponge or handkerchief."

In the spring of 1846 Morton tested his theory: "I tried an experiment upon a water spaniel, inserting his head in a jar having sulphuric ether at the bottom. . . . After breathing the vapor for some time, the dog completely wilted down in my hands. I then removed the jar. In about three minutes he aroused, yelled loudly, and sprung some ten feet, into a pond of water."

Now convinced that using ether to produce unconsciousness was safe, Morton found a patient named Eben Frost to whom it could be given: "I . . . waited impatiently for some one upon whom I could make a fuller trial. Toward evening, a man, residing in Boston . . . came in, suffering great pain and wishing to have a tooth extracted. He was afraid of the operation and asked if he could be mesmerized. I told him I had something better, and saturating my handkerchief, gave it to him to inhale. He became unconscious almost immediately. It was dark, and Dr. Hayden held the lamp, while I extracted a firmly rooted bicuspid tooth. There was not much alteration in the pulse, and no relaxation of the muscles. He recovered in a minute, and knew nothing of what had been done to him. This was on the 30th of Sept., 1846."

Morton was certain that he was going to make a fortune from his discovery, and so obtained from Eben Frost a signed statement that the extraction had been painless. As an extra precaution, Morton had his assistants, Horace Hayden and A. G. Tenney, also sign. The next day an account of the procedure appeared in the Boston *Daily Journal*. On the same day, Morton went to see Richard Eddy, the Boston commissioner of patents, to apply for a patent on his method.

Patients soon began flocking to Morton's office, though other dentists did not approve what they heard about the new technique, and with good reason. There was some difficulty involved in administering the ether—particularly in controlling the amount inhaled. One woman became only slightly drowsy when Morton gave her ether on a sponge. But when he substituted for the sponge a new instrument he had devised, she almost suffocated. Rumors began to circulate that Morton had nearly killed a few patients in his chair.

Within a week of pulling Eben Frost's tooth, Morton decided to test ether publicly. He approached Dr. John Collins Warren, the same eminent Harvard surgeon who had watched Wells make a fool of himself, and asked to be allowed a demonstration; a few days later, he received this note:

> Dear Sir:
>
> I write at the request of Dr. J. C. Warren, to invite you to be present on Friday morning at 10 o'clock, at the hospital, to administer to a patient who is then to be operated upon, the preparation which you have invented to diminish the sensibility to pain.

The date was October 14, 1846, and the signature was that of C. F. Heywood, house surgeon to the Massachusetts General Hospital.

Within hours of the scheduled operation, Morton had designed a new, safer inhaler and consigned its construction to a Boston instrument maker. On the morning of Friday, October 16, the device was still not finished; the anxious dentist was forced to wait impatiently while the last touches were added. Finally he grabbed the inhaler and ran to pick up Eben Frost, who would testify before the audience of the preparation's effectiveness should the procedure be a failure.

In his pocket Morton carried a bottle of ether, with aromatic oils and opium added to disguise the characteristic odor. He did not want the audience to guess the nature of the preparation before a patent was granted. He clutched at the bottle as he rushed down Cambridge Street, his head bent, his cloak billowing out around him, while Frost followed behind, puffing. Through Blossom Street and Fruit Street the two men ran, to the huge hospital with its Bulfinch dome that dominated the Charles River. With a final burst of energy, Morton bounded up the plain granite staircase to the small surgical amphitheater.

Inside the room, everyone had been waiting for more than fifteen minutes. The rows of seats were jammed with students and eminent Boston medical men. Dr. Warren, ready to perform the operation, stood near the patient, Gilbert Abbot, a consumptive young man with a tumor at the angle of the jaw. In his high-pitched but brusquely commanding voice Warren had already announced that a new pain-killing preparation was to be tested. Now, after a glance at the clock, the dignified surgeon picked up his scalpel and remarked, looking at the assembled audience with a sarcastic smile, "As Dr. Morton has not arrived, I presume he is otherwise engaged." A burst of derisive laughter emerged from the crowd as attendants began to strap down the patient.

Suddenly Morton burst into the room, followed by Frost puffing after him. When Morton began to murmur an apology for being late, Warren cut him sternly short with an imperious "Well, sir, your patient is ready."

"Are you afraid?" Morton asked the patient.

"No," the man replied, "I feel confident and will do precisely as you tell me."

Morton inserted a tube from the inhaler between the patient's lips and ordered him to breathe in and out through his mouth. After a few spasmodic movements of his arms and legs, Gilbert Abbot sank into unconsciousness.

"Sir," said Morton as he bowed to Warren, "your patient is ready."

The surgeon seized the tumor with one hand and made his first incision. The growth was removed. The wound was closed. The patient did not utter a cry, though he did move his legs a bit and make a few incoherent sounds. After his face was washed, he awoke from the effects of the ether. When questioned, he affirmed that he had felt no pain, only a vague blunt scratching of his cheek.

Warren turned to his students. "Gentlemen," he said, "this is no humbug."

Within days, news of the painless operation performed with ether created a sensation throughout the world, levitating William Morton to the high point of his career and his life. But only for a moment, for soon the fight for priority sank him into an abyss worse than he had ever known.

This fight resulted from advice Morton had sought from Charles Jackson, about administering ether. Morton recalled: "I said, in as careless a manner as I could assume, 'Why cannot I give the ether gas?' He said that I could do so, and spoke again of the students taking it at Cambridge. He said the patient would be dull and stupefied, that I could do what I pleased with him, that he would not be able to help himself. Finding the subject open, I made the enquiries I wished as to the different kinds and preparations of ether. He told me something about the preparations and thinking that if he had any it would be of the purest kind, I asked him to let me see his. He did so, but remarked that it had been standing for some time, and told me that I could get some highly rectified at Burnetts."

Morton had been having difficulties consistently producing anesthesia, and this conversation gave him the reason for his failure—he had been using impure ether. The highly refined Burnetts ether obtained on Jackson's recommendation was subsequently used at the Massachusetts General demonstration. The apparent caution Morton employed in soliciting his former preceptor's advice was well-advised, for Jackson was an insanely vicious, unscrupulous man.

Jackson had studied medicine at Harvard but became more interested in chemistry, mineralogy, and geology. He went to Paris to study at the Sorbonne, making there a good name for himself in the French scientific community. After returning to America in 1833, he had set up a medical practice. Patients were quickly driven away, however, by his unpleasant personality.

Just at this time, an army doctor, William Beaumont, had published a report of an extraordinary medical case. A decade before, he had been called to attend the abdominal gunshot wounds of a young man, Alexis St. Martin. St. Martin survived, against all odds, but with a fistula or opening from his stomach to his skin. Beaumont immediately recognized his unique opportunity and made the first accurate observations of the living stomach digesting food by lowering meat and other substances attached to a thread through the fistula.

As might be expected, St. Martin was not happy with this life; he was expected to act as Beaumont's servant while he also served as guinea pig. Eventually he ran away, but being too weak to continue in his old job of fur trapping, he was forced to return to Beaumont and undergo more tests. Among the further indignities he had to endure was exhibition at medical colleges as "the man with the window in his stomach."

Jackson saw one of these exhibitions at the Connecticut Medical College in 1833 and begged Beaumont to give him a vial of gastric fluid for chemical analysis. After receiving this, he tried to get Beaumont stationed in Boston in order to use St. Martin for his own experiments, petitioning the Secretary of War and obtaining signatures of two hundred members of Congress. There was, however, no way he could steal credit for the digestion experiments, since Beaumont had already published a book on the case that remained unrivaled until Pavlov began work on digestion toward the end of the century.

Though unsuccessful with Beaumont, Jackson soon became involved in a more serious dispute. When returning to America from France in 1832, he had sailed on the packet steamer *Sully,* making the acquaintance of Samuel Morse, a portrait painter and gadgeteer. Morse had the bad luck to tell Jackson of his ideas for sending messages by electrical impulses. In 1837, after Morse had built the first telegraph, Jackson tried to claim credit for it, and was very nearly successful. Only after a bitter battle that raged for seven years was Morse able to prove the falsehood of Jackson's outrageous assertions. Morton was not to be so lucky.

On December 21, 1846, Jackson sent two letters to a geologist friend in Paris, L. Élie de Beaumont, requesting that they be read to the French Academy of Sciences. Without even mentioning Morton, these letters claimed that Jackson was the discoverer of surgical anesthesia. Once this had been done, Jackson pressed Morton for a share of the patent rights, and, because of bad legal advice, Morton agreed. Then on March 2, 1847, Jackson read a paper before the American Academy of Arts and Sciences in which he again proclaimed himself as the discoverer of anesthesia. Jackson had his paper reprinted in the Boston *Daily Advertiser* and sent copies to European colleagues the next day on the mail packet. This action made it ap-

pear that the Academy itself had sanctioned Jackson's claim. Thereafter, for a considerable time in Europe, the impression prevailed
that Jackson was the discoverer of anesthesia, though the Academy
did everything possible to contradict this view.

Jackson eventually became totally insane, spending the last seven
years of his life in the McLean Asylum, but not before he had managed to use his influence to ruin Morton's dental practice. The bankrupt Morton applied to Congress, and finally a bill was written
awarding him $100,000 for his discovery. But the bill became mired
in committee when rival claims were entered by Jackson and Crawford Long. As a result, Morton never received a penny. He died at
the age of forty-nine in severe mental anguish and dire poverty.

Morton's patent proved to be of no value, for doctors soon discovered that they did not need his complicated inhaler for ether administration; a soaked sponge would work just as well. But for many years
the second plane of anesthesia, the stage of delirium, remained a
problem. Hugh Hampton Young, the Johns Hopkins surgeon who
founded the specialty of urology, wrote this account of his experiences about 1895:

"One day I was giving ether to a burly, six-foot Irishman whose
red face gave indication of many years of heavy drinking. These patients are invariably hard to anesthetize, and in some instances ether
has very little effect. I filled and refilled the sponge with large dashes
of ether. Still the patient could not be got under and fought desperately. Finally, when I took the cone off to add more either, he seized
upon that moment to get away. With one violent movement he raised
his knees and broke the strap across them. In another desperate
surge with his hands he tossed the orderly over on the floor, and before I could get hold of his head he had tumbled off the stretcher
with the board fastened to his back. Regaining his feet, out of the
room he dashed, his only covering being the board that was strapped
to his back. Down the hall he went in a drunken fury, scattering
nurses and patients as he went on his way, and finally ran out into
the street, where a policeman caught him.

"Another time I was giving ether to a young mulatto girl. . . .
She had taken [it] over and over again and was hard to get under.
As I took off the cone to add more ether, she rolled her black eyes
and said, 'Kiss me again, Dr. Young.' If only she hadn't said 'again.'
I had been on the staff only a short time, and this occurrence worried
me no little."

Because of the difficulties associated with ether administration, other anesthetic agents were sought. And within a year one was found—chloroform.

Chloroform had been discovered independently in 1831 by three investigators: Justus von Liebig in Germany, Eugène Soubeiran in France, and Samuel Guthrie in America. Guthrie had, furthermore, observed his little granddaughter fall asleep next to his tubs of chloroform, yet failed to recognize its anesthetic properties, believing instead that it was nothing more than an all-purpose elixir.

On November 4, 1847, James Young Simpson, an English obstetrician, inhaled chloroform and noted that its effects were similar to those of inhaled ether. A few days later he successfully used chloroform to relieve the pains of labor and delivery. But the British public became incensed over this tampering with nature because of the famous passage in Genesis 3:16 that contains God's punishment of Eve for her part in the Temptation: "I will greatly multiply thy sorrow and thy conception; in sorrow thou shalt bring forth children."

Something of a Bible expert himself, Simpson countered with the fact that God was the first anesthetist, as reported in Genesis 2:21: "And the Lord God caused a deep sleep to fall upon Adam, and he slept: and he took one of his ribs, and closed up the flesh instead thereof." Simpson finally won out by gaining an ally considerably more influential in Britain than God—Queen Victoria. After chloroform had been successfully used during her royal accouchement, Simpson, a baker's son, was knighted for his great discovery, and the biblical proscription was forgotten.

Today, chloroform and ether have been replaced by less toxic, less flammable agents. Nitrous oxide is used somewhat more frequently, though not extensively. Yet these anesthetics still stand as great milestones in the science of healing. Dr. Oliver Wendell Holmes, addressing his medical class at Harvard in the fall of 1847, put it best: "The fierce extremity of suffering has been steeped in the waters of forgetfulness, and the deepest furrow in the knotted brow of agony has been smoothed forever."

CHAPTER FOUR

Infection

The discovery of ether anesthesia created a sensation in Europe. Only days after the announcement from Boston, the first European trial was held. On Monday, December 21, 1826, the procedure, an amputation, was performed at the University College Hospital of London.

The surgeon was Robert Liston, one of the great scalpel speed demons. Liston was an enormous man, who would amputate a thigh by compressing the artery with his powerful left hand while cutting and sawing with his right. It was said that when he took up his knife, the spectator who sneezed, winked, or turned his head for an instant missed the operation. Once, during an especially quick amputation, legend has it that he accidentally took off one of the patient's testicles and two of his assistant's fingers.

Yet even the speedy Liston had his share of horrible recollections: patients screaming, tearing madly at their restraints, held down only by brute force. One man to be operated on for a bladder stone had lost his nerve on the operating table, rushed down the long corridor, and locked himself in a lavatory. Liston tore out after him, battered down the door with his powerful shoulder, carried the petrified patient back, and operated successfully.

But this amputation was different. After the patient, a butler named Frederick Churchill, had been anesthetized, Liston removed the diseased leg without hearing a cry. When the butler awoke, he said, "When are you going to begin? Take me back, I can't have it done." He had not the slightest memory of suffering any pain.

Unfortunately, Liston had also unknowingly caused Frederick Churchill's problem. The butler had fallen, sustaining an injury to his tibia. As infection set in, pus began to discharge from the wound. Yet if left alone, the infection might have cleared up spontaneously.

Instead, the butler was brought to the University College Hospital of London. Liston, who usually wore an old stained frock coat spattered and encrusted with blood, examined the injury. First he probed it, then made an incision into which he inserted his dirty finger. After feeling the bone and thoroughly disseminating the infection, he plugged the wound. The inevitable signs of sepsis occurred: fever, sweating, rapid and feeble pulse, headache, nausea, twitching, exhaustion. Amputation was the only recourse.

In the audience watching Liston remove Frederick Churchill's leg was a young student, Joseph Lister. Within a few years, Lister was to make one of the great discoveries in the science of healing by learning how to prevent wound infections. This finding allowed the crude operative techniques of Robert Liston to be transformed into the sophisticated, life-saving science of surgery that exists today.

A Few Words About Wounds

As far as wounds are concerned, man is not one of nature's more favored creatures. The wounded salamander, for example, does much better. If it loses a whole limb, it can grow another one. Scientists say that it has a great capacity to regenerate. Only a few mammalian tissues can regenerate so well: epidermis, bone, occasionally nerve. But a severed muscle can never grow back. Even such a modest structure as a hair root—to the dismay of many older men—cannot be reconstructed.

For this reason, man's wounds heal by a patching up with connective tissue, a biologically simple, cheap, and handy substance filled with organic fibers and specialized cells called fibroblasts. When a wound occurs, millions of fibroblasts begin to generate new connective tissue. In the meantime, spilled blood, dead cells, foreign material, and bacteria are eliminated in a process known as inflammation. Extra blood flows around the injured area while temporary leaks develop in the smallest vessels so that antibacterial proteins and other useful substances can flow out. White blood cells migrate through the walls of capillaries into the wound, where they set about killing bacteria and ingesting debris. This entire inflammatory process is triggered by chemicals released from damaged tissue.

When not enough bacteria are around to cause trouble, the cleaning and rebuilding of the wound go on at the same time. Fibroblasts multiply, closing the defect with fibers. New blood vessels also grow into the area. This mass of new material is called "granulation tissue," because it appears red, fleshy, bumpy, and granular. The wound is, at the same time, being pulled closed by the fibroblasts. Such repair is known as "healing by primary intention."

But if many bacteria are introduced into the wound, healing takes place by slow "secondary intention" or not at all. Suppuration, the flooding of bacteria-killing white cells into the infected wound, is a common response. If the white-cell-filled pus is whitish and creamy, the outcome will probably be more favorable than if the pus is thin and malodorous. For this reason, whitish, creamy pus was long identified with the venerable Latin term, *pus bonum et laudabile* or "good and laudable pus."

If the infection spreads superficially further, a red halo develops around the wound, for which the Greeks coined the term *erysipelas*. Should infection spread deeply into the tissue, blood vessels leak excessively and the wound swells. As the bacteria continue to gain territory, the wound becomes a spreading ulcer. A worse calamity, the massive destruction of tissue, was known as *melasmos* or "blackening" to the ancient Greeks; it is now called gangrene. And at any time, the bacteria may gain a foothold elsewhere in the body. This catastrophe, known as sepsis, was almost invariably fatal before the days of antibiotics. So characteristic are all these manifestations of infection that ancient physicians mistakenly believed that each represented a separate, distinct disease.

An even greater error was the old conviction that pus could not be entirely bad. Greek physicians, convinced that the formation of whitish, odorless pus was the most favorable event possible, did their best to encourage it—a grievous mistake. Only after Joseph Lister's work in the late nineteenth century was it apparent that pus in a wound was an undesirable complication indicating bacterial infection.

Today it is easy, in light of modern bacteriologic knowledge, to fault ancient physicians for their ignorant belief in the value of laudable pus. But there were some rather deceptive, convincing truths upon which this belief was based:

First, as was mentioned, wounds exuding laudable pus were known to be much more likely to heal than those with thin, malodorous pus.

Second, suppuration partially cleans out of a wound the pieces of dead or dying tissue that would otherwise keep it from closing. Modern surgeons help by washing the wound and picking out extraneous matter—a process called *debridement*. Ancient physicians preferred to let the pus accomplish this.

Third, the Hippocratic corpus clearly states that "if swellings do not appear on severe wounds, it is a great evil." The grain of truth in this essentially correct observation is that total absence of swelling and pus may signify the body's defenses to be so poor that healing is not possible. Then, a little shaky logic leads to the obvious conclusion: "No pus is bad, so pus is good."

Fourth, the Greeks believed that "good, white pus" prevented worse complications. The logic here is questionable, since it probably derives from the fact that laudable pus is the least of the evils.

Fifth and last, the idea of laudable pus fitted into a hoary theory of disease known as the doctrine of the four humors. Since pus was believed to form as a wound "ripened," then this ripening must be the setting aside of a bad humor. The Greeks named this process *apostasis,* and from it is derived the old English *apostem* for abscess.

Yet, even in the face of these pro-pus arguments, the Greeks had noticed that many wounds healed quite adequately without suppuration. The physician, therefore, was forced to decide whether the wound should be helped to suppurate. This decision was influenced by the presence of bruised tissue; if it was present, he tried to encourage healing "by taking the wound rapidly through suppuration." To do this, a favorite preparation was applied:

> Wool as greasy as can be procured,
> dip it in very little water,
> add 1/3 wine, boil to good consistency

No doubt the presence of greasy wool in a wound did encourage suppuration.

To prevent suppuration, special drugs known as *enhemes* were used, particularly on fresh wounds. The dry, powdered variety of enheme could contain combinations of lead oxide, powdered lead metal, zinc oxide, copper oxide, copper sulfate, and alum. When sprinkled on a wound, these crude antiseptics did kill some bacteria, but unfortunately killed healthy tissue as well. Other enhemes were liquid preparations also having antibacterial properties. One contained strong white vinegar, honey, alum from Egypt, roasted sodium carbonate, and a little bile all boiled together. An enheme recommended after nasal surgery was composed of honey and copper oxide.

That these and other enhemes were of value could not be doubted by the Greek physicians who recorded their effects in the Hippocratic corpus: "Billos had been wounded in the back; much air came out of the wound, with noise; he bled; he was treated with enhemes and healed. The same happened to Dyslytas."

The Greeks favored still another wound wash: wine. This was one of the most efficacious of all treatments, because wine contains a polyphenol called malvoside that is thirty-three times stronger than the phenol used by Lister as an antiseptic. Though the enhemes did not survive beyond Greek times, treatment of wounds with wine continues in some places to the present day.

A more drastic antiseptic, fuming nitric acid, is fortunately no longer in use, though until the end of the nineteenth century it was popular—among physicians but not patients—for infected wounds and dog bites. Hugh Hampton Young, the Johns Hopkins surgeon, describes its use on his father's leg wound inflicted by a Yankee bullet during the Civil War battle of Kennesaw Mountain: "After days of suffering and lack of medical attention, Father finally reached a hospital. By that time the shattered left leg, with splintered bones and a large flesh wound, had become gangrenous. . . . Father told how he was strapped to a stretcher and, without anesthesia, nitric acid was poured into the rotting flesh, which crackled until the smoke reached the ceiling."

The elder Young somehow managed to survive this treatment, though not without a large, ugly, depressed scar on his leg. But most patients with serious wounds were not this lucky. Especially vulnerable were young women after giving birth. The severe lacerations resulting from delivery were susceptible to infection that rapidly spread. The outcome, puerperal sepsis, or childbed fever, was almost uniformly fatal.

A Hungarian physician, Ignaz Philipp Semmelweis, was responsible for the elimination of puerperal sepsis epidemics from maternity hospitals. In doing so, he became a pioneer in the use of the methods of epidemiology. Though at the time scorned and reviled for his techniques and his findings, Semmelweis is now regarded as one of the great figures in the science of healing.

Epidemiology and Semmelweis

Epidemiology, the study of the incidence, distribution, and control of disease in a population, is one of the most valuable tools for understanding illness. A recent example of its use was the analysis of the legionnaires' disease.

In the summer of 1976, a mysterious malady killed 29 people and hospitalized 151 others after an American Legion Convention in Philadelphia. The symptoms were similar in all affected cases: muscle pain, shaking chills, and high fever. Since the victims stayed in one building, the Bellevue Stratford Hotel, state epidemiologists examined every possible avenue along which disease might have been spread. The water supply, the air ducts, the food were unrevealing; puzzled scientists could not even decide whether a toxic substance or a micro-organism was at fault. Admitted Dr. William E. Parkin, chief epidemiologist of the Pennsylvania State Health Department: "It may be one year, five years, or a hundred years before our technology becomes efficient enough to cope with it."

Then in October 1976 a pathologist who had examined some of the victims became seriously ill with symptoms that looked strikingly like those of the legionnaires' disease. Convinced that an organism must be responsible for the illness, scientists at the U. S. Public Health Service's Center for Disease Control in Atlanta tried a new approach: to look for a strange bug rather than a familiar one.

One researcher, Dr. Joseph McDade, finally found the answer. After he inoculated guinea pigs with tissue from the lungs of two patients afflicted with the disease, the animals developed the characteristic signs within a day: fever, lethargy, watery eyes. Chick embryos infected with the same material died within six days. Microscopic examination of the embryo yolk sacs revealed clusters of a hitherto unknown rod-shaped bacteria that also might have caused an unexplained outbreak of a pneumonia-like illness that killed at least sixteen people in 1965 in St. Elizabeth's Hospital in Washington, D.C. This was shown when blood from the survivors of legionnaires' disease and the St. Elizabeth's epidemic demonstrated identical antibodies to the bacterial strain.

Semmelweis reached his conclusions about puerperal sepsis by using statistical methods that were also employed at the outset of the legionnaires' disease. Yet in spite of the fact that the germ theory of disease was unproven, he managed to guess correctly the means of spread and probable cause of this devastating illness of young mothers, thereby achieving the ability to prevent future outbreaks. In doing so, he showed an uncanny insight that allowed him confidently to reject many old, widely accepted ideas about infection, some of which had been postulated by the Greeks two thousand years before.

The high incidence of puerperal sepsis in Vienna's Allgemeines Krankenhaus prompted Semmelweis to confront the problem. This institution, founded by the Empress Maria Theresa at the close of the Seven Years' War in 1763, had become the world's largest obstetrical hospital during the reign of her son and successor, Joseph II. To make it also the best, the emperor had sent the chief obstetrician, Lucas Johann Boër, on a tour of all lying-in hospitals in France and Great Britain. When he returned, Boër became the ablest obstetrician of his time and a pioneer of the "natural method."

Trained as he had been among the English, who were strongly convinced of the contagiousness of childbed fever, Boër immediately introduced scrupulous care, cleanliness, and isolation of sick cases in the face of great staff hostility. He also shunned the use of corpses for obstetrical demonstrations, employing instead a mannequin or "phantom." Though antipathy toward these practices—quite radical by most European standards—continued to grow, the chief obstetrician would not relent. But finally, during the period of general reactionary sentiment that spread through Austria after the French Revolution, the government and numerous enemies coerced Boër to resign. He was replaced by Johann Klein, his former assistant, who had no regard whatever for the methods of his English-trained predecessor.

Naturally, the death rate from puerperal sepsis immediately shot upward. While Boër's death rate had averaged about 1 per cent, under Klein this rose at once from 0.84 per cent in one year to 7.8 per cent in the next year. During epidemics it sometimes reached nearly 50 per cent. Pregnant women among Vienna's poor were well aware of this and so had a mortal fear of the great lying-in wards, often seeking to avoid the hospital until their babies were born.

The government and the hospital authorities were also deeply disturbed. Committee after committee met and suggested remedies. But current medical thought was dominated by the ancient epidemic theory of the cause of puerperal sepsis, which held that atmospheric-cosmic-telluric influences were responsible for the disease. Since no one had the faintest idea what these influences might be, no solution could be hoped for.

About 1840 Klein made a redistribution of his pupils according to sex. Until that time, the first obstetric clinic and the second obstetric clinic had been attended by both midwives and medical students. Now, the first clinic was given over to students while the second one was reserved for midwives.

In a short time the mortality rate among the patients in the midwives' clinic had dropped considerably below that of the patients in the students' clinic. Two peculiar characteristics of this mortality incidence were also noted. First, the mortality in the students' clinic showed a seasonal variation while that in the midwives' clinic did not change. Second, in the students' clinic the patients often became sick in rows, while in the midwives' clinic the cases were scattered throughout the ward.

Another enigma lay in the mortality rate of prolonged labor. The chances for survival were decreased only in the students' clinic, not in that of the midwives. As for the case of premature births, these appeared to be of no benefit in the midwives' clinic, though in the students' clinic the incidence of puerperal sepsis was lower. Finally, women who had street births when taken to the midwives' clinic had no advantage over women who were delivered in the clinic, but when admitted to the students' clinic they did much better than women delivered there.

Ignaz Semmelweis would seem to have had no particular educational advantages that contributed to his solution of this classic problem in epidemiology. He had left his affluent Hungarian family to read law in Vienna, but then switched to medicine, graduating from the medical school of the University of Vienna at the age of twenty-six. Shortly afterward he became an observer, and in 1846 an assistant in the first obstetric clinic of the Allgemeines Krankenhaus. Klein, still clinic director, would live to rue this particular appointment.

Semmelweis was a heavily built, prematurely bald man with a great air of dynamic authority about him. With his intense ambition, he seemed the type of man who could go into a revolving door behind you and come out in front. He was also extremely truculent, without the slightest pretense of tact, and despite his neophyte status, he had no qualms about lecturing his superiors in matters of obstetrics. They in turn retaliated by disdaining his thickly accented speech and flawed command of written Germany.

Yet despite his brusque, overbearing nature, Semmelweis did manage to make a few important friends: Ferdinand von Hebra, the founder of dermatology; Joseph Skoda, who improved physical examination methods of the heart and lungs; and the famous pathologist, Karl von Rokitansky, whose discoveries contributed to making Vienna the premier medical center of mid-nineteenth-century Europe. These men were later the first to recognize the importance of Semmelweis's work and lend much-needed support.

In February 1846, after being appointed provisional assistant at the first clinic, Semmelweis began to make early morning rounds with the students, examining each patient and later reporting his findings to the chief of service. In the afternoon, as assistant, he gave the students bedside instruction by examining every patient in labor. In the evenings he was always on call to assist the midwives in his division.

The enormously high incidence of puerperal sepsis in his clinic seems to have begun to distress Semmelweis during the time of his assistantship. A reasonably well-adjusted physician can usually become inured to the repetitive appearance of even the most grotesque manifestations of illness and death; if this were not true, there would be no cancer specialists today. But Semmelweis, besides his other peculiarities, had a personality type that would now be called cyclothymic because of his periodic alternation between moods of elation and depression. While his older colleagues had long before accustomed themselves quite well to the decimated rows of young mothers under their care, these repeated deaths threw Semmelweis into fits of deep despair. Discovering their cause became an obsession.

Almost immediately, he recognized that the division of the clinic into two parts provided him with a control group against which changes in the condition of the other group could be measured. To accomplish this measurement, he began by constructing a mortality table from the exacting records of admissions, deaths, and causes of death kept by the hospital. The table was unambiguous. In the first clinic, where the medical students worked, 1,989 women or 9.9 per cent of the total admissions had died over a six-year period. In the midwives' clinic the record was substantially better—691 women dead, or 3.4 per cent over the same six-year period. And Semmelweis knew that the results were actually worse than they appeared, for it was customary at that time to transfer very sick women from the students' clinic to the wards of the general hospital so that their deaths would not appear in the clinic record.

The discovery of a control group and the application of simple statistical methods were in themselves landmarks in the study of disease. But a solution to the problem was still far from apparent, because there was no clear indication what caused puerperal sepsis or how it was spread. Besides the cosmic-telluric-influence theory which has already been mentioned, a number of other ideas were also current. Some authorities believed that the malady occurred frequently in cases of stillbirths, that it depended on whether a woman was married or single, that it was caused by a mysterious halo clinging to the obstetrician. For many years one school of thought had held that it was a fever of the milk; a Frenchman even claimed to have found milk in the peritoneal cavity of a victim. Still other physicians maintained that scarlet fever, measles, and smallpox were related to childbed fever, and that one could turn into the other. An especially popular notion, the fear theory, was the first that Semmelweis set out to test.

A robed priest and a bell-ringing attendant daily walked through the wards to administer last rites to the dying. The women lying in their beds were petrified with fear by this doleful ritual. Semmelweis quietly urged the cleric to approach the dying by a roundabout route and without the bell. The death rate was totally unaffected, but the simplicity of the technique encouraged Semmelweis to try other approaches.

By April 1847 the death rate in the first clinic had climbed to a staggering all-time high of 18 per cent. The sensitive, unstable Semmelweis was plagued by women crouching at his feet, clinging to his trousers, begging not to be sent to his ward. Just when he was plunged into an especially deep fit of depression by these unsettling circumstances, he noticed a difference in the method of delivery used in the two clinics. While in the first clinic the procedure was performed with the woman on her back, in the second clinic she was on her side.

Though he did not believe that position made a difference, Semmelweis ordered that his ward should adopt the method of the second clinic. He was right. The death rate remained unaltered.

In the meantime, Dr. Joseph Skoda had seen a copy of his friend's obstetric mortality table and proposed that another commission should meet to take some sort of remedial action. Thus threatened, Klein was able to delay the meeting by invoking the protection of the minister of education. But when the death rate in the first division soared to four times that in the second, a commission did meet. The conclusion: Puerperal sepsis was the result of injury to the genital organs inflicted by students during their course of instruction—particularly foreign students. Therefore, the number of these foreigners should be reduced. After this burst of xenophobia, the mortality dropped slightly, then rose again as the last foreigners were excluded.

One of the final foreigners to leave was Semmelweis himself, though not because of the exclusion rule. His position, only a temporary one, had lapsed. Thoroughly depressed and disillusioned, he decided to take a brief vacation before going to England to resume his career. Instead, the departure of a permanent hospital staff member left a vacancy. After a brief holiday in Venice, Semmelweis resumed his old duties.

He had hardly returned when a freak accident provided him with the critical clue needed to solve the problem of puerperal sepsis. Just as happened in the legionnaires' disease epidemic more than a century later, a pathologist examining the body of a victim became infected. This man, Jakob Kolletschka, had received a puncture wound of the finger from an assistant's knife during an autopsy. He thereupon developed a disease identical to puerperal sepsis, and a few days before his death the infection had spread or metastasized to one of his eyes, as sometimes also happened in puerperal sepsis.

In a flash, Semmelweis grasped the significance of what had occurred, and wrote, "In the excited condition in which I then was, it rushed into my mind with irresistible clearness that the disease from which Kolletschka had died was identical with that from which I had seen so many hundreds of lying-in women die."

Now the cause of puerperal sepsis could be deduced with ease. Kolletschka had died because a poisonous substance from the cadaver he was examining had entered his body through the puncture wound in his finger. This same poisonous substance was introduced into the wounded genitalia of women after childbirth by the hospital physicians, including Semmelweis, who came to examine them with unwashed hands directly after performing autopsies on puerperal sepsis victims.

Nothing demonstrates the risky, double-edged nature of valuable medical research better than this disastrous situation. In the mid-eighteenth century an Italian anatomist, Giovanni Battista Morgagni, had demonstrated conclusively that diseases were not generally dispersed throughout the body; rather, they often began locally in specific organs or tissues. Morgagni was able to show, for example, that apoplexy or stroke primarily resulted from changes in blood vessels and not from lesions in the brain itself; that cerebral abscess was the result, not the cause, of a discharging ear; that cerebral lesions on one side of the brain affected movements on the opposite side of the body. These important discoveries were made by correlating good clinical histories with meticulously detailed autopsies. When France became the great center of medical research in the early nineteenth century, a new understanding of tuberculosis and chest diseases resulted from correlating the sounds heard through the stethoscope with pathologic changes in the lungs found on autopsy.

But since no one was certain how disease was spread, no precautions were taken to protect live patients from indirect contact with cadaveric material via the hands of physicians. So from the valuable technique of autopsy came the terrible epidemic scourge of puerperal sepsis.

An analogous situation occurred after the discovery of X rays. These wonderful new rays could be used to see changes within the living body that previously could be seen only on autopsy. Diagnoses could be made that were never before possible in a live patient. But at first the hazards of X rays remained totally unappreciated. Only after many serious injuries resulted from X-ray overexposure were adequate safety precautions instituted. Unfortunately for Semmelweis, the cause of puerperal sepsis was less immediately obvious to most members of the medical profession than was the cause of X-ray burns.

Semmelweis immediately put his theory to the test. Beginning in May 1847 all medical students and physicians wishing to examine women in his ward were required to wash their hands—not merely in soap and water, but in chlorinated lime solution, thoroughly scrubbing with clean sand until all odors of the dissecting room were removed.

Since two decades were to pass before the germ theory of disease was understood, these new rules provoked enormous hostility and bitter protests from other physicians and students. Yet during the seven months that followed, the death rate dropped from 12 per cent to 3 per cent. In 1846 it had been 11.4 per cent in the students' clinic and 2.7 per cent in the midwives' clinic. During 1848 it decreased even further to 1.27 per cent in the students' clinic, slightly lower than the 1.33 per cent of the midwives' clinic.

Then suddenly an outbreak of puerperal sepsis recurred, killing eleven of twelve women in the students' ward. The outbreak began shortly after a pregnant woman with an infected cervical cancer was put into bed number one. Immediately realizing that infective material from this patient must have caused the epidemic, Semmelweis insisted that the hand-washing in chlorinated lime must be carried out between each examination.

Within a month, a second infected woman was admitted to the ward, this time with a draining left knee joint, whose stench filled the entire room. Despite hand-washing between every patient examination, the ward was again decimated. Semmelweis concluded, "The air of the labor room, loaded with putrid matter, found its way into the gaping genitals just at the completion of labor, and onward into the cavity of the uterus where the putrid matter was absorbed, and puerperal fever was the consequence." From then on he kept out any badly infected cases, and the low mortality rate continued to prevail.

Had Semmelweis been a stable, likable, tactful individual, no doubt he could have achieved immediate recognition for his tremendous discovery, now regarded as one of the great contributions to the science of healing. But he had begun to remain more continuously depressed than before, constantly haunted by overwhelming feelings of guilt.

"God only knows the number of women I have consigned prematurely to the grave," he would cry to his colleagues, making them feel guilty, too.

Soon the guilt feelings turned into ideas of persecution. When the suggestion was made that a simple investigation of his results be carried out, Semmelweis reacted angrily and in a deeply offended manner. He even refused an invitation to address the Vienna Medical Society on his work.

In December 1847 Ferdinand von Hebra, as editor of *The Vienna Medical Journal,* published an article describing Semmelweis's work and "cadaveric poison" theory of puerperal sepsis. Though this paper caused great excitement, Semmelweis maintained an inexplicable silence. Other colleagues did not, however, and sent letters to eminent obstetricians throughout Europe. Professor Michaelis of Kiel, whose work on the "obliquely contracted pelvis" is still famous, received one of these letters; he subsequently eliminated puerperal sepsis in his clinic by instituting the chlorinated lime handwash.

The general revolutionary upheaval in Europe of 1848 drowned out for a time the hand-washing controversy. When Hungary rose in revolt against Austria, Semmelweis joined the "Academic Legion," performing deliveries while fully attired in uniform and plumed hat. Hebra, though more accustomed to dermatologic eruptions than to political ones, joined also. The year 1848 may have been a bad one for revolutionaries on the barricades, but it was a good one for lying-in mothers in the Allgemeines Krankenhaus. The general excitement in Vienna caused the hospital physicians so to ignore their routine duties that during one month not a single case of childbed fever occurred.

By 1849 the armed fighting had subsided, and Semmelweis was again battling with colleagues over his methods. His friend Hebra published a second article, this time comparing him to Jenner, the discoverer of smallpox vaccination. But Klein had now determined to rid his clinic once and for all of this obstreperous obstetrician.

Summarily firing Semmelweis was out of the question because of the remarkable results he had obtained. So impressed was the Vienna Academy of Science that it subscribed money to enable continuation of the study. With his usual lack of tact, Semmelweis refused the contribution with the statement that the clinical evidence was, or should be, quite sufficient.

Klein's opportunity came when Semmelweis made application for elevation to the position of privatdocent in midwifery. The application was ignored. In 1850, with his position as assistant about to lapse, Semmelweis applied for an extension. Again Klein ignored him. As though to retaliate, Semmelweis presented papers before the Vienna Medical Society in which he pointedly noted the low incidence of childbed fever during the tenure of Professor Boër, the previous chief obstetrician, and for the first time mentioned the dangers of unclean utensils, soiled instruments, and dirty fingers. Hebra, Skoda, Rokitansky, and other famous Viennese physicians lent strong support, but to no avail.

The *coup de grâce* came in October 1850. After having waited nineteen months, Semmelweis received the appointment as privatdocent of theoretic midwifery. In this appointment Klein had included the humiliating restriction that only an anatomical model could be used in teaching. Semmelweis was strictly prohibited from instructing students at live deliveries. So effective is this method for getting rid of faculty undesirables that its variations are still in use at medical schools today.

Had Semmelweis been a less sensitive and temperamental individual, he might have been able to accept the new appointment as a challenge. And had he persevered, very likely his influential supporters would have moved to intercede on his behalf. Even Dr. Johann Chiari, Klein's own son-in-law, had spoken highly of the beneficial effects of the chlorinated lime handwash.

But Semmelweis was totally mortified. Deeply embittered and disappointed, he stormed out of Vienna without a word of explanation or farewell to anyone. Skoda, hurt by this conspicuous show of ingratitude, never spoke again of his erstwhile colleague and friend.

Once back in Hungary, Semmelweis found life little more agreeable than it had been in Vienna. The only position he could find was as an unpaid senior physician in the obstetric clinic of a hospital in Pest, across the river from Buda, where he was born. His father and mother were dead, and the country was in a state of upheaval from the 1848 rebellion. Now thirty-eight years old, he married a girl of eighteen. Tragically, his first child was born with hydrocephalus—a severe brain abnormality—and was dead within forty-eight hours. A year later, a second child died within a few months of peritonitis.

Despite these misfortunes, Semmelweis continued his efforts to promulgate his doctrine. In the hospital where he worked, he was able to reduce the incidence of puerperal sepsis drastically. And finally—ten years too late—he decided to organize and publish all of his findings. He spent three more years writing his *Aetiology, Conception, and Prophylaxis of Childbed Fever,* a rambling, repetitive, polemical, and egotistical treatise, filled with such sentiments as, "Fate has selected me as the champion of truth . . . a duty laid upon me which I cannot refuse to perform." Yet within this mass of self-serving verbiage lay camouflaged the brilliant guess—arrived at a full twenty years before germs were discovered to cause disease—that puerperal fever results from transmission of organic particles to the open wounds of a woman after delivery.

Semmelweis had completed the book in an almost manic state, furiously writing and rewriting chapters, which were then packed off to the printer uncorrected. When finally published, it understandably produced no reaction at all, since the dense, repetitious prose made it almost unreadable. Its author's behavior then took a decidedly pathologic turn—perhaps due to a disease contracted years before.

No record survives of Semmelweis's health in his early years, but there is strong reason to suppose that he may have developed syphilis as a young man. A man who examines female bodies and genitalia all day long certainly could be expected to seek some sexual outlet, and an unmarried one—as Semmelweis was through much of his career—might have frequently engaged the services of prostitutes. Alternatively, syphilis could have been contracted during the bare-handed examination of an infected woman's genitalia. The disease was quite a common one and, before the effective forms of treatment discovered in the twentieth century, was a frequent cause of early organic brain deterioration. When he died at the age of forty-seven, Semmelweis's brain did show just such extensive deterioration at autopsy, and this was mirrored in the behavior of his last years.

Realizing that his book was a failure, Semmelweis began to dash off long, emotionally charged letters to influential physicians and opponents. The bitter, irrational, accusatory nature of these letters is typified by one to a professor of midwifery in Vienna: "In this period of ten years at least 1,924 patients lost their lives from avoidable infection. . . . In this massacre you, Herr Professor, have participated."

By mid-1865 Semmelweis's actions had become so eccentric and bizarre that the presence of mental illness could no longer be doubted. His lectures to the local medical society had become a source of acute embarrassment to his colleagues. The therapy he received was standard for the day: bloodletting and cold-water dousing.

Finally, he was taken back to Vienna, where one of his few remaining friends from his early years, Ferdinand von Hebra, persuaded him to enter a mental institution. On examination after admission, an infected, gangrenous wound was found on a finger of Semmelweis's right hand, probably inflicted during his last obstetric operation. A few days later, he died, like Kolletschka, of a puerperal-type sepsis—a final irony, since just such a wound years earlier had made the young Semmelweis comprehend the mechanism of infection.

The Germ Theory

In 1865, the year Semmelweis died, the germ theory of disease gained its earliest acceptance. Though Semmelweis himself had made the remarkable guess that wounds become infected by organic particles, some of his difficulties may be laid to the fact that he had no proof. The great French chemist Louis Pasteur was responsible for this proof with his discovery that bacteria cause disease—a finding made possible by the microscope.

The observation that curved surfaces can magnify is an old one. Seneca, among many others, was aware of this phenomenon, writing in A.D. 63 that "letters, however minute and obscure, are seen larger and clearer through a glass bulb full of water." In the thirteenth century Roger Bacon, an English monk, first used a curved crystal lens to magnify objects, recording the results in his *Opus Majus,* written for Pope Clement IV: "If the letters of a book or any minute object be viewed through a lesser segment of a sphere or crystal whose plane base is laid upon them, they will appear far larger and better. For this reason, such an instrument is useful to old men and to those with weak eyes, for they may see the smallest letters sufficiently magnified." Bacon was imprisoned and his writings hidden until 1733, so that his contributions to the science of optics did not influence the development of the microscope, though there is evidence that he did foresee the possibility of this device.

The first useful microscopes were direct descendants of the magnifying lenses made for spectacles by two Italians, Salvino degli Armati and Alexander Spina, between the years 1285 and 1313. By the early seventeenth century the art of lens-grinding had reached the point where accurately made lenses could be used as simple or one-lens microscopes. Compound or two-lens microscopes, more powerful than the one-lens variety, were devised during this period by a Dutch spectacle-maker, Zacharias Janssen. Galileo is known to have made a number of microscopes, and Robert Hooke, using an elegant compound microscope of his own design, was the first to observe the cells contained in cork.

The greatest of all the early microscopists was Anton van Leeuwenhoek. Though possessed of no formal scientific training, he is credited with conceiving the sciences of bacteriology and protozoology. Regarded as a mere curiosity for more than a hundred years after his death, his work was to lead to the revolution that took place in late-nineteenth-century medicine and surgery.

Leeuwenhoek was born at Delft, Holland, October 24, 1632, the son of a basketmaker and grandson of a brewer. After a scant education, he was sent at the age of sixteen to a linen draper's shop in Amsterdam to learn the business. Here he worked for six years before returning to his native town.

Mid-seventeenth-century Holland had risen to a peak of wealth and prosperity. Amsterdam was a money center comparable to New York or London today. The Bank of Amsterdam was a financial power such as the world had never known before, remaining so until its collapse during the Napoleonic wars. The general affluence provided support for the artists Rembrandt and Hals; Jan Vermeer was Leeuwenhoek's good friend, and on the artist's death, the draper found he had been named executor of the insolvent estate, which consisted mostly of paintings.

In Delft, Leeuwenhoek prospered in the affluent climate. He married twice, bought a house and shop in which he set up a drapery and haberdashery business. Esteemed by his fellow townsmen, he was elected alderman and official wine gauger, as well as being licensed as a surveyor.

Some time after his return to Delft, this apparently busy man acquired an unusual hobby: lens-making. How he learned to grind the glass and mount the lenses will never be known, since throughout his life he was quite secretive about his techniques, perhaps with good reason. Because of his skillfully made lenses, his simple, one-lens microscopes were vastly superior to those of all other early workers.

Each of Leeuwenhoek's microscopes consisted of a single, tiny lens, laboriously mounted between two thin sheets of silver or brass with small openings masking all but the central area. In so masking the lens, he vastly improved the resultant image by taking advantage of the optical principle that the least light distortion occurs close to the central ray. How he managed to learn this important principle, unknown to most of his colleagues, remains uncertain.

The majority of his microscopes were no more than two to three inches in height, an inch or less in width, and—excluding the thumbscrews—less than a half inch in depth. Solid specimens were held before the lens on needle points adjustable with thumbscrews for both height and distance. Small glass vials and capillary tubes were examined by means of special holders. At his death he had built 247 complete microscopes and 419 lenses; most were capable of magnifying 40 to 160 diameters, though one in the collection of Utrecht University Museum is reported to magnify 275 diameters.

Using these simple but powerful instruments, Leeuwenhoek meticulously examined every conceivable substance from his surroundings: rainwater, scum from the surface of ponds, unborn mussels, animal and human tissues, scrapings, excreta of all sorts, infusions of peppercorns—even his own semen. When he found a particularly interesting specimen, he left it attached to the microscope and built another instrument. A great number of these was placed in small lacquered boxes, one or two dozen boxes to the case. A bequest of one such case was made to the Royal Society in London.

Through his microscopes, Leeuwenhoek became the first to see and describe protozoa and bacteria, which he named "animalcules." To estimate their sizes, he employed a grain of sand as his standard, equating the organism's volume with one thousandth, one hundred-thousandth, or one millionth of a grain. Some of these crude measurements of known species show a surprising correspondence with modern measurements. He also observed the very rapid multiplication of the animalcules when samples remained standing for a few days. His records contain drawings of berry-shaped and corkscrew-like forms that today can be recognized as distinct bacterial types: cocci and spirochetes.

Leeuwenhoek reported his findings in letters written in simple, naïve conversational Dutch—the only language he knew. The grammar was not always good and the prose was often frank and earthy. Here, for example, are his comments after entertaining curious visitors: "I have had several gentlewomen in my house, who were keen on seeing the little eels in vinegar; but some of 'em were so disgusted at the spectacle, that they vowed they'd ne'er use vinegar again. But what if one should tell such people in future that there are more animals living in the scum on the teeth in a man's mouth, than there are men in a whole kingdom? Especially in those who don't even clean their teeth? . . . For my part, I judge . . . that all the people living in our United Netherlands are not as many as the living animals I carry in my mouth this very day. . . ."

These gentlewomen comprised only a small part of the horde of ordinary visitors who came to look through Leeuwenhoek's lenses after he had become famous. Many celebrities also wanted a peek at the wonderful, new little world, including kings, queens, noted statesmen, and Czar Peter the Great of Russia. But kibitzers offering advice were resented by the secretive microscopist, who would neither disclose his methods nor sell a single instrument.

Leeuwenhoek was fortunately undisturbed by the jealous attacks of contemporaries and unbelievers. Of such criticism, he once wrote, "I am well aware that these my writings will not be accepted by some. . . . They're still saying . . . I'm a conjurer, and that I show people what don't exist. . . . I well know there are whole universities that don't believe there are living creatures in the male seed: but such things don't worry me; I know I'm in the right."

Certainly he was right in his meticulous observations, but he somehow lacked the imagination to draw rather simple conclusions. For example, he saw young mussels being attacked and devoured by legions of tiny bacteria, yet failed to investigate or even guess at the possibility that similar animalcules might cause illness by attacks on human tissues. Yet this possibility seems obvious only in retrospect; a century after Leeuwenhoek's death in 1723 it had occurred to no one else either.

The Dutch microscopist also did not investigate the origin of the animalcules, probably because the question of how such life forms came about had a well-accepted answer: spontaneous generation. Maggots were believed to originate in the rotten meat from which they squirmed. Crocodiles, seen pushing themselves up from the warm mud banks of the river Nile, were assumed to arise from their surroundings. And everyone knew that mice grew from sacking, flour, dust, and other ingredients to be found lying about the floor of a baker's shop.

The naïveté of the concept of spontaneous generation now seems laughable, but at first the theory actually appeared to be validated by observation and experiment. An early eighteenth-century French naturalist, Georges Buffon, claimed the small organisms Leeuwenhoek had seen in putrefying material and in scum from ponds were but particles of matter arising from the disintegration of previously existing matter. He felt these possessed the property of movement and termed them "organic molecules."

At about the same time John Needham, another naturalist, boiled a beef infusion and placed it in a stoppered vial, only to find that putrefaction later took place. Since boiling should have killed the animalcules, and since the vial was kept well-closed, Needham believed he had verified experimentally the phenomenon of spontaneous generation. The error here was finally rectified by Lazzaro Spallanzani, one of the most innovative and productive of all eighteenth-century physiologists.

Spallanzani, the son of a distinguished Italian lawyer, was educated at the Jesuit College at Reggio, where he was ordained as a priest. Then, to indulge his father, he became a law student at the University of Bologna. Biology, however, was his true interest, and just before he was to take his law degree, a friend and naturalist, Antonio Valisneri, intervened. The elder Spallanzani was quickly convinced, and soon his son had taken up with his microscope where Leeuwenhoek left off.

In 1762 Charles Bonnet, a close friend, prompted Spallanzani to consider the problem of spontaneous generation, pointing out that in Needham's experiment the vials could not be considered adequately sealed. Also, organisms in the fluid might have resisted the high temperature of boiling for a short period.

Almost immediately Spallanzani was able to show that living organisms always emerge in boiled infusions introduced into stoppered bottles. He also found that even though the bottles were sealed airtight, organisms appeared in the infusion. Suspecting that these bacteria might exist on the inner surface of the bottles, he flamed the glass before introducing the infusion. Still organisms were detected. Could they have entered with the air in the process of cooling?

To test this final supposition, Spallanzani put an infusion into the flasks, sealed them airtight, and subjected them to the heat of boiling water for an hour. No organisms appeared. If, however, the seal were disturbed so as to let in a bubble of air, organisms were soon found.

The conclusion to be drawn from these experiments was inescapable: Living organisms were necessary for putrefaction. Spontaneous generation was a myth.

Unwilling to stop here, Spallanzani carried the work still further, testing the effect of different temperatures and various substances such as oil of turpentine, camphor, sulfur, brandy, and wine. He even subjected one infusion to electric shocks. Examining broth that had become contaminated, he noted that some bacteria reproduced by splitting, others by making eggs or spores.

A most resourceful experimenter, Spallanzani continued to make contributions to physiology. In order to test whether spermatic fluid was essential for the fertilization of ova in amphibians, he fitted silk trousers to a group of male frogs. To see whether digestion resulted from grinding or the action of gastric juice, he fed meat contained in small metal cages to a pet hawk, then noted correctly that a chemical process was involved. But his remarkable conclusions regarding spontaneous generation failed even to dent the surface of this firmly entrenched popular theory. In the mid-nineteenth century, several eminent scientists still supported it. One of them, Felix Pouchet, director of the French Natural History Museum at Rouen, announced to the Academy of Sciences that animals and plants could be generated in a medium absolutely free from atmospheric air.

The theory of spontaneous generation was finally laid to rest by Pasteur. Though an extraordinary feat, it was only one among many that this unusually gifted man achieved.

Pasteur

Of all the contributors to the science of healing, none initially showed less promise than Louis Pasteur. The son of a tanner in Arbois, he initially showed a pronounced bent for drawing—but not much else. Some of his pastel portraits have a quaint and primitive charm, though they by no means suggest the early work of a great artist.

Perhaps aware of this deficiency, Pasteur decided to study science —at first, apparently halfheartedly. In 1842 he received a certificate in mathematical sciences at Dijon with a grade of "mediocre" in chemistry, meanwhile continuing to spend his time drawing in pastels. When he sat for his entrance examination to the École Normale Supérieure in Paris, he again made a mediocre showing, placing fifteenth out of twenty-two candidates.

Pasteur's interest in chemistry was finally stimulated by Jean Baptiste Dumas, one of the most eminent chemists of the day. After contact with Dumas and private lessons from Barruel, Dumas's assistant, Pasteur passed to fourth in the list of the École Normale Supérieure, graduating in 1846 at the age of twenty-four.

The path that led Pasteur from chemistry to spontaneous generation and bacteriology was a fortuitous, indirect one. After developing an interest in crystals and studying the crystallization of sulfur, he became involved in a problem concerning tartaric acid. In 1800 an Alsatian industrialist, Kestner, had noted the appearance in his tartaric acid factory at Thann of an acid he had never seen before. Though its chemical composition was identical to that of tartaric acid, its physical properties were different. One property in particular the new acid, which was eventually named racemic acid, lacked was the ability tartaric acid possesses to rotate polarized light to the right. Pasteur solved this puzzle by demonstrating that racemic acid crystallizes into two chemically identical but physically different forms. The right-faceted crystals were recognized as ordinary tartaric acid. A second type of crystal, a left-faceted crystal, which could rotate polarized light to the left, was perceived by Pasteur as being a chemical mirror image of the right-faceted form. Mixed together in solution, the rotatory properties of the two forms cancel each other to produce the optically inactive racemic acid again.

When these results were published in 1848, the elegant, carefully worked out presentation immediately won Pasteur the attention and respect of leading French scientists. By December, the young chemist had been appointed assistant professor of chemistry at the Faculty of Sciences at Strasbourg. And in May 1849 he married Marie Laurent, the daughter of the rector of the college. Marie, a tolerant, devoted person, was strongly convinced of her husband's genius, assisting him with his notes and records throughout an active, hectic career.

This career turned toward bacteriology during the autumn of 1856. Pasteur, now dean of the Faculty of Sciences at Lille, was consulted for advice by a Monsieur Bigo, a Lille industrialist. It seemed that many manufacturers in the region—Bigo included—were experiencing much difficulty in their production of alcohol from beets.

Pasteur had been interested in the properties of alcohols since 1849, and his previous studies had revealed that amyl alcohol had two chemical components, one of which rotated polarized light to the left and the other of which had no rotatory property at all. To study the alcohol and alcohol production at Lille, he brought with him a coke-heated oven and a microscope.

By the mid-nineteenth century, the microscope had undergone considerable evolution since Leeuwenhoek's time. Early lenses had the annoying habit of surrounding objects in the field of view with distracting fringes of color, a defect known as chromatic aberration. Because these fringes were more marked in the more powerful compound microscopes than in the weaker simple ones, useful high magnification was difficult to achieve. In the late eighteenth century Dutch designers were able to overcome chromatic aberration by combining a convex (outward curved) lens made of crown glass with a concave (inward curved) lens made of flint glass. Additionally, the stability and focus precision were increased by substituting all-brass construction for the wood and cardboard that had been used earlier.

In 1830 a second important defect in the microscope was overcome. Though the new Dutch achromatic lenses were useful at lower magnifications, at higher powers a new distortion, spherical aberration, was introduced by curvature in the lens glass. Often spherical aberration negated completely the benefits of the achromatic lens. This problem was solved when an amateur English microscopist, Joseph Jackson Lister, found that if two separate achromatic lenses were combined as a single lens, the outcome was complete freedom from both chromatic aberration and spherical aberration. The resulting lenses opened the way to the construction of high-power microscopes and vastly facilitated the investigations made by Pasteur and his contemporaries.

In studying the fermentation of beet sugar with his microscope, Pasteur identified tiny globules in the fermenting juices. If the process were proceeding normally to form only alcohol, the globules had a configuration resembling brewer's yeast. Chemists at the time held that living organisms were not necessary for fermentation; Pasteur disproved this notion by showing conclusively that sugar never underwent alcoholic fermentation unless living globules of yeast were present.

On ferments that became contaminated with lactic acid, Pasteur noted a peculiar gray substance in suspension in the liquid. This unwanted gray substance, seen microscopically to be rod-shaped organisms, could change sugar to lactic acid in an environment containing no air. Pasteur then discovered that the addition of a salt, tartrate of ammonia, would prevent lactic acid contamination, thus solving the brewers' problem.

In reality, much more had been accomplished. For the first time, minute living things, some capable of surviving without oxygen, had been shown to play tremendously important roles in chemical processes. The science of bacteriology was born.

Pasteur returned to Paris in October 1857 to accept the post of director of scientific studies and administration at the École Normale. The school, once France's most famous, had fallen on scientifically unproductive hard times. Never a modest man, the new director immediately affirmed that he had accepted the job in order to restore the school to its former greatness.

This he managed to do through his own researches, though as an administrator he was a disaster. He dealt harshly with childish complaints about the food and meted out overly severe punishment to cigarette smokers. Needless to say, such strict disciplinary measures made him thoroughly unpopular among his students—a genuine surprise to Pasteur, for he had used the same rigor successfully in training young minds to cope with scientific problems.

Another surprise may have been the laboratories the now-famous chemist was assigned at the École Normale. The only available space consisted of two small rooms in the school attic—hot and dark in summer, cold in winter. A year later he was given a suite of five slightly better rooms. He was forced to install his incubator under a stairway and could approach it only on his knees. His research was financed almost wholly from his own pocket. Yet such circumstances were traditional for nineteenth-century French scientists; in fact, many chemists and physicists were proud to have made their discoveries in similar dark little garrets using apparatus that cost only a few pence. Pasteur was likewise to triumph over such unprepossessing surroundings, but not before his life was struck by a series of personal tragedies.

The first was the death of his nine-year-old daughter, two years after the move to Paris in 1859. The child had been staying in Arbois with her grandfather when she became one of the victims of a typhoid fever outbreak in the district. Pasteur was devastated. "I cannot keep my thoughts from my poor little girl," he wrote to his father three months after she died.

But within a few weeks he had begun to study the theory of spontaneous generation in order to try to refute it. The impetus for this work was his discovery during the fermentation research that outside, unwanted organisms could "disease" the alcohol-forming process. Could other unwanted organisms also cause animal disease?

Pasteur was not the first individual to consider this possibility. In 1546 Girolamo Fracastoro, the physician who named syphilis, published *De Contagione,* concluding that epidemic diseases were produced by imperceptible *seminaria* or seeds that multiplied in the patient's body. Carl von Linné (Linnaeus), inventor of the present system for classifying plants and animals, mentioned "argillaceous particles" in his 1753 doctoral thesis as a possible explanation for certain recurrent fevers. And Semmelweis also suspected organic particles as the cause of puerperal sepsis.

To verify this notion of a germ theory of disease, Pasteur realized he would have to prove conclusively that life could not form spontaneously out of suitable media but could only arise from parent organisms. Spallanzani had attempted this proof a hundred years before, yet the scientific community remained unconvinced. Even earlier, Francesco Redi, a seventeenth-century Italian scientist, had demonstrated that maggots hatched from flies' eggs and could not arise spontaneously from putrid meat. Redi's results, however, were received even more scornfully than were Spallanzani's. Well aware of the entrenched nature of the theory of spontaneous generation, Pasteur was nonetheless determined to refute it beyond question.

To accomplish this refutation, Pasteur began by examining atmospheric air, and found that microscopic organisms were contained in it. Then, by using various liquid culture media, he proved that the appearance of organisms could be provoked at will when atmospheric air was let into the flasks. To show that screening out germs, rather than preheating the air, was responsible for absence of organisms in the culture media, he employed balloon flasks with long swan necks. Germs in the air settled in the bends and could not enter the interiors of the flasks, thus allowing the liquid within to remain perfectly clear and free of bacterial growth.

Proponents of spontaneous generation were still not convinced. They argued that if the air contained enough germs to cause fermentation, as Pasteur suggested, then "a crowd of them would produce a thick mist as dense as iron."

Pasteur answered this argument by showing that the air was not equally thick with germs. In the company of assistants, he climbed the Jura mountains with seventy-three sterile, sealed flasks, which he opened and resealed at various elevations. As the party climbed higher and higher, the percentage of flasks that became contaminated grew smaller. Eight out of twenty flasks opened at Mount Poupet, 850 meters above sea level, showed bacterial growth. Only one of twenty opened near the Mer de Glace at 2,000 meters above sea level, in a high wind, became contaminated.

The results of these experiments were presented publicly in a lecture at the Sorbonne on April 7, 1864. Pasteur was known to be a skilled showman, and he attracted an audience filled with celebrities: Alexandre Dumas, Sr., George Sand, Princess Mathilde, and others. After showing his swan-neck flasks to his audience, demonstrating the material, and explaining what he had proved, the famous chemist eloquently concluded: "And, therefore, gentlemen, I could point to that liquid and say to you, I have taken my drop of water from the immensity of creation, and I have taken it full of the elements appropriate to the development of inferior beings. And I wait, I watch, I question it, begging it to recommence for me the beautiful spectacle of the first creation. But it is dumb, dumb since these experiments were begun several years ago; it is dumb because I have kept it from the only thing man cannot produce, from the germs which float in the air, from Life, for Life is a germ and a germ is Life. Never will the doctrine of spontaneous generation recover from the mortal blow of this simple experiment."

Pasteur was right; it never did.

At the same time that he had been involved in this work, he also took up the problems of vinegar-makers in Orleans. With his usual thoroughness, Pasteur showed that the "little eels" first seen in vinegar by Leeuwenhoek, a genus of threadworm called *Anguillula,* were detrimental to the vinegar fermentation process because they interfered with *Mycoderma aceti,* the vinegar-forming organism. He then worked out a practical, standardized process for accurately controlled vinegar-making. Singularly devoid of an itching palm, Pasteur patented his process and immediately made it public property so that everyone could profit from it.

His growing fame as an industrial troubleshooter brought Pasteur one of his most well-known and important commissions. In 1863 Napoleon III personally commanded the chemist to investigate a disaster in the wine industry that threatened to upset the whole French economy. Many vintners throughout the country were producing enormous quantities of diseased wine. At the time, two million hectares of French soil were involved in the making of five hundred million francs' worth of wine. The grave threat to this enormous investment and premier French industry explains the imperial concern.

Pasteur found that he could tell by microscopic examination whether the wine had spoiled even without tasting it. The trick was again the identification of disease-producing organisms. And the solution to the problem was elegantly simple: Heat the fully fermented wine gently to kill off the bacteria. Dubious but desperate, the vintners tried the method. Thus was pasteurization born—in wine, not milk.

Napoleon III was overjoyed. For a week he entertained Pasteur at the Château de Compiègne, and asked his honored guest to explain to the court in drawing-room language how tiny organisms could cause so much trouble. But this triumph of imperial recognition was soon marred by tragedy.

First Pasteur's father died. Then his two-year-old daughter, Camille, succumbed to an inoperable tumor. In the spring of 1866 typhoid fever killed his twelve-year-old child, Cécile. All three were buried in the small cemetery at Arbois.

Finally Pasteur himself became ill. At the age of forty-five, on the morning of October 19, 1868, he suffered a severe chill which progressed to a left-sided paralysis by the end of the day. A leading doctor from the Académie de Médecine applied leeches to the patient's forehead, and somehow his condition improved.

News of the illness afflicting France's greatest scientist spread throughout the country. The deeply concerned emperor sent a liveried footman each morning to the Pasteur home for a progress report, which was carried back to the palace in a sealed envelope. The emperor's aide, General Favé, paid the invalid a visit to bring a translated English book, Samuel Smile's biographies of courageous lives entitled *Self-Help*. But soon, in spite of the leeches and the pessimism of the doctors, the frequency of the imperial footman's visits decreased. Pasteur was recovering.

From Lister to Listerine

Pasteur's germ theory of disease was first applied to human illness by an English surgeon, Joseph Lister. Unlike Pasteur, whose scientific career was filled with numerous discoveries, each more important and elegant than the one before, Lister made but one great discovery—how to prevent wound infection. Yet so monumental was Lister's finding that he is acknowledged to be the founder of modern surgery.

Joseph Lister was born April 5, 1827, at Upton, Essex, England, the fourth child and second son of Joseph Jackson Lister. The elder Lister, comfortably fixed because of a prosperous family wine business, devoted much time to his favorite hobby, microscopy; for his discovery of how to eliminate spherical aberration from an achromatic lens, the Royal Society awarded him a fellowship in 1832.

Young Joseph, raised in the surroundings of a quiet Quaker family, adopted his father's scientific interests and decided early that surgery should be his life's work. After receiving a Bachelor of Arts degree from London's University College in 1847, he continued to study medicine at the same institution and was awarded a Bachelor of Medicine degree in 1852. In this year his first scientific publication, "On the Contractile Tissue of the Iris," appeared in the *Quarterly Journal of Microscopical Science,* followed a few months later by another, "The Muscular Tissue of the Skin."

In September 1853, with a letter of introduction from a former teacher, Lister called on James Syme, a professor of clinical surgery in the medical school of the University of Edinburgh. The young man intended to visit several medical centers in his search for a position, but so impressed was Syme that he made a job offer which Lister accepted on the spot.

And Lister was indeed an impressive man: nearly six feet tall, handsome, upright, deep-chested, and compactly built. His manner was always restrained and his bearing dignified. The strongest expression anyone ever heard him utter was, "It's an infamous shame." This gracious demeanor was complemented by his impeccable Victorian attire of black frock coat, waistcoat, and chimney-pot silk hat.

Though conventional in dress, Lister was quite innovative as a surgeon. He is credited with inventing several ingenious instruments during his career, including a needle for silver suture wire, a hook for removing foreign bodies from the ear, a forceps for use in sinuses, and a screw tourniquet for compressing the abdominal aorta. The blunt-pointed Lister bandage scissors are still in wide use today.

These contributions were rewarded when the professorship in surgery at Glasgow University was vacated. Lister was chosen from among seven applicants for the appointment, assuming his new post on March 9, 1860. In another year he was placed in charge of the surgical wards of the Glasgow Royal Infirmary.

Surgery at this time was a last resort, attempted infrequently. In the 1860s one leading London teaching hospital, University College, performed only about two hundred operations annually. The infamous complications of infected surgical wounds—erysipelas, gangrene, sepsis—killed most patients and made surgical wards nightmares of smell and suffering.

Over the years, Lister had puzzled at surgical wound infections. His initial conviction was that lack of cleanliness might be in some way causative, and he immediately insisted on introduction of ordinary cleanliness at the Glasgow Royal Infirmary. The liberal use of soap and water was strongly resisted at first, but unlike Semmelweis, Lister was a gentle, kind, tactful man—and so he soon got his way.

Unfortunately, infections continued to occur, and in a rather peculiar distribution. Why, Lister wondered, should a simple fracture heal when a compound fracture, in which the ragged bone ends break the skin, proved almost always fatal? Why was mortality greater among hospitalized patients than among those in private homes? What causes wounds to suppurate?

The answer came when Dr. Thomas Anderson, a professor of chemistry, drew Lister's attention to the writings of Pasteur. At once Lister grasped the fact that germs causing putrefaction might cause suppuration by gaining access to an open wound. Repeating some of Pasteur's experiments, Lister became even more strongly convinced that micro-organisms produced wound infections. No doubt infections were more common in hospitals than homes because in the former they were transmitted from one patient to another.

But how to combat the germs was a problem. Certainly a patient could not be pasteurized like a bottle of Montrachet.

Then Lister remembered reading in a newspaper that the sewage at Carlisle had been successfully treated with carbolic acid, and that this compound had also been used to get rid of certain parasites on cattle. Carbolic acid—also called German creosote, or phenol—was a sweet-smelling, very impure, dark liquid that was easily obtainable. After securing a bottle from Dr. Anderson, Lister determined to test his theory on a case of compound fracture, an injury almost always terminating in fatal infection.

The first trial was a failure, but on August 12, 1865, James Greenlees, an eleven-year-old boy, was admitted to the Glasgow Royal Infirmary with a compound fracture of the left lower leg. Though a sizable wound was present, little bleeding had occurred.

Lister first applied carbolic acid to the wound directly, then dressed the area with a lint cloth soaked in the solution. A tin-foil covering was used to prevent evaporation, and the leg was splinted. Periodically the leg was redressed with a freshly soaked bandage. In six weeks the bones had reunited and the wound was entirely healed. Lister reported, "The remarkable retardation of suppuration, and the immediate conversion of the compound fracture into a simple fracture with a superficial sore, were most encouraging facts." Ironically, Semmelweis died in Vienna of septicemia August 13, 1865, a day after Lister had begun this first successful antiseptic treatment.

On March 16, 1867, Lister's first series of eleven cases was published in *The Lancet*. The paper, entitled "On a New Method of Treating Compound Fracture, Abscess, etc." revealed that one patient required amputation, another died of hemorrhage, but nine recovered completely—a remarkable record in that era.

Lister soon began to explore the "etc.", turning his attention to treating suture materials. Surgeons had habitually carried silk suture threads in coat lapel buttonholes for convenience. After experiments on animals, Lister found that silk sutures soaked in antiseptic could be left in wounds without suppuration, unlike the buttonhole variety. Tests of suture materials from animal sources showed that sterile catgut not only worked as well as silk but was absorbed *in situ*.

Experimenting further, Lister discovered even more measures to assure an infection-free surgical wound. Instruments were immersed in carbolic acid solution for twenty minutes before use. Operators and assistants were required to scrub their hands with soap and water, dipping them frequently into carbolic acid solution. The skin of the operative field was scrubbed with soap, water, and carbolic acid solution; towels soaked in the solution were used to surround the operative site.

Concerned that germs floating in the air also might pose a hazard, Lister developed a spray technique. By means of a sprayer which became affectionately known as "the donkey engine," a 1:1000 dilution of carbolic acid in water was disseminated as vapor in the operating room. Later, the hand sprayer was replaced by a steam sprayer. But the spray was annoying to everyone exposed and, before it was discarded as useless, engendered much professional hostility to the new antiseptic technique.

The greatest resistance occurred among British surgeons, who were the last to adopt antisepsis. Perhaps this relative tardiness occurred because Lister was never an impressive figure in the operating room. One surgeon who watched him described him as the worst practitioner imaginable of the doctrine he preached. Before operating, he doffed his coat, rolled up his shirt sleeves, and pinned an unsterilized towel over his waistcoat to keep bloodstains off his clothes. Then, after washing his hands in carbolic acid (they were by that time quite chapped from the repeated chemical irritation), he would begin.

But French and German surgeons began to use Lister's methods almost immediately, and with spectacular success. In America, Dr. William S. Halsted of Johns Hopkins added a further refinement by introducing rubber gloves. Yet because of ignorance in the medical community, even Dr. Halsted sometimes had difficulties maintaining sterility, as Dr. Hugh Hampton Young described:

"There were many regions in which the surgeon operated with trepidation. One of these was the knee joint, as infections at such operations usually meant loss of the leg. Up to 1895 few such cases had been operated upon. A Negro woman came to the hospital with fracture of the patella, that flat, oval bone which works up and down when our knees are in motion, commonly called the kneepan. Owing to the fear of opening the knee joint, great precautions had been taken to get the region absolutely sterile. We had begun three days before in the ward by shaving and cleaning the region of the operation. This was repeated on the second and third days. Then the patient was brought to the operating room. The wet bichloride dressing was removed. With a sterile razor the skin was shaved and then abundantly lathered. This was washed off with sterile water, and ether followed by alcohol was applied to get every remnant of the soap and grease away. The limb was carefully stroked with a sponge red with a saturated solution of potassium permanganate. This in turn was dissolved with the oxalic acid. Abundant libations of 1:1000 bichloride of mercury were then applied and sterile towels placed around the knee, leaving only a slit through which Dr. Halsted was to operate.

"The occasion was considered so important that rubber gloves had been sterilized for Dr. Halsted and his entire operating team. A few feet away from the table stood an old bearded practitioner, Dr. Crim. With his knife poised, Dr. Halsted turned to Dr. Crim, who had referred the patient, and said, 'When you first saw this girl, how far apart were the two fragments of the fractured patella?'

" 'The upper fragment was right here,' said Dr. Crim, as he placed his large, dirty hand on the limb we had spent three days in cleaning for operation. With a cry of anguish, Dr. Halsted stepped back, nurses rushed in, pulled off the draping, and the ritual of cleaning up the field of operation was begun again—soap, ether, alcohol, permanganate, oxalic acid, and bichloride."

The almost unbelievable results obtained by surgeons such as Halsted finally won over to antisepsis the last doubters. In his later years Lister was showered with honors. His visits to Continental Europe resembled triumphal marches. Yet this reserved, dignified Englishman was not above a little capitalizing on his fame. When approached by two Missouri businessmen, he permitted his name to be used on a patented concoction in exchange for a royalty—which is still being paid. As a consequence, the great surgeon is an integral part of an advertising campaign that has produced such gems as the following:

> He said that she said
> That he had halitosis,
> Here's what she said to do,
> Buy Listerine, try Listerine
> Keep breath fresh
> Gargle Listerine
> Buy Listerine, try Listerine
> Keep breath clean with antiseptic Listerine!

CHAPTER FIVE

The Rise of the Scalpel

The practice of surgery is ancient, having begun well before the advent of recorded time. Castration of a bull to form an ox was probably the first intentionally performed operative procedure; when it initially occurred, however, is difficult to determine. But the domestication of animals is known to have begun around 8000 B.C. and the first castrations were probably done at about the same period.

The man who had the idea of making a hole in the head vies with the castrator for the honor of being the first surgeon. Evidence of this procedure, called trepanation, has been found in skulls that may date back as far as 10,000 B.C. The evidence is sometimes ambiguous, since some skulls may have been perforated by birth defects, tumors, the teeth of mice and rats, or the abrasion of wind-blown sand. But if the patient died soon after the procedure—by no means the rule—the marks of the instrument are so clear that the basic operative techniques may be deduced. Skulls from such cases have been found throughout the world: in France and other parts of Europe, in northern Africa, Asia, New Guinea, Tahiti, and New Zealand. The ancient Peruvian Incas were master trepanners, performing the operation with knives of glass-hard obsidian after narcotizing the patient, perhaps with coca leaves.

What were the indications for trepanning? One was skull fracture or head injury. In 1913 a British anthropologist working in the mountains of Algeria reported, "The native surgeons . . . are unanimous in declaring that injuries resulting from a blow are the sole cause of the favourite operation. . . . Women . . . have been known to undergo trepanation in order to support fictitious charges of assault against husbands from whom they were seeking grounds for a divorce." In ancient skulls, too, holes have been found clearly placed along a fracture line.

Trepanning for head trauma is, surprisingly, a life-saving procedure. When performed today for subdural hematoma—a collection of blood between the dural membrane and the brain just beneath—it can prevent brain injury, as well as death, by relieving pressure on the cranial contents. But ancient man also probably trepanned for less valid reasons, including epilepsy and insanity.

Chances of surviving the trepanning were good. In practically all the series of cases studied, survival can be inferred to approach 100 per cent, the criterion being extensive bony healing around the hole. One modern native surgeon in East Central Africa claimed to have done over a hundred cases without a single fatality. Such amazing records may have been achieved in part by the use of dressings to prevent exposure to the surrounding air, since trepanned skulls have been found with dressings in place. Another protective factor may have been the absence of hospital physicians carrying virulent strains of bacteria from one patient to the next.

Besides castrating and trepanning, primitive man also cut off fingers. On a wall of the Gargas cave in southern France ancient imprints of mutilated hands have been found. Some are lacking more than one finger, though the thumb seems to have been spared. Similar handprints have also turned up in the Maltravieso cave of central Spain.

The reason for these amputations is unknown. Perhaps they represented a form of surgical treatment for crushed fingers. Another explanation: ritual sacrifice. Several Indian tribes of northwestern Canada amputate the little finger at the first joint and place it on a coffin edge, in order, as they say, to "cut off the deaths" in a family. The Dugum Dani tribe of New Guinea are known to do the same, using little girls as the sacrificial victims. Almost all Dani girls lose several fingers, yet maintain a high degree of manual skill.

Ancient ritual amputations, like modern ones, were no doubt per-

formed by priests or tribal chieftains who acted as part-time surgeons. The first full-time surgeons appeared in Mesopotamian civilization sometime after 3100 B.C. While the perfume-makers and
the glass-makers left detailed cuneiform-on-stone records of their
methods, the surgeons did not—probably because their technical rep-
ertoire was so primitive that it was hardly worth mentioning.

Not so their malpractice statutes. The Code of the Babylonian
king Hammurabi—282 laws found engraved on a huge black polished
stone, eight feet high, by a French expedition in 1901—included
provisions regulating physicians and surgeons. The king himself was
pictured receiving these draconian laws from Shamash, the sun god,
about 1700 B.C.

The Code did not hold a physician responsible for an illness due
to an outside cause, such as an evil spirit, a god, cold, dust, or a bad
smell. But if the complication had resulted from the surgeon's knife,
penalties could be harsh indeed: "If a physician operate on a man
for a severe wound with a bronze lancet and cause the man's death;
or open an abscess of a man with a bronze lancet and destroy the
man's eye, they shall cut off his fingers."

Making the same mistake, or worse, on a slave, was not as serious: "If a physician operate on a slave of a freeman with a bronze
lancet and cause his death, he shall restore a slave of equal value."

The code must also have diminished inflationary pressures on the
Babylonian economy by setting physicians' fees: "If a physician performed a major operation on a man with a bronze lancet and has
saved the man's life, or he opened the eye-socket of a man with a
bronze lancet and has saved the man's eye, he shall receive ten
shekels of silver. If he was a member of the commonalty, he shall receive five shekels. If it was a man's slave, the owner of the slave shall
give two shekels of silver to the physician."

A thousand miles, as the crow flies, from the legal jurisdiction of
Hammurabi, Egyptian civilization arose around the Nile valley.
Here, a more advanced brand of surgery was used. The first known
practitioner, Hesy Re, chief of dentists and physicians to the pyra-
mid-builders of the Third Dynasty (c. 2600 B.C.) may have drilled
bones to drain dental abscesses, though this is uncertain. Evidence of
definite surgical activity was found in Fifth Dynasty tombs: fractured
limbs set with splints and bandages spotted with the world's oldest
bloodstains.

The most important record of Egyptian surgery is a papyrus probably recovered from a tomb by one Mustapha Aga. On January 20, 1862, Aga sold the document to Dr. Edwin Smith, an American scholar visiting Thebes. Two months later Aga came up with another papyrus, again bought by the acquisitive Dr. Smith. This second scroll was actually made up of three papyri pasted together. Realizing that two of these formed a battered page of the papyrus he had bought in January, Smith carefully separated the fragments and attached them to his earlier purchase. After Smith's death, his reassembled document was donated by his daughter to the New York Historical Society.

In 1920 Dr. James Henry Breasted, director of the University of Chicago's Oriental Institute, agreed to look at the still-untranslated Smith Papyrus. So absorbed did Breasted become that he spent the next ten years producing the most elegant, thorough, critical English version of any ancient text. The meaning of each word and sentence is carefully analyzed, and in such detail that the entire work fills two enormous volumes.

The Smith Papyrus author's name is unknown. There is good internal evidence, however, that the document was a manual of war surgery, implying that the author was a surgeon who had followed an army in time of war. Two observations, especially, support this hypothesis. First, the sex of patients described is designated as male or not at all. Second, the wounds—particularly the head wounds—seem to have been caused by weapons. The language is that of the Old Kingdom, implying that the author must have lived roughly between 2600 and 2200 B.C.—so far off in time that he never even saw the wheel.

The papyrus itself is a large one, 4.68 meters long. The 21½ columns of cursive hieroglyphs actually contain the fragments of two books. One is anatomical, the *Book on the Vessels of the Heart*. The second is surgical: the descriptions of forty-eight cases, including injuries, wounds, fractures, dislocations, and tumors—in other words, the types of troubles that fall into the realm of a surgeon. These descriptions are arranged from the head downward, in order of severity within each group. The cases are given one of three labels, depending on the chance of successful treatment:

> An ailment which I will treat
> An ailment with which I will contend
> An ailment not to be treated

The last and most ominous label reflects a view widespread in antiquity, that a hopeless case should not be touched. Commenting on his translation, Breasted wrote that the hopeless group "evinces the surgeon's interest in the human body quite apart from any thought of healing or treating it." More likely, the segregation of a hopeless group evinced the surgeon's interest in appearing to be a successful healer—an appearance that could only be damaged by taking on lost causes.

Several centuries after the death of the original author, the Smith Papyrus was modified by a commentator. By this time, several of the terms must have appeared so obsolete that the information could no longer be medically useful without clarification. This the commentator added in sixty-nine short explanations. For example, case four discusses splitting a skull. In his gloss, the commentator writes that "it means separating shell from shell of his skull, while fragments remain sticking in the flesh of his head, and do not come away." Case five, "smashing his skull," is clarified, "It means a smash of his skull into numerous fragments, which sink into the interior of his skull."

The hand that wrote the Smith Papyrus belonged neither to the author nor to the commentator but to a scribe working about 1650 B.C. This fellow had a beautiful script, though he was rather careless —not unusual for Egyptian scribes. As was customary, he alternated between red and black ink, without much method, correcting in black the mistakes made in red, and vice versa. Once, after forgetting a word, he inserted the world's first asterisk. Finally, partway through his work, he stopped copying in the middle of a word for reasons that will never be known.

Yet despite the unfortunate absence of a portion of the text, the Smith Papyrus gives a good picture of Egyptian surgery. We know that the author examined all his cases carefully, recording the pulse, which he realized might be affected by a head injury. He was as ignorant of the nature of infection as was his nineteenth-century counterpart, Robert Liston, exploring with his dirty fingers the depths of wounds he treated. He knew that a patient might sustain a depressed fracture of the skull vault even though the scalp was not torn, and that such an injury, if it involved the brain, might lead to loss of speech and paralysis of the limbs. He seems to have recognized traumatic aneurysms—a local ballooning of injured arteries. And though he did not diagnose tuberculous abscesses as such, he correctly advised that they not be incised. Today we know that without antituberculous drug treatment, such incised abscesses will often continuously drain pus and never heal.

As a therapist, the author of the Smith Papyrus would receive fair marks. He reduced dislocations of the jaw in the same way we do today. He closed wounds with adhesive plaster, a technique far superior to the use of unsterile sutures. He reduced fractured collarbones in a sound manner, though his method for retaining the fragments in position would not seem to be as good as the presently employed figure eight bandage. He writes: "If thou examinest a man having a break in his collar-bone . . . thou shouldst place him prostrate on his back, with something folded between his two shoulder-blades; thou shouldst spread out his two shoulders in order to stretch apart his collar-bone until that break falls into its place. Thou shouldst make for him two splints of linen, thou shouldst apply one of them both on the inside of his upper arm and the other on the under side of his upper arm. Thou shouldst bind it . . . treat it afterwards [with] honey every day until he recovers."

In 1872, ten years after Dr. Smith had reassembled the fragments of his scroll, George M. Ebers, a German Egyptologist, acquired a second Egyptian medical text, written in the same language and script as the Smith Papyrus at about the same time. Both papyri are believed to have been found in the same tomb, but there are considerable differences between the two.

The Ebers Papyrus is composed of 108 columns, and at 20.23 meters is almost five times as long as the Smith Papyrus. Within this added length is contained a complete medical compendium consisting of monographs and excerpts devoted to a variety of subjects: internal diseases, eye diseases, skin diseases, diseases of women, and surgical diseases. The surgical section, dedicated mostly to plastic surgery, demonstrates the great concern the Egyptians must have had for improving cosmetic appearance. Considerable space is devoted to methods for removing wrinkles and moles, dying the hair and eyebrows, correcting squints, and generally beautifying the body. Home improvement instructions are also given: how to expel fleas from the house; how to prevent a snake from coming out of its hole; how to prevent a fly from biting; how to sweeten the smell of the house or the clothes.

The First Advance

The ancient author of the Ebers Papyrus should have stopped at body improvement. Home improvement soon led surgeons almost entirely out of the medical mainstream. By late antiquity, learned physicians more and more frequently abandoned surgery, leaving operations to manual workers—especially barbers. The separation of surgery from medicine was essentially complete in the Middle Ages.

Not surprisingly, the surgeon's functions were severely limited. Performing bleedings and draining abscesses were his more common chores. He was also called upon to treat syphilis, miscellaneous skin conditions, fractures, and dislocations. Wounds, too, both civilian and military, were considered part of his domain, and it was in the treatment of these that the first significant advance was made—the ability to control surgical bleeding.

Hemorrhaging from a wound had been a concern of medical men since antiquity. Though ignored by the author of the Smith Papyrus, the problem was recognized as formidable in the Ebers Papyrus. One paragraph deals with a "lump of ukhedu," described as a pocket full of gum water—perhaps a cyst or abscess: "You should give it the cutting treatment; beware of the 'mt' [blood vessel]."

How should bleeding from the "mt" be coped with? We are told a few lines later during instructions for treating a "vessel tumor": "It comes from a wound of the vessel. Then you should give it the cutting treatment. It [the knife] should be heated in the fire; the bleeding is not great."

Thus burning appears as the first recorded hemostatic method, and not only for the treatment of abscess. Recounting a reed operation on the "sft" of a vessel, a nondescript lump, the author writes, "If it bleeds a lot, you must burn it with fire."

While burning is an effective method for controlling tiny bleeding vessels, it leaves much to be desired when larger arteries are involved. Extensively burned tissue, as might be expected, just will not heal.

The obvious alternative is ligation or tying, a technique described in the writings of Galen and Celsus. Yet long after ligatures were known, surgeons remained unenthusiastic about undertaking the one procedure where ligation was most indicated—amputation. And amputations were avoided with good reason. Whether ligatures were used or forgotten, the results were uniformly disastrous, since the battered stump of the limb was always smothered in scalding oil or roasted with a red-hot iron, then often coated with a favorite Galenic "styptic": frankincense, one part; aloes, one part; mixed with egg white to the consistency of honey, to which was added a pinch of clippings from the fur of a hare.

Few amputees managed to survive such ministrations, but up until the Middle Ages amputation was a rarely indicated procedure. The invention of gunpowder, however, changed all this. A gunshot wound of an extremity often becomes infected, and without antibiotics, amputation is the only way to stop a spreading infection.

During the early sixteenth century, when gunpowder came into use, the frequent fatal infections in gunshot wounds were a perplexing problem. Knowing nothing of the germ theory of disease, medical authorities surmised that the gunpowder itself was a poison. The only effective antidote was believed to be boiling oil.

A young French army surgeon, Ambroise Paré, was the first to abandon this horrendous form of treatment. Paré had learned his trade as apprentice to a Paris barber-surgeon before going off to one of the many French wars as surgeon to Maréschal de Montéjan, colonel-general of the French Infantry. During his first campaign in 1536, the twenty-six-year-old Paré made the accidental discovery upon which most of his fame rests—that boiling oil not only was of no use, but actually was harmful in the treatment of gunshot wounds. Here, in his own words, is how this came about:

"Now all the soldiers at the Château, seeing our men coming with a great fury, did all they could to defend themselves, and killed and wounded a great number of our soldiers with pikes, arquebuses, and stones, where the surgeons had much work cut out for them. Now I was at that time a freshwater soldier, I had not yet seen wounds made by gunshot at the first dressing. It is true that I had read in Jean de Vigo, first book, 'Of Wounds in General,' chapter eight, that wounds made by firearms participate of venenosity, because of the powder, and for their care he commands to cauterize them with oil of elder, scalding hot, in which should be mixed a little theriac; and in order not to err before using the said oil, knowing that such a thing would bring great pain to the patient, I wished to know first, how the other surgeons did for the first dressing, which was to apply the said oil as hot as possible, into the wound with tents and setons, of whom I took courage to do as they did."

Then, like the United States and Western Europe in 1973, Paré suddenly ran out of oil: "At last, my oil lacked and I was constrained to apply in its place a digestive made of the yolks of eggs, oil of roses, and turpentine. That night I could not sleep at my ease, fearing that I should find the wounded on whom I had failed to put the said oil dead or empoisoned, which made me rise very early to visit them, where beyond my hope, I found those upon whom I had put the digestive medicament feeling little pain, and their wounds without inflammation or swelling, having rested fairly well throughout the night; the others to whom I had applied the said boiling oil, I found feverish, with great pain and swelling about their wounds."

Above all a humane and compassionate man, Paré immediately modified his treatment method: "Then I resolved with myself never more to burn thus cruelly poor men wounded with gunshot."

Encouraged by favorable results, Paré in 1552 abandoned the traditional hot cautery iron to stop bleeding in cases of amputation, substituting his "new method"—the age-old ligature. The outcome was dramatic. For the first time in the history of surgery, amputations could be performed with a good chance for success.

Jealous medical contemporaries, especially Dr. Étienne Gourmelen, a professor of medicine, bitterly criticized Paré and his new method. In reply, Paré wrote The Apology and Treatise, in which his adversaries' objections were answered by citing specific examples of successful ligations. The book also gives an account of its author's surgical experiences in various campaigns.

Paré wrote two other important and influential books. One, The Method of Curing Wounds Made by Gunshot, was published in 1645. Besides presenting the new manner of treatment, it also describes an effective means of locating the ball responsible for the wound: If the victim could reassume his position at the time when wounded, a careful search in the direction of entry might reveal the bullet.

The second book, a handbook on anatomy, was written in a simple French text intended for surgeons ignorant of the customary Latin and Greek. While some dissections had been made by the author himself, credit for others was generously given to the Italian anatomist Vesalius. In addition to anatomy, obstetrics was also discussed, including Paré's method of changing the position of a child *in utero* to prevent a difficult delivery.

His discoveries and his writings brought the once-obscure barber-surgeon into the service of four French kings. While acting as surgeon-in-ordinary to the first, Henri II, husband of Catherine de Médicis, Paré was captured by the Spanish. Hoping to escape a long captivity, he disguised himself in the dirty clothes of a common soldier, but gave himself away in prison when he could not resist showing off his surgical skills. So awed were his captors that he was invited to enter the service of the Spanish emperor. When Paré declined, he was set free after he cured Seigneur de Vaudeville of a leg ulcer which had plagued the nobleman for six years.

Upon returning to Paris, Paré became a trusted surgeon of the king, and despite little formal education was elevated to the rank of master surgeon by the Collège de Saint Côme. But life at court was not pleasant, being riddled by intrigue, dread, and suspicion. France had been ravaged by war, then divided into hostile factions by the rapid spread of the Protestant faith among the well-to-do middle classes. Yet Paré managed somehow to remain so determinedly neutral that to this day his real sympathies—if indeed he had any—are unknown.

In 1559 King Henri was accidentally struck in the head with a lance while hunting, and the point of the lance remained imbedded within the skull. Paré was called, and even Andreas Vesalius was said to have been summoned to act as a consultant. The two eminent physicians dissected the heads of two executed criminals to decide on the best form of treatment, but to no avail. After the king died, Paré was appointed surgeon to Henri's son, François II.

The new king, only sixteen years old, was frail in both body and intellect. When he died not long after ascending the throne, the court began to whisper that Paré had poured poison in his ear. Fortunately for the surgeon, the queen mother, Catherine, never believed these whisperings.

Charles IX, a beastly boy with a violent temper, succeeded his brother. Like many other sovereigns, the new king was fearful of assassination—especially by poison. Mithridates, an ancient king of Pontus, had confronted this problem by immunizing himself with the blood of poisoned ducks. But Charles thought he had found a better antidote: a small gray stone called a *bezoar,* for which he had paid an enormous sum. Bezoars are hardened collections of undigested material from animal stomachs and were at the time believed to possess magical properties.

When Charles showed the bezoar to Paré, the surgeon was skeptical and suggested that the stone be tested on a criminal about to be executed. The chosen experimental subject was a cook to be hanged for stealing two silver plates from his master. A royal pardon was offered to the man if he would take poison and then swallow the bezoar.

The poor cook had little faith in the stone, but preferred a private poisoning to a public execution. An apothecary mixed the poison, the cook took it, and then swallowed the stone. Paré describes what happened:

"Having these two good drugs in his stomach, he took to vomiting and purging, saying that he was burning inside, and calling for water to drink, which was not denied him. An hour later, having been told that the cook had taken this good drug, I prayed the provost to let me see him. I found the poor cook on all fours, going like an animal, his tongue hanging out of his mouth, his eyes and face red, retching and in cold sweat, bleeding from his ears, nose and mouth. I made him drink oil, thinking to aid him and save his life, but it was no use because it was too late, and he died miserably, crying that it would have been better to have died on the gibbet."

The stone, carefully removed from the dead victim's stomach, was returned to the king, who threw it into the fire when he heard what had happened.

The next ten years of French history, from 1562 to 1572, were filled with many more equally violent deaths, but these were in the name of God rather than science. Paré entered the bloody civil war with the king on the side of the Catholic forces, and was present at the sieges of Bourges and Rouen. Finally, at the battle of Montcour, he saw the Huguenots, commanded by Admiral Coligny, defeated.

A truce was negotiated in 1572, when the leaders arranged a marriage between the king's sister Margaret and the Huguenot leader, Henri of Navarre. With a show of friendliness, both factions assembled in Paris for the ceremony, though enmity seethed just beneath the surface.

On Friday, August 22, four days after the wedding, Admiral Coligny was shot in the finger and arm as he returned from watching the king play tennis. The would-be assassin, a man named Maurevel, was in the employ of the dukes of Anjou and Guise. These noblemen were quite possibly in league with Catherine de Médicis, who was insanely jealous of Coligny's influence over the king.

After the admiral had been taken to his own house, his friend Paré was sent for. The surgeon amputated the damaged finger and removed the bullet from Coligny's arm, but with much pain since the surgical instruments were not in good condition.

Various versions of subsequent events have been recorded, all of which have been contested by scholars, but here are the facts in essence. Paré remained with Coligny. A short distance away, at the Louvre, the thwarted queen was fearful that the Huguenot leaders, incensed by the assassination attempt, would strive for revenge. On Sunday, August 24, 1572, the Feast of St. Bartholomew, at half past one in the morning, Catherine ordered the bell in the tower of Saint Germain l'Auxerrois be rung to signal the beginning of a prearranged massacre of the Huguenots.

Hearing the signal, the Duc de Guise, leader of the Catholic faction, assembled a large mob before the door of Coligny's house. When "Open, in the King's name" was shouted, house servants obliged.

Rushing in, the assassins immediately killed the man who had unlocked the door. Other servants were also slain. The admiral, realizing there was no escape, put on a long robe and sat in a chair to await his fate with dignity, Paré at his side. The door was opened suddenly, and Cornation, one of the admiral's men, dashed into the room. When Paré demanded the meaning of the commotion, Cornation replied, "Sir, it is God calling us to himself."

Some of the servants managed to escape, including Cornation. Though Paré, suspected of being a Huguenot, knew he was in great danger, he stayed with his friend as the chamber door was thrown open a second time. In rushed a group of men, including one with a bloody sword. Then a German named Behm approached the admiral, put the point of a sword to his chest, and asked whether he was Coligny.

"Yes," was the reply, "but you cannot shorten my life except by the permission of God."

The German, an impatient man, could not wait for that, and after he had finished with his victim, the rest of the mob fell on the admiral with swords and daggers until he fell to the floor. Behm went to the window and reported to Guise, that the job was done. The skeptical duke demanded proof, however, and when Behm tried to raise the body, the still-living Coligny braced himself with his feet against the wall. Crying out with rage, Behm then drew his dagger and stabbed the admiral again. An instant later the body was finally dumped out the window into the stone courtyard below. Paré, alone with the mob and the other corpses, somehow remained untouched, and apparently was escorted safely to the Louvre.

Guise gave the admiral's remains one good swift kick before he left. Someone else cut off the head. The body was played with by children, dragged through the streets, burned, doused in the river, and eventually dragged up the hill to Montfaçon, where it was hung by its feet to a gallows. When it had begun to decay, the whole court went to see it, and the king remarked, "The smell of a dead enemy is always sweet."

Throughout the riots, the king worked himself into a frenzy of excitement, using his arquebus to take potshots from his window at fleeing Huguenots. Just before breaking down emotionally, he sent for Paré and remarked to him, "I do not know what ails me. . . . I burn with fever; all around me grin pale, bloodstained faces. Ah, Ambroise, if they had but spared the weak and innocent." After this remorseful interlude, the monarch grew wild and boisterous, cavorting like a buffoon.

Having survived the St. Bartholomew's Day massacre, Paré continued to work and accrue honors. The last historical record of him is at the siege of Paris in 1590. The eighty-year-old surgeon, walking through the streets, saw a crowd of starving peasants begging the Archbishop of Lyons for bread. Paré interceded eloquently, saying, "Monseigneur, these poor people whom you see about you are dying of the cruel rage of hunger, and demanding pity of you. For God's sake, Monsieur, give it to them."

The Corpse Crunch

The innovations of Ambroise Paré and the increased demand for military surgeons brought about a rebirth of surgery in the seventeenth century. Surgeons became respected members of the community. More and more young men were attracted to surgery as a career. The art was becoming a science.

But surgery requires a more detailed knowledge of anatomy than does any other medical specialty, and the teaching of anatomy demands a continuous supply of bodies for dissection. A few cadavers became available for legitimate dissection in 1540 when London barber-surgeons were given the right to four bodies a year—the bodies of executed criminals. At the same time, Edinburgh surgeons were granted the remains of "ane condampnit man."

Criminals were aghast that their bodies might be dissected. The loudest protests were raised by those guilty of the most fiendish crimes: Nicol Brown, who forcibly held his wife upon an open fire until she was roasted to death; Sarah Metyard and her daughter, proprietors of a millinery shop in Hanover Square, who flogged to death orphan girls apprenticed to them; the egregious Joseph Wall, lieutenant-governor of Senegambia, who watched one of his soldiers die from his sentence of eight hundred lashes.

These criminals and others employed any means they could to prevent their remains from reaching the dissecting table, perhaps because they feared the possibility that they might be cut up alive. Hanging was not as effective then as it is today, since there was no drop. Not uncommonly, therefore, the friends of the condemned assembled at the foot of the gallows and suspended their weight from the victim's kicking legs, assuring a speedy demise. Then a full-scale riot would ensue to prevent the corpse from falling into the anatomist's hands.

Such tactics and the skyrocketing demand for cadavers soon produced what might be called a "corpse crunch," as the supply was rapidly outstripped. Bodies began to disappear from graveyards. In England riots broke out. Medical school windows were smashed. Professors of anatomy and surgery were attacked by incensed mobs.

Alarmed, the British government decreed in 1751 that all murderers executed in London and Middlesex be either publicly dissected or hung in chains on gibbets. Though this act helped increase the supply of cadavers, there were still not nearly enough. As a result, "resurrection men"—professional grave robbers—moved in to fill the gap. Many graves were guarded by an angry citizen with a bell-mouthed pistol in one hand and a grog bottle in the other, but more still were not, allowing the grave robbers to carry on a profitable business. Undertakers and sextons were paid off so that bodies could be filched from their coffins even before burial. Those corpses that did make it into the ground were often raised the same night.

But as the demand for cadavers continued to grow, a few enterprising tradesmen discovered a better method of obtaining them than robbing graves. The most notorious was William Hare, proprietor of a flea-bitten Edinburgh flophouse frequented by vagrants and aged prostitutes. After one penniless guest had died owing four pounds, Hare and two assistants—William Burke and Burke's mistress, Helen McDougal—pilfered the corpse from a parish coffin, selling it at a profit to Dr. Robert Knox, a professor of anatomy at the University of Edinburgh.

Burke and Hare had never made money so easily before. They waited impatiently for other guests to die, but the old men and women remained obstinately alive. So the two innkeepers began bringing in impoverished strangers from the streets of Edinburgh. After getting the intended victim quite drunk, Hare would sit on him while Burke held both his hands over the victim's nose and mouth—a procedure which soon became known as Burking. Since no marks of violence were left on the bodies, Knox purchased them eagerly, apparently not suspecting that foul play was involved.

All went well for a while until some well-known characters turned up on Dr. Knox's dissecting table: Abigail Simpson, a notorious old drunkard, and Daft Jamie, a favorite town imbecile. But when Mary Paterson's remains fell into Knox's hands, the news spread throughout the city. Miss Paterson, one of the most beautiful whores in Edinburgh, was shortly followed by another missing woman, named Dougherty.

Within a few hours, Burke, Hare, and Helen McDougal were arrested and narrowly escaped death at the hands of an angry mob as they were taken to prison. Another group of enraged citizens broke all the windows in Knox's house and threatened to set fire to it.

At the trial of the three conspirators on December 24, 1828, Hare turned king's evidence and was acquitted. Helen McDougal was also freed for lack of evidence. But on Christmas Day Burke was found guilty. Thousands saw him hanged and then publicly exhibited in the anatomical lecture theater of the University of Edinburgh. His skeleton, labeled "William Burke, the Murderer," was preserved in the school's museum.

Yet even public recognition of this and other bizarre crimes did not ease the corpse crunch, and anatomists continued to receive material from unusual sources. For example, during the building of the first railroad across the Isthmus of Panama, between 1850 and 1855, six thousand laborers died of malaria, dysentery, cholera, sunstroke, and yellow fever. The sheer number of bodies that had to be disposed of made burial impractical. But since a large percentage of the dead men had no known next of kin, no permanent address, often not even a known last name, the construction company decided to pickle the bodies in large barrels, then sell them in wholesale lots. The result was a thriving trade with medical schools throughout the world, the proceeds going to finance a small Panamanian railroad hospital.

Early Aseptic Surgery

In 1855 a small railroad hospital or even a large hospital could boast of few more surgical techniques than had been known to Ambroise Paré or even the author of the Edwin Smith Papyrus. True, an early-nineteenth-century American surgeon, Ephraim McDowell, had successfully removed ovarian tumors from the abdomen in a small number of cases, but the risk of fatal infection was so great that McDowell was bitterly criticized. After Lister's work, however, the whole situation changed. Surgeons using aseptic or sterile operating technique quickly made the abdominal cavity their playground.

The most outstanding of the early abdominal surgeons was Christian Albert Theodor Billroth. Born on the North German island of Rügen in 1829, Billroth was only five years old when his father, an impoverished preacher, died and left him, with four other siblings, in the care of a tuberculous mother. At the University of Greifswald, young Theodor was an average student scholastically, though he had a great musical aptitude. In deference to his mother, however, he abandoned a musical career to study medicine at the University of Göttingen, one of the pre-eminent institutions in Europe. During his first year of medical school he rarely attended medical lectures, preferring to pursue his musical hobbies, but during the second term an old doctor friend of the family aroused a latent interest in medicine.

After graduation from Göttingen, Billroth first took a clinic job, then entered a disappointing period of private practice. This ended when by great good fortune he received an appointment as assistant to Dr. Bernhard Langenbeck, one of the most well-known German surgeons of the era. The young man's gifts as a surgeon were immediately recognized, and in 1860, at the age of thirty-one, he was offered and accepted a professorship of surgery at the University of Zurich.

In Zurich, Billroth's restless energy allowed him to pursue both medicine and music. Three years after his arrival he published *General Surgical Pathology and Therapy,* a textbook which went through eleven editions and was translated into many languages. Although it was a well-written, well-researched work, only the later editions made a real contribution to the science of surgery. Billroth also composed a string quartet, a piano quintet, and three trios, but later destroyed them, remarking, "It was awful stuff and stank dreadfully as it burned." His conducting, however, was not so bad, and on two occasions he served as guest conductor of the Zurich music society.

At the age of thirty-eight, Billroth came to Vienna as professor of surgery. No doubt, as a Prussian, he had some misgivings. The Prussian army had just defeated the Austrians at Sadowa, and the Viennese were usually none too friendly toward anyone with North German speech. But Billroth, already recognized as one of the brilliant young surgeons of Europe, found the city so congenial that he stayed for the remainder of his life. He was an extremely hard worker and probably something of an insomniac who spent very little time in bed. Once he had accepted Lister's methods, his industry and drive allowed him to develop surgical techniques that are still used today.

In 1873 Billroth was the first surgeon to remove completely a larynx for cancer, though preceded by Patrick Watson, an Edinburgh surgeon, who had performed a similar operation for syphilis. But this feat is minor when compared to his most famous work—the development of stomach surgery. Billroth had predecessors here too, but their results had been dismal.

In 1879 Jules Emile Péan, a Paris surgeon, had opened the abdomen of a patient and found a cancer of the pylorus or far end of the stomach. Péan cut out the diseased section and sewed the remainder to the duodenum, but the patient died five days later. A year afterward another surgeon, Ludwig Rydyger, did the same thing. Though this time the procedure had been planned in advance, the patient again died within twelve hours of "exhaustion."

Billroth was initially more fortunate. In 1881 he operated successfully on a forty-three-year-old woman, though she died four months later when her stomach cancer spread to the liver. But his next two stomach cancer operations were failures, and when this news leaked out, he was actually stoned in the streets of Vienna. He did not give up, however, and soon devised an ingenious improvement.

In his first cases, Billroth simply stitched the cut ends of the duodenum and stomach together, a procedure now called the Billroth I operation. Unfortunately, leakage was very prone to occur at the junction. Then in 1885 Billroth was forced to operate on the pyloric cancer of a very debilitated patient. Fearing to perform his usual operation because of the risk of operative shock, he decided simply to make one opening in the stomach, another in the small bowel, and connect the two, thus bypassing the malignant tissue. When the patient remained in a fair state, he went on to cut out the growth, stitching closed the stump of the duodenum and the cut end of the stomach. This method, now called the Billroth II operation, is still in widespread use, especially for peptic ulcer. The great advantage of the Billroth II: the openings in stomach and intestine can be tailor-made for an exact fit. When joining the stomach directly to the duodenum, as in the Billroth I, the surgeon must close part of the cut stomach to accomplish a perfect fit; even the slightest miscalculation can lead to leakage. While modern techniques have reduced the chances of leakage in both operations to practically nil, the Billroth II is still preferred in most cases.

Throughout his life, Billroth remained as devoted to music and food as to surgery. He developed a close friendship with Johannes Brahms, and it is said that he was once offered a post in Germany but declined because Brahms would not leave Vienna. After the composer had dedicated two string quartets to the surgeon, Billroth remarked that these would allow his name to outlast his medical fame. Out of gratitude and because of the rivalry between Brahms and Wagner, the corpulent Billroth would stomp majestically out of any concert that contained an unexpected Wagnerian composition. In his own mansion outside the Vienna Woods, Billroth gave private concerts conducted by himself, Brahms, or his other great friend, Johann Strauss. These soirées filled with the rich delicacies and wine that he loved no doubt aggravated the illnesses that beset the famous surgeon: gallstones, kidney stones, bronchitis, pneumonia, and heart disease.

Among Billroth's most eminent pupils was a Pole, Johann von Mikulicz-Radecki, who became professor of surgery at Breslau. Mikulicz not only performed and modified many recently devised operations but also introduced new techniques. In 1880 he sewed up a perforated gastric ulcer for the first time, but nonetheless the patient died three hours later of shock. In an attempt to prevent surgical wound infection from the hands, Mikulicz introduced sterile white linen gloves; these were not received with enthusiasm, however, and were eventually replaced by rubber gloves that did not interfere with the surgeon's sense of touch. Mikulicz was also the first to make extensive use of the gastroscope, a rigid, angulated tube with mirror optics, through which the inside of the stomach could be seen. Gastroscopy, which was once said to require a surgeon with the instincts of a sword swallower and the eye of a hawk, was raised to a high art by Mikulicz.

After Billroth's death in 1894, Mikulicz became one of the most famous surgeons in Europe, and physicians from many countries flocked to see him in the operating room. But Mikulicz was not always as fastidious dressing himself as he was dressing wounds. During one operation witnessed by Dr. J. M. T. Finney of Johns Hopkins and recorded in his autobiography, the great surgeon's trousers fell down. Mikulicz managed to comport himself with considerable dignity while assistants scurried to fasten them up again.

Halsted

One of the most innovative surgeons who studied with Billroth was not a European but an American, William Stewart Halsted. In the mid-nineteenth century American surgeons often would spend a year or two in Viennese or German clinics, as most medical education—particularly surgical education—in the United States was quite unsatisfactory. The majority of American medical schools were nothing more than highly profitable diploma-mills. But in 1890 at the newly founded Johns Hopkins University in Baltimore, Halsted and three colleagues—William Osler, an internist; William Welch, a pathologist; and Howard Kelly, a gynecologist—became the first to pattern American medical education on the German model.

William Halsted was born in 1852 to socially prominent, well-to-do parents with houses on Fifth Avenue and at Irvington, New York, where the family spent summer months. Young William had the quintessential patrician education and upbringing: governesses until he was ten, then Phillips Academy at Andover, and from there to Yale.

At Yale, Halsted showed little interest in his studies, and in fact was indifferent to many aspects of college life but sports, becoming captain of the football team in 1873. Though popular, he had the arrogance of a New York Brahmin, and his sarcastic wit made him many enemies, both while a student and throughout the rest of his life. Another trait, his desire to appear impeccably dressed, turned almost into a fetish later on.

In his last year of college Halsted bought a copy of Gray's *Anatomy*. Now at last he seemed to have found something besides clothes and sports which interested him. By his graduation at age twenty-two, he had decided to become a physician.

The medical school he chose was the one most in keeping with his character—New York's College of Physicians and Surgeons. This school more than any other, even today, has a reputation for producing "the gentleman physician," often preferring a liberal arts background to a scientific one. Yet Halsted must have applied himself more ardently than most gentlemen would, for he finished in 1877 first in his graduating class.

During his last year before graduation and first year after, Halsted began his hospital training. The first part of this was received at Bellevue, where to his surprise and great delight he was accepted after passing a competitive examination. Only two Bellevue surgeons at the time were convinced of the value of asepsis. The rest still operated in bloody butchers' aprons or old frock coats after giving the dirty scalpel one or two perfunctory wipes. Halsted, however, was certain that Lister was correct, and the mania he developed for sterile technique was to stand him in good stead during his career.

The last of his American training was received at the New York Hospital, where again he was accepted after a competitive examination. Here he showed himself to be not only a brilliant surgeon but a curious one as well. He would put any tumor he found in a jar and examine it in Dr. William H. Welch's makeshift pathology laboratory in an old morgue on the East River. Welch, teaching the first pathology course in America, quickly made Halsted realize how valuable a pathologist and laboratory could be for a surgeon. The two men became the closest of friends—a relationship that was to have a more profound effect on Halsted's life and career than any other.

In 1878 Halsted traveled to Europe. Besides his studies with Billroth and other eminent surgeons, he learned anatomy, embryology, and histology with Albert von Kölliker and Karl Weigert, whose tissue-staining method is still used. Another tutor gave him private lessons in dissection of the brain. These took place at six in the morning in the professor's bedroom. But Halsted soon found waking the teacher and getting him out of bed to be so repugnant that the lessons were abandoned.

Upon returning to New York, Halsted achieved immediate success as a surgeon. American surgery was still a very bloody affair, as the importance of stopping bleeding to prevent surgical shock was not recognized. But in Europe, Halsted had watched Mikulicz operate while more than a dozen clamps were left hanging in the wound. Though the other Americans in the audience were greatly amused, Halsted immediately grasped the significance of what his colleagues thought a merely untidy, uncouth technique. Thereafter his operations became models of perfection and safety, and he achieved results in his meticulous, unhurried way that other New York surgeons could not.

As a surgeon, Halsted's *sang froid* made him almost legendary. In 1881 his sister was moribund from hemorrhage after giving birth. Without hesitating, Halsted withdrew blood from his own vein and injected it into her. A year later his mother became critically ill with gall bladder disease. When consultants refused to operate, Halsted saved her life by removing multiple gallstones, though he had never before operated on a gall bladder.

Occupied as he was with a growing surgical practice, Halsted still found time to teach anatomy at the College of Physicians and Surgeons. In shirt sleeves and shiny silk hat, he would move from table to table to inspect each student's work. Though growing bald and nearsighted, he was becoming a good teacher, and conducted for his students a special quiz course of private lessons for which each paid a hundred dollars. Here they often learned more medicine than at the school lectures.

Halsted rapidly became so busy that his trips as attending surgeon to the hospitals on Ward's and Blackwell's Islands had to be made at night. Yet he continued to visit Welch's grubby laboratory in the ancient morgue and also managed an active social life.

With a friend, Thomas McBride, Halsted shared a fashionable house on Twenty-fifth Street filled with fine furniture, antiques, and rugs, of which he was a connoisseur. The two bachelors gave supper parties and musicales, in addition to entertaining any unexpected guests. In the midst of all this activity, the energetic Halsted managed to work in yet one other pursuit: anesthetic research.

In 1884 Carl Koller, a German ophthalmologist, reported his success anesthetizing the cornea and conjunctiva of the eye with cocaine. This drug was known to the Incas of ancient Peru, who chewed coca leaves for stimulation and applied the spittle to the skull to reduce the pain of trepanning. By 1855 Albert Niemann, a German chemist, had isolated and named the white crystalline powder that Koller employed.

After reading of Koller's work, Halsted correctly guessed that cocaine might be used to produce local anesthesia by regionally blocking individual nerves. To test this hypothesis, he and a colleague at Roosevelt Hospital, Richard Hall, injected themselves with cocaine solutions. Out of this work has evolved the valuable nerve-blocking techniques now widely used in dentistry and surgery.

While experimenting with cocaine, Halsted discovered that he felt wonderful under its influence. His head seemed to become clearer, he needed little sleep, and fatigue was almost banished from his busy life. Soon he was sniffing the drug as well as injecting it.

Around the time of his cocaine experiments, Halsted developed a drug addiction, believed by all previous biographers to have been cocaine addiction. But in 1969 a secret record of the early days at Johns Hopkins written by Halsted's colleague William Osler was published. Osler had kept his record in a small black book with a little silver lock and key. At his death the book had been entrusted to a cousin and literary executor, Dr. William Francis, with the understanding that its contents not be published until the hundredth anniversary of the Johns Hopkins Hospital in 1989.

Francis, however, after reading this "secret history," decided otherwise, writing in 1958, "Now that everyone mentioned in it is dead, it should be published." Unfortunately, Francis died in 1959, and ten years elapsed before the section on Halsted finally appeared in the *Journal of the American Medical Association.*

The "secret history" reveals that Halsted was addicted to morphine, not cocaine. Osler learned this after developing a close relationship with Halsted. This relationship probably was reflected when Osler came to write the section on opiate addiction in his famous textbook, *The Principles and Practice of Medicine,* in 1892:

MORPHIA HABIT (Morphiomania; Morphinism).
This habit arises from the constant use of morphia—taken at first, as a rule, for the purpose of allaying pain. The craving is gradually engendered, and the habit in this way acquired. The injurious effects vary very much, and in the East, where opium-smoking is as common as tobacco smoking with us, the ill effects are, according to good observers, not so striking.
The habit is particularly prevalent among . . . physicians who use the hypodermic syringe. The symptoms are at first slight, and moderate doses may be taken for months without serious injury and without disturbance of health. There are exceptional instances in which for a period of years excessive doses have been taken without deterioration of the mental or bodily functions. As a rule, the dose necessary to obtain the desired sensations has gradually to be increased. As the effects wear off the victim experiences sensations of lassitude and mental depression. . . . Occasionally there are profuse sweats, which may be preceded by chills. . . .
The treatment of the morphia habit is extremely difficult, and can rarely be successfully carried out by the general practitioner. . . .
It is essential in the treatment of a case to be certain that the patient has no means of obtaining morphia. Even under the favorable circumstances of seclusion in an institution, and constant watching by a night and day nurse, I have known a patient to practice deception for a period of three months. After an apparent cure the patients are only too apt to lapse into the habit.

Biographers, incorrectly believing that Halsted was addicted to cocaine, attributed the condition to "the courageous . . . striving to relieve human suffering . . . ignorant of the terrible danger." Since cocaine was actually not the addicting agent, an interesting question arises: How did Halsted become hooked on morphine?
The answer is the old one known to Osler in 1892. "The habit is particularly prevalent among . . . physicians who use the hypodermic syringe," just as the textbook says. Many doctors, crushed like Halsted under a heavy burden of work and long hours, are prone to turn to the medicines in their little black bags for surcease. There is

no possibility that Halsted, a well-educated physician, could have been ignorant of the terrible danger of addiction, since this was pointed out in medical textbooks written even before Osler's.

Once addicted, Halsted no doubt endured the symptoms that Osler describes: lassitude, mental depression. Once gay and gregarious, the surgeon's whole character changed. He became gloomy and withdrawn. Finally, urged by friends, he entered a mental hospital in Providence for a year. One wonders whether he was the institutionalized patient mentioned by Osler in his textbook who obtained morphine by deception in spite of constant watching by a night and day nurse.

After being discharged from the hospital in Providence, Halsted returned to New York City, abandoned by all his former friends except Welch. He tried to work, but the drug craving soon became too great for him. The result was the common one Osler predicted. After an apparent cure, he lapsed back into the habit.

Welch in the meantime had moved to Baltimore to accept a position at Johns Hopkins, though neither the medical school nor hospital had yet been opened. Knowing about Halsted's addiction, he nevertheless arranged to employ him in his laboratory. Welch even took Halsted to live in his own home, perhaps hoping that his influence and presence could prevent morphine use.

Over the next two years, from 1887 to 1889, Halsted made a great effort to break himself of the drug habit. One ploy was a trip to South America, on which he took along less narcotic than he was accustomed to using. This resulted in a frightening, degrading incident. Half mad during the subsequent period of withdrawal, he broke into the captain's cabin to steal narcotics from the medicine chest. By a stroke of good fortune he was not arrested or shot, and the story was hushed up until after his death.

In mid-May 1889 the Johns Hopkins trustees decided to ask Halsted to act as chief surgeon pro tempore. They knew of his addiction and uncertain cure, but were impressed because he had opened an office and had quickly become well known in the city after several successful operations. But his great snobbishness and arrogance were also well known, as Osler described in his secret record:

"[Halsted] was very much 'verdeutsched' and held that there were only three or four good surgeons in the world and they were all Germans. . . . Mixing but little with the local profession he never acquired a large consultation practice. In fact, he cared so little for it that he did not keep office hours nor had he a door plate. He secured

a very good income from a very few patients as his fees were enormous—at least they were so regarded. He was not very popular with
the trustees at first, partly on this account, as they heard so many
comments on his high charges. The natives were simply aghast at
them—in fact I used to think them high, but I never went back on
him though he often got me into trouble.

"He charged a patient of mine $10,500 for a gallstone operation—
a most serious and protracted case, with two operations—but the
woman got well. The people were wealthy, and I stood by him and
told the artist story to the old man, who at the last felt thankful that
the fee was so small. He really had not much conscience in the matter of charges, but he had the feeling of a high class artist about the
value of his work."

Halsted used the enormous fees he collected, in part, to support an
increased fastidiousness in dress. He had always been careful about
his appearance, but now his closets began to fill with expensive suits,
some of which he wore only a few times. Unhappy with the local
laundry, he had his expensive shirts sent to Paris for washing and
ironing. His elegant shoes were made by a Paris bootmaker.

It was not long before the immaculately dressed surgeon acquired
an ardent admirer, a young nurse named Caroline Hampton. Miss
Hampton had been born into an aristocratic South Carolina family
impoverished by the Civil War. Forced to work, she attended the
Mount Sinai and New York Hospital nursing schools in New York
City, then came to Baltimore to become head nurse in Halsted's operating room. Osler describes an incident in the courtship that probably occurred around 1890:

"Dr. Halsted . . . had very advanced ideas of teaching the nurses
bacteriology, and it was soon evident that he was becoming very interested in his pupil. One Sunday morning I went into a room in the
Pathology Laboratory and found Dr. Halsted teaching her Osteology
—demonstrating the fibula. I then knew all was 'up with him.' I sat
down and chaffed them for a few minutes, and on leaving wrote on a
slip of paper the following lines:

> 'But what delights can equal those
> That stir the spirit's inner deeps
> When one who loves, but knows not, reaps
> A Truth from one who loves and knows.'

The engagement was announced within a week."

Halsted's concern for his fiancée prompted him to introduce rubber gloves in the operating room. When he learned that Miss Hampton's delicate hands were being chafed by the strong, highly irritating mercuric chloride disinfectant solution, Halsted had plaster casts of her hands prepared, then took them personally to the Goodyear Rubber Company in New York to have the gloves made. The first ones were thick and clumsy, but also boilable. A young intern in charge of instruments soon also began to use them, and in 1896 Halsted himself finally sent bronze casts of his hands to the Goodyear Company, ordering gloves that were thin, pliable, and close fitting.

A few months after the first gloves had been made, Halsted and Caroline Hampton were married. But Osler quickly learned that his colleague still was not well:

"They had no family, cared nothing for society but were devoted to their dogs and horses. The proneness to seclusion, the slight peculiarities, amounting to eccentricities at times . . . were the only outward traces of the daily battle through which this brave fellow lived for years. When we recommended him as full surgeon to the hospital in 1890, I believed, and Welch did too, that he was no longer addicted to morphia. He had worked so well and so energetically it did not seem possible that he could take the drug and do so much.

"About six months after the full position had been given, I saw him in a severe chill, and this was the first intimation I had that he was still taking morphia. Subsequently I had many talks about it and gained his full confidence. He had never been able to reduce the amount to less than three grains daily;* and on this he could do his work comfortably and maintain his excellent physical vigor (for he was a very muscular fellow). I do not think that anyone suspected him, not even Welch."

Halsted proved to be a typical case of morphine addiction. The severe chills are just as Osler described them in *The Principles and Practice of Medicine*. The three-grain dose is a very large one, six times the usual amount needed for analgesia, and would probably be lethal for anyone without tolerance for opiates. But as the textbook said, "There are exceptional instances in which for a period of years excessive doses have been taken without deterioration of the mental or bodily functions."

The asterisk after "three grains daily" is a reference to a footnote added sometime between 1912 and Osler's death in 1919: "*Subse-

quently, 10 Jan. 1898, he got the amount down to 1½ grains, and of
late years (1912) has possibly got on without it." Evidently Halsted
must have consulted Osler on Jan. 10, 1898. But Osler left Baltimore in 1905 to become regius professor at Oxford, and so his later
speculation that his friend may have possibly got on without morphine is no doubt wishful thinking. Such a long-standing addiction
rarely can be overcome.

The Halsteds' entire domestic life appears to have been tainted by
the opiate addiction, and it can only be described as grim. Contacts
with the outside world were few and formal. The rare dinners that
the couple gave were unpleasant at best. Conversation was desultory,
since the host and hostess were totally incapable of relaxing enough
to make small talk. And after the days of preparation for the affair—
the whole household was invariably involved—Mrs. Halsted would
take to her bed with a severe attack of migraine headache.

Perhaps to escape this dreary life, the couple purchased a country
place, High Hampton, in North Carolina. Mrs. Halsted would arrive
in the early spring. Dressed in whatever worn clothing was available,
she would care for her dogs and horses, or work in the fields helping
to plant and harvest crops.

Halsted, however, would not join his wife until after an annual trip
abroad. Part of the time in Europe he spent inspecting clinics and attending professional meetings. But the rest he would pass shut up in
some small hotel in Paris or Folkestone or Brighton.

His professional life is quite well documented, and reveals him to
be one of the giants in the history of surgery. Far more scientifically
inclined than any other surgeon of his day, Halsted improved the
operations he performed by means of meticulous laboratory research.
He is held in high regard especially for his studies on wound healing,
his work on breast cancer, and his technique for repairing inguinal
hernias.

Inguinal or groin hernia, the most common form of "rupture," has
long been a terrible problem. The condition causes pain and discomfort in the groin, made worse by any form of straining. And sometimes a loop of bowel will become stuck (incarcerated) or even
strangulated within the hernia. In the absence of surgical intervention, strangulated hernia is almost always fatal.

Inguinal hernias occur in men because the testicles, which develop
inside the abdominal cavity of the fetus, migrate before birth into
the scrotum outside the abdomen through an opening called the in-

ternal inguinal ring. They are followed by an important structure, the spermatic cord, through a muscular tunnel, the inguinal canal, finally emerging into the scrotum, where they are covered only by skin and fat. Sometimes, though, the lining of the abdominal cavity, the peritoneum, bulges into the inguinal canal and forms a hernial sac containing loops of bowel. The problem cannot simply be remedied by sewing closed both ends of the canal, since this would mean sacrifice of the spermatic cord and testicle.

Surgeons since antiquity had struggled with inguinal hernias, but, ignorant of the correct anatomy of the area, they could achieve nothing. Trusses, which have been known since ancient times, are of value only in hernias not incarcerated or strangulated. Surgical intervention was considered so dangerous that it was rarely attempted.

After the introduction of aseptic technique, a number of surgeons tried to devise an effective hernia repair. In America, Halsted reported the first good method in 1889. Using silk stitches, he reconstituted the ligaments and fascia of the area, while tightening the inguinal canal by sewing its walls together beneath the spermatic cord. As in all his operations, Halsted took great care to tie off every bleeding point. But at the same time that Halsted's report appeared, an Italian surgeon, Edoardo Bassini, published an account of a somewhat similar method devised independently.

Though the Halsted hernia repair is still considered a good technique, the radical mastectomy Halsted devised to treat breast cancer is falling into disuse. Before Halsted, surgeons either refused to treat such tumors, amputated the breast with a clean sweep of the knife, or employed a cautery. But Halsted, believing in the importance of an extensive operation, would excise not only the breast but also the underlying muscle and the nearby lymph nodes. The entire procedure could last more than four hours, once leading Halsted to remark to an assistant, "Would you mind moving a little? You've been standing on my foot for the last half hour." Years later, simple removal of the tumor combined with radiation therapy was shown to give a woman the same chance to survive the cancer while preserving her breast.

As he aged, Halsted became unable to tolerate the long hours at the operating table. First he began leaving more and more of the work to assistants, and finally he stopped operating entirely. But by this time he had trained a number of fine disciples. The most eminent of these men, Harvey Cushing, extended the surgeon's range in another formerly inaccessible area: the cranial cavity.

Harvey Cushing and Neurosurgery

While skull operations are one of the oldest surgical procedures, successful trepanners were well aware of the hazards of breaking through the dura mater, the tough membrane which lines the interior of the cranial cavity and covers the brain. A British anthropologist questioning medicine men from the mountains of Algeria discovered "all . . . agreed that on no account must the dura mater be disturbed, as death will inevitably result should this be done." As the nineteenth century drew to a close, however, the new aseptic techniques made the brain and spinal cord beneath the dura mater surgically accessible.

At the same time, a series of discoveries paved the way for the development of neurosurgery. In 1870 Gustav Fritsch and Eduard Hitzig found that the cortex or outer layer of a dog's brain was electrically excitable. Soon investigators were using electrical stimulation and other methods to determine which parts of the brain and spinal cord controlled particular organ and body functions; Sir Charles Sherrington is especially well known in this regard for his work on anthropoid apes. At the same time, Sir William Macewen and Sir Victor Horsley began removing brain tumors. Horsley introduced bone wax to help control the fearsome bleeding, but bleeding was only one of the problems that plagued neurosurgeons until the innovations introduced by Harvey Cushing.

Cushing was born on August 8, 1869, the youngest of ten children of a Cleveland physician, Henry Kirke Cushing, and his wife Betsy. The father, "Dr. Kirke," was a stern, unbending, God-fearing man; yet even he, with his iron discipline and tight fist, could not entirely subdue his mercurial youngest son. No amount of rebuke served to curb Harvey's terrible fits of temper. This trait earned the nickname "Pepper Pot" for the child, and made him many enemies throughout his life. Harvey was an adequate student, though he never managed to master the intricacies of spelling.

In 1887 the young man entered Yale, renting a room with his

cousin, Perry Harvey. Letters home to Dr. Kirke were full of complaints. "We have a terrible time," Cushing wrote, "with the dust which rises off this matting. Everything is just covered with it. My last bottle of ink got so full of it that I had to buy another which is rapidly being spoiled. I have to stand on a chair when I put on my pants in the morning for if they touch the floor they get covered with matting dust."

Though the rugs young Cushing wanted were soon forthcoming, no regular allowance was. Every penny first had to be meticulously accounted for. Because the good doctor could never comprehend that Yale should be so expensive, his son acquired painfully an undergraduate preoccupation with financial deficits. These were especially bothersome when his father discovered they resulted from frivolities rather than necessities.

"Dear Father," Cushing wrote during his first year, "I was very sorry to have received such a letter from you as I did last week. . . . I don't know as you have any reason to think that I have not been studying, and do not intend to study faithfully, I am sure you know I always did at home and I don't see why you should suspect I do not here. As for repenting that you sent me here I am very sorry if I have been the cause but if you are afraid I won't study here I don't see why you should suppose I would elsewhere. I went up to N.Y. to spend Thanksgiving . . . but did not go expressly to see a football game although we did go to see the game, and I am sure from the accounts of one of the boys who stayed here that the excitement in New Haven was as great as in New York, if not more so, with bonfires and so forth. I believe you went to college once, and although one has to grind the greater part of the time, there are times when one doesn't. I don't know whether I will make the first division or not as there are a great many remarkably bright men in our class but I have studied hard for it. I hope I haven't said too much but I was surprised and disappointed very much. . . ."

Actually, Cushing was a creditable student and diligent worker. Because learning did not come easily to him, he acquired the perfectionism that became so marked later on. Yet he still had time to participate in sports, and sometimes made his father quite angry doing so. Once, after he had gone to Cambridge with the baseball team, Dr. Kirke wrote, "It looks to me as if in the glamor and excitement of College sentiments and surroundings, you have reasoned yourself into feeling that if you only keep in the first division, it was none of my business what else you did. . . ."

Consistent spelling problems and increased demands for money also irked the elder Cushing. In one letter he said, "Please buy a dictionary and consult it as you write. In almost every letter I note misspelt words. . . ." When the son had been elected to a sophomore society, the disapproving father replied, "I trust you will critically examine your Society relations and calmly judge if you do not think the price asked for its blandishments [an initiation fee of thirty-five dollars] is not large for its worth."

In his senior year young Harvey began to think about his future. First he considered taking up architecture or chemistry, but finally turned to medicine. This was partly a result of the influence of his brother Ned, who was an intern at the Massachusetts General Hospital in 1888. Mostly, though, the decision seems to have been shaped by a course in physiological chemistry with Dr. Russell Chittenden. Chittenden had a deep effect on Cushing, and also on other Yale undergraduates: Elliott Joslin, who became a world-famous diabetes specialist; Graham Lusk, who took over the Department of Physiology at Yale; and Lafayette Mendel, who succeeded Chittenden in the chair of physiological chemistry at Yale.

Cushing graduated in June 1891 and entered the Harvard Medical School that autumn. Immediately he distinguished himself in anatomy class. The arm is traditionally the first part of the body to be dissected. Cushing accomplished this so skillfully that students and teachers came to watch. Thereafter he remained a prominent figure while at school.

In his first year at Harvard, Cushing found time for girls—in particular, one from Cleveland named Katharine Crowell, who was staying with friends in Boston. When she left, Cushing took her to the train, and was nearly carried off during a prolonged good-bye.

Work on the wards in the Massachusetts General Hospital began for Cushing in his second year, and it was during this period that he introduced one of the many innovations for which he is now known. While substituting for a classmate at the hospital, he was to administer anesthetic to a woman undergoing surgery for a strangulated hernia. At that time, the necessity of closely monitoring an unconscious patient was unrecognized. The ether was given in a large single dose rather than continuously, and the surgeon hoped that the patient did not wake up in the middle of the procedure.

On this particular morning, the surgeon, Dr. Porter, was in a rush, forcing Cushing to etherize the woman as quickly as possible. Shortly after the cutting began, the patient died suddenly. Though Cushing had given ether before, death had never been the result, and now he was tortured by remorse and anguish. He wandered aimlessly through the streets of Boston and finally went to see Dr. Porter at his house. When he told the surgeon that he was going to give up medicine, that he was unfit to be a doctor, Porter insisted that the patient had no chance of surviving and that certainly Cushing was not at fault. In fact, he said, deaths from ether were fairly common, and Cushing should not give a moment's consideration to abandoning medicine on account of this unfortunate incident.

But Cushing kept brooding until finally a solution occurred to him. With a friend, Amory Codman, he devised charts for continually recording pulse and respiration during an operation. Using these, the surgeon and anesthetist could tell at a glance the condition of the patient. After the charts had been adopted at the Massachusetts General, ether deaths dropped dramatically, and the method soon spread to other hospitals.

By 1895, during his fourth and last year of medical school, Cushing had begun to show a keen interest in neurological surgery. One case that he followed especially closely was that of William N. Conant, a man who had sustained a compound fracture of the skull. Cushing's notations on the chart exemplify the bleeding problem that he later did so much to ameliorate:

"Patient had fearful hemorrhage from brain sinuses. Pulse kept along very well and finally went out all at once and could not be felt at wrist. With pressure which checked the hemorrhage the pulse finally came back a few beats at a time, as an Indian starts up from a way station, and finally became pretty regular 120-110-100." On the front of the record is another scribbled note, "Bled enormously," and a follow-up note indicating that Cushing had gone to the trouble of visiting the patient at the Waverly Convalescent Home outside Boston, learning there that the man ultimately was discharged well.

Under the strain of the last year of medical school, Cushing began to demonstrate more prominently the unpleasant traits that were so evident later in his life. To patients he was invariably kind and courteous, but to other interns and nurses he showed a tense reserve that could momentarily turn into vicious anger. In the diary that he began keeping at the time, he noted periods of depression reminiscent of those that affected Semmelweis.

But another trait, common to successful men, was also in evidence: the desire to add extra work to what an ordinary person would consider a full-time load. In spite of all his other duties, for example, Cushing began to experiment with X rays. Shortly after Roentgen announced his discovery in Germany, December 28, 1895, American medical journals began to carry X-ray photographs. Seeing these, Cushing contributed out of his small funds for an X-ray machine, with which he worked as much as possible. Yet he was quite lucky to be otherwise so fully occupied. His friend Codman, who had more time to spend with the new machine, eventually suffered from serious X-ray burns.

As his fourth year at Harvard drew to a close, Cushing determined to secure an appointment at Johns Hopkins, though positions on Halsted's surgical house staff were not easily obtained. After several months' negotiations filled with hope and despair, his wish was granted. Yet initially he was rather dismayed with what he encountered.

Baltimore was a sleepy, dusty southern town when the twenty-seven-year-old Cushing arrived in the autumn of 1896. The monotony of the famous blocks of row houses depressed him—they were "as alike as streptococci," he said. Even the southern custom of serving sausage with griddlecakes seemed annoying. But these shortcomings were minor when compared with those Cushing perceived in the chief of surgery.

Halsted, fully occupied trying to wean himself from morphine, was moody, taciturn, and difficult. He was frequently absent from the hospital, and Cushing, unaware of the addiction problem, was prone to regard the chief's dereliction of duty with some scorn. When Halsted wrote him, "Dear Cushing, You may have the operating room tomorrow for I should like to watch the cases which interest me for a day or two longer. P.S. I send you over some papers for the one-armed boy in D," Cushing noted sarcastically in the margin, "Characteristic note of the Professor—not operated for a week. One-armed boy left hospital a week ago."

Yet Halsted's benign neglect proved to be Cushing's good fortune. "Here I am," he wrote to Katharine Crowell in Cleveland, "a youth, doing surgical work that not one of my school confreres will hope to do for years. It frightenes me sometimes. The Chief rarely operates. Today I did all his private cases."

Miss Crowell—Cushing called her his "Puss Cat"—eagerly awaited such letters, since marriage had been foremost in her mind for quite some time. She came to visit shortly after Cushing arrived in Baltimore, and—after seven years of waiting—was finally able to stir her reluctant suitor into a belated course of action. When she left again for Cleveland, he wrote Mrs. Crowell (the father was dead) asking for permission to marry Kate. Immediately after mailing the letter, poor Cushing was seized by a paroxysm of terror. Had he been too impulsive?

Two years after the affirmative reply from Mrs. Crowell, the Puss Cat was still waiting, and was not happy about it. Her fiancé by this time had gone to study in Europe. Upon receiving one dunning notice from her, he replied, "My dear child, Your letter troubles me a wee bit. When your flag is not flying I always feel that I must chase home and marry you instanter. It's wicked of me to have made you wait." But, he explained, "I want you to move in with the house furnished and the carpets down and a warm fire burning for you."

Cushing stayed abroad for fourteen months, finally returning to Baltimore in August 1901. Now his surgical training was completed, and Halsted suggested that he take up the new specialty of orthopedics. But Cushing had become fascinated with surgery of the brain though methods used were still crude. In England he had watched Horsley operate on a woman for tic douloureux, a nervous condition in which the face is convulsed by periodic painful spasms. After seeing Horsley cut the patient's Gasserian ganglion, Cushing was so unnerved that he decided the refinements in neurologic surgery could not be learned there.

Nor anywhere else, for that matter, since the mortality rates in most neurosurgical operations approached 100 per cent. Until 1905 about half of the patients died right on the operating table from shock or hemorrhage. In a third of the cases, the surgeon couldn't even find the growth, and if he did there was only a fifty-fifty chance that it could be removed. Most surgeons liked to take the tumors out with their bare fingers, assuring that the patient would die of infection should he by chance emerge from the operating room alive.

An English brain operation performed in 1884 serves as an example of the state of the art. A young man of twenty-five was admitted to the Hospital for Epilepsy and Paralysis in Regent's Park, London, complaining of twitchings, weakness of his left arm and leg, vomiting, and headache. After the diagnosis of tumor in the motor area of the right side of the brain was made, Rickman John Godlee, Lister's nephew, decided to operate. Though the patient was immediately relieved of his original symptoms, the surgeon's close relationship to the father of antisepsis did not prevent a wound infection, and the man died twenty-eight days later.

Cushing was certain that he could consistently obtain better results than this, and strongly believed that improved techniques could drastically reduce the hazards of brain-tumor operations. Such improvements would encourage general practitioners to recognize these lesions at an earlier stage when the chance of cure was better.

Halsted was antagonistic to Cushing's point of view and hesitant to give the young surgeon a full-time appointment. The uncertainty of waiting was almost unbearable for Cushing, who grew morose, ill-tempered, and despondent. But finally the appointment was made, with the proviso that part of the time be spent in the neurological division of the surgical clinic.

Immensely pleased, Cushing found, with two other bachelors, a comfortable house at 3 West Franklin Street, just next door to the Oslers. The three were given latchkeys to the Osler household, and all remained on intimate terms during the four years before Osler left for England. It was this experience that gave Cushing so much of the personal material included in his two-volume *The Life of Sir William Osler,* a Pulitzer Prize–winning biography that has stayed in print since 1925.

In addition to his gift for writing, Cushing had a great deal of personal charm that he could radiate when he wished to. A talented artist, he made many excellent sketches and anatomical drawings. He even composed clever verses for children; these, for example, describe his appendectomy in 1897:

DEAR CHILDREN

To pay up for his many sins
In cutting deep holes through your skins—
And tieing you to Bradford frames
And other things which have no names
   Dr. "Cushong" took some "Efur."

II

He screamed and made a dreadful fuss,
And wrung his hands and made a muss
Of everything in reach. " 'Cause why?"
Just 'Cause. It was quite wrong to cry
    For nothing more than "Efur."

III

They took him down upon a truck
Like any one of you, whose luck
That day might have been ill. "Dear me,"
He cried, "Quite scared am I." You see—
    Like you he feared the "Efur."

IV

He had to breathe it just as you
Have done and slept and never knew
A thing until at last, awake, he found
Miss "Sherring" there, and safe and sound
    He'd come out from his "Efur."

V

And now he thanks you one and all
From Mary short to Claude so tall
For those pink roses, a delight
They were, so sweet and fresh they quite
    Make up for taking "Efur."

Unfortunately, Cushing chose to display his charm all too seldom,
substituting instead the more vituperative side of his personality. One
operating-room nurse whom he had repeatedly abused composed the
following:

"C" is for Cushing
So Cussedly Clever
He can be polite
But he hardly is ever.

"C" is for Cushing
So cleverly cussèd
If he ever gets sick,
He never will be nussèd.

Reports of Cushing's bad temper soon reached Osler, who wrote the young surgeon this warning letter:

Dear Cushing:

I arranged with Dr. Hurd—he did not understand that they were your private patients. He must have you put on the hospital staff in some way officially.

You will not mind a reference to one point. The statement is current that you do not get on well with your surgical subordinates & colleagues. I heard of it last year & it was referred to by a strong admirer of yours in New York. The statement also is made that you have criticized before the students—the modes of dressings, operations, &c of members of the staff. This, I need scarcely say would be absolutely fatal to your success here. The arrangement of the Hospital staff is so peculiar that loyalty to each other, even in the minutest particulars, is an essential. I know that you will not mind this from me as I have your interest at heart.

Sincerely yours,
Wm. Osler.

Receiving this letter, Cushing became frantic and offered to resign. Osler, however, mollified him. For a short time afterward, Cushing tried to keep his temper in check, but soon he became as difficult as before. Though he always frowned upon vacations as a waste of time, he was never reluctant to take an ego trip whenever the opportunity arose.

One record of these trips was made by Dr. William Sharpe, who came to Baltimore to study neurosurgery with Cushing in 1911. Sharpe had been counseled by an older colleague not to get too upset by Cushing's temper tantrums, because this particular creative genius worked under such severe tension that even trivialities assumed overwhelming proportions. But the young resident soon discovered that he had chosen to work for a hard man indeed.

Arriving on New Year's Day, Sharpe found Cushing excising the pituitary gland of a dog. Without stopping his work, Cushing ordered his new assistant to rush to a Washington, D.C., funeral parlor, and there remove the ductless glands—pituitary, thyroid, parathyroids, and adrenals—from one of his former patients, a pituitary giant. In addition, the brain, heart, lungs, kidneys, pancreas, and testicles were also to be brought back. A Polish priest, who had influenced the family to permit the autopsy, was to be given fifty dollars. Since funeral services were scheduled for two o'clock that afternoon, there was no time to lose.

Sharpe reached the funeral home shortly after eleven, and was led by the priest to the seven-foot three-and-a-half-inch corpse, dressed in formal attire and boiled shirt, reposing deeply within an enormous coffin. Sharpe and the undertaker tried to lift the body out but could not. The priest refused to help, informing the exasperated surgeon that the relatives hadn't even given permission for a post mortem.

So, without removing the body from the coffin, Sharpe raised the boiled shirt over the corpse's face and removed the neck, chest, and abdominal organs with a long, curved knife. As a few of the mourners had begun to gather in the front room, the young resident started noisily sawing off the vault of the skull to retrieve the pituitary gland. But this proved to be a difficult task, and the front room had soon filled with people wanting to view the body and curious about the sawing noises. Just in time, Sharpe was able to finish and jump into a waiting cab the frantic priest had summoned. Someone threw a rock at the car just as it pulled away.

Once back at the hospital, Sharpe placed the organs in a refrigerator and telephoned Cushing. The new resident went to bed that night quite satisfied with the performance of his first assignment. But before daylight his shoulder was shaken roughly by an angry Dr. Cushing.

"I thought I told you to get every ductless gland in that man's body!" he said. "Did you understand me?"

"Yes, Dr. Cushing, and I did."

"You did not. You missed the left parathyroid body."

Sharpe tried to explain the difficulty of the procedure and the fact that he had never before seen a parathyroid gland. The annoyed Cushing would have none of this.

"When I tell you to do a job," he said, "you are to do it!" He then rudely informed Sharpe that he had chosen the wrong profession and fired the young surgeon on the spot. Sharpe began to cry as Cushing stormed out of the room. But a few hours later Cushing rehired him.

Within a week, a much more serious episode occurred. Cushing ordered Sharpe to wait in the room with a private patient—a hopeless case with a large, protruding brain tumor. Cushing said that he would return in a few minutes to dress the lesion. Two hours later there was still no sign of Dr. Cushing, and so Sharpe asked a nurse to stay with the patient while he went to search for the chief. The nurse, however, was called away for an emergency in an adjoining room.

After ten minutes' futile search, Sharpe returned to the patient's room to find Cushing there—enraged.

"Didn't I tell you to remain here until I returned?" the angry chief roared.

"Yes, sir, you did," Sharpe admitted. "I did remain here for almost two hours. Then I asked the nurse to remain while I—"

"Don't blame it on the nurse," Cushing retorted. "You're yellow!"

"With that," Sharpe writes in his autobiography, *Brain Surgeon,* "I forgot all about the great Dr. Cushing and my ambition to become a neurosurgeon. Impulsively I grabbed his right shoulder with my left hand and almost struck him with my right fist. Thank God, I restrained myself, or I would have regretted it to my dying day. Dr. Cushing, of slighter build and of shorter stature, looked up at me with ashen pallor. As I released his shoulder he turned about to finish the patient's dressing. He did not utter a single word."

The nurse, who had collapsed in tears on a chair, now assisted with the last of the dressing. Sharpe followed Cushing dejectedly to the front door of the hospital, but the chief did not turn or utter a word. Still, he later forgave Sharpe, who somehow managed to stick out the year.

Sharpe apparently left Johns Hopkins on reasonably good terms with Cushing. But a much more eminent neurosurgical resident, Walter Dandy, did not. Dandy first battled with Cushing over experimental results he had obtained that contradicted those about to be published by Cushing.

"Dandy, nobody could think of such a thing as that but you," Cushing said.

"I was only trying to check results," Dandy replied.

Later, as Cushing was leaving to accept a position at Harvard, he came to see some of Dandy's other experimental results. "I showed them to him," Dandy said, "and he put them in his box of materials. . . . I took them out and told him they were going to stay there as they were mine and he had nothing to do with them. He flared up, quickly calmed down and said he guessed they did not amount to anything anyhow."

Cushing, who could never stand to allow anyone else to get credit for work done, retaliated by canceling an appointment he had obtained for Dandy at Harvard. The lateness of this cancellation almost deprived Dandy of the chance to retain his position at Johns Hopkins. Luckily, Halsted recognized Dandy's great ability and subsequently managed to find a place for him on the surgical staff.

Dandy fulfilled Halsted's expectations. In 1918 he introduced ventriculography, an important technique that allows X-ray localization of brain tumors. Cushing, however, remained quite reluctant to utilize this new diagnostic aid even after its wide acceptance; no doubt this reluctance stemmed from the older man's jealousy of his young trainee's superb accomplishment.

Cushing continued to fight with Dandy, though the two maintained outwardly a gentlemanly attitude toward each other. In September 1922 Dandy published a note in the *Johns Hopkins Hospital Bulletin* describing a method for removing acoustic nerve tumors. This irritated Cushing because he had described the same operative approach previously, though Dandy had not cited the description in his note. Cushing sat down and wrote an angry letter to Dr. Winford H. Smith, the director of the Johns Hopkins Hospital, in which he said, "I have been very much disturbed by seeing an article by Dandy in the last issue [of the *Bulletin*] which, in the shape of a preliminary report, consists of nothing more than a promise, so far as I can see, that he is going to describe in the future an operation for a certain kind of brain tumor. It is exceedingly bad for me, inasmuch as many people know that I had something to do with Dr. Dandy's training; it is equally bad for Dr. Dandy himself, inasmuch as general professional esteem is concerned; but what affects all of us still more is that it is very bad for the Hopkins to have the *Bulletin* accept and permit the title of such an incomplete and promissory article to get into the literature. . . ."

Later, having decided to send this letter directly to Dandy, Cushing added the following note in longhand: "Dear Dandy, I have cogitated over this letter a good deal. I think I will send it to you instead of to Dr. Smith. Perhaps you will wish to show it to him and get his advice. . . . I think you are doing yourself a great deal of harm by the tone of some of your publications. . . . You must not forget your manners, and this last note of yours is in extremely bad taste. . . ."

Dandy was greatly offended by this attack. He was not by custom required to cite the literature; this would be done when the final paper was published. Submitting Cushing's letter to the *Bulletin*'s board of editors, he wrote that he was "absolutely at a loss to discover the point for such a letter other than personal animus," also noting that neither Cushing nor anyone else had reported a procedure for the safe total removal of acoustic nerve tumors.

Subsequently a penned letter to Dandy written by Cushing but never mailed was found in the Cushing papers of the Yale Library of Medicine. Jealousy and bitterness have never been more clearly expressed: "Everyone knows that you were once a pupil of mine, and though most of them know that you have far surpassed your teacher, there are at the same time certain amenities which most of us try to observe."

Dandy, as might be expected, never forgave Cushing. In 1945 he wrote to Cushing's biographer, John F. Fulton, "I think he realized his unfairness in later life and in some slight way tried to make amends, to which I did not at all reciprocate. . . . Cushing certainly was not a big man; he was a selfish one and certainly not the type who wished his pupils to excel." Then Dandy added, in a final slap, "I have never felt that his scientific contributions were trustworthy."

Tragically, Cushing's relations with his own son were no better than those with Dandy. In 1902 he married Katharine Crowell after a ten-year courtship, and in 1903 William Harvey Cushing was born. When the father, an iron disciplinarian like his father before him, demanded complete subjugation to his will, Bill resisted. Especially trying were summer vacations, when Bill was at home with his father while Kate and the other children were away. Cushing's notes to his wife are full of complaints about the son's behavior: "Bill blew in last night an hour late for dinner with that defiant look of his. I told him what I thought of it and subsequently apologized, but he was still sulking this morning and got up an hour late. . . ."

The bitterness between the two became so great that it must have approached hatred. The son would defy the father in whatever way he could. After the inevitable explosion, the father would brood. By the time Bill was ready for Yale, father and son could hardly even look at one another without fighting.

The separation brought about by college produced a surprising improvement in the relationship. The more mature son gradually developed affection for his famous father. The father reciprocated by being less domineering. Then one Saturday morning in June 1926 Cushing was about to leave his office for the operating room when he received word that the twenty-three-year-old Bill had been killed in an automobile accident.

Cushing was more fortunate with his three daughters than with his son Bill. All the girls were beautifully brought up and very attractive. The youngest, Barbara, made headlines in the New York *Daily News,* which reported from Reno in late July 1947:

"This rough and ready divorce capital gasped tonight when it learned that William S. Paley, president of the Columbia Broadcasting System, had given his wife a check for $1.5 million as a settlement in the divorce she obtained today. . . .

"The CBS president is reported planning to marry Mrs. Barbara (Babe) Mortimer, a willowy socialite eyeful from Boston. Barbara, chosen by the New York Dress Institute in 1945 as the best-dressed woman in the world, is the youngest daughter of the late surgeon, Dr. Harvey Cushing. She is the sister of Mrs. Vincent Astor and Mrs. John Hay Whitney. Barbara also got a Nevada divorce when she parted company with Stanley G. Mortimer, Jr."

But none of his children achieved the enormous world acclaim that Dr. Cushing himself was accorded, which began to accrue when he attempted to achieve good results in removing brain tumors. At the time, as has been mentioned, very few patients survived such operations. Cushing immediately realized that it would be far better to devise a procedure to decompress the brain than to attempt total removal of the tumor. His simple solution: Remove a flap of bone from under the muscles of the temple or those of the back of the skull. The ugly bulging of the tumor was then prevented by the muscles, yet the brain could still expand enough to relieve symptoms. This "palliative decompression" soon became the accepted procedure and stimulated Cushing to seek good methods for taking out tumors completely.

In 1910 Cushing reported his first promising series of operatively removed brain tumor cases. Unlike other surgeons, who used their fingers, he dissected the growths out gently with a piece of gauze—a method that often prevented shock and hemorrhage. The dissections were done with infinite pains, leading observers to marvel at Cushing's endurance. He could stand motionless, pressing a piece of cotton to a tiny bleeding point for thirty minutes if necessary. But the overall mortality of 10 per cent, though much better than in previous reports, was still mainly due to that old neurosurgeon's nemesis—

bleeding. One particularly tragic result serves to underscore the point.

In this case, the patient had only local anesthesia and was fully conscious as Cushing incised the scalp and turned back the bone flap. As everyone in the operating room watched, a firm, golf-ball-sized tumor emerged from the brain and was extirpated without any problem. But left behind was a stalk from which the tumor seemed to have grown. Cushing, eager to be thorough, seized the stalk with his forceps and cut it off.

The stalk proved to be a small artery, which immediately began to gush blood profusely. Unfortunately, Cushing's technique had not evolved to the point of coping with such bleeding vessels. As the rest of the operating room looked on horrified, Cushing put down his instruments, walked to the side of the table, and leaned over the conscious patient, who was—without knowing it—quickly bleeding to death.

"You must not worry now," Cushing told the man. "In a very few minutes you are going to feel better."

By 1911 Cushing had devised two almost foolproof methods to control bleeding and prevent such needless operative deaths. In one, tiny silver wire clips were picked up with forceps and permanently applied to compress the bleeding point. For hemorrhage in the dura mater, where clips could not be used, he introduced small pieces of muscle tissue. When he published a case series employing these techniques in 1915, his operative mortality had dropped to an astounding 8 per cent. Sir Victor Horsley and other surgeons of the day were still blundering along with rates of 40 to 50 per cent.

A final refinement was added ten years later. At an American Medical Association meeting in 1925 Cushing observed a demonstration of a diathermy used to cut up a piece of beef with an electric current. Electricity had been employed in surgery before, but never in surgery of the brain. When he returned to Boston, Cushing commissioned a physicist, Dr. W. T. Bovie, to build a machine with two currents—intense for cutting, weaker for coagulating bleeding points.

In October 1926 the Bovie apparatus was used for the first time on a patient. The cumbersome machine, wheeled to the hospital from a laboratory one block away, had to be overhauled on the spot because of the bumps and jolts it had received. Since no one trusted the new device, a medical student was sent for to act as blood donor.

Cushing was especially edgy because a delegation of French doctors, all with head colds, was there to witness the operation.

The surgical exposure of the tumor went smoothly, but as Cushing picked up the electric device, there was a loud thump. Everyone turned to see the medical student, who had fallen from his corner stool in a dead faint. The strain became too much for Cushing's new assistant, who announced he could not go on and left the room. Aides rushed out to find the regular assistant while everyone stood around waiting. Then the patient took a turn for the worse. But finally things got started again, and the Bovie device worked superbly. As a result, Cushing was able to reoperate successfully on many other patients whose tumors could not be removed before.

His highly sophisticated operative techniques allowed Cushing to pursue an interest in a part of the brain that had attracted little previous attention—the pituitary gland. Osler, even in later editions of his textbook, makes no mention of pituitary disorders, though in 1901 Alfred Frölich, a Viennese physician, had reported the association of obesity, lack of sexual maturation, and pituitary tumor. At the same time, Cushing had also encountered a similar case in a fourteen-year-old girl.

After becoming director of surgery at Peter Bent Brigham Hospital in Boston, Cushing published his first important work on pituitary disorders in 1912. This monograph was based on his extensive animal experiments and on surgical procedures he devised to remove pituitary tumors. The early cases had a mortality rate of 14 per cent, but when he changed his operative approach and entered the skull through the nose instead of the forehead, mortality decreased to 4 per cent—a truly remarkable result.

In his monograph on the pituitary, Cushing recognized that tumors made up of cells which stained with the dye eosin produced the growth hormone. If this hormone appeared in excess before adulthood, gigantism was the result. But if too much growth hormone was elaborated during adulthood, acromegaly occurred, a condition of localized bony overgrowth. Cushing also noted a second type of pituitary cell, the basophil, and speculated that it probably elaborated some other essential secretion. This extraordinary guess was validated twenty years later, when he produced his most original contribution to the science of healing: the description of a new disorder.

Cushing's syndrome, a disease entity that is now one of the most well known in all endocrinology, was considerably more difficult to characterize than gigantism or acromegaly. While eosin-staining tumors often came to surgery because they interfered with vision, basophil tumors did not. Not until he was sixty years old did Cushing begin to suspect that a basophil tumor could produce the set of symptoms that had previously been given the vague name of "polyglandular syndrome."

Reading a European report of one case of basophil tumor, Cushing recognized that the manifestations were quite similar to those shown by one of his own patients. While this man was being closely followed, three other patients with the same signs appeared, and all had basophil tumors at autopsy. Cushing did not learn of the death of his original patient until three days after the funeral, but using his considerable charm, he was able to persuade the family to have the body exhumed. It, too, showed a basophil tumor.

Now, from observation alone, Cushing was able to deduce that the pituitary was a master gland capable of influencing the function of the other endocrine glands—the thyroid, the gonads, the adrenals. His first official presentation of his findings was made on February 29, 1932, before the Johns Hopkins Medical Society. The full text then appeared in the March issue of the *Johns Hopkins Hospital Bulletin*.

Syndromes, or groups of signs and symptoms characterizing a particular disease entity, were more unfamiliar then, and Cushing managed to mispronounce the word "syndrome" throughout his talk. After the presentation was finished, Dr. William Welch, who had sat listening closely in the first row, took the podium. Obviously not appreciating the enormous significance of what Cushing had found, Dr. Welch proceeded for the next forty minutes to trace the derivation of the word syndrome, and then pedantically informed Cushing that the accent should be on the first syllable.

The day after the lecture, Cushing was observed walking down the hall with one of the professors of surgery. After every few steps he would stop and look out the large windows along the corridor of the hospital into the courtyard. He would continue to talk and after one to two minutes of standing proceed down the hall only to stop short at another window.

This peculiar behavior is characteristic of severe intermittent claudication, a condition caused by blood-vessel disease and painfully insufficient circulation in the muscles of the legs. Cushing probably brought this problem on by smoking heavily for many years. After his compulsory retirement from Peter Bent Brigham Hospital at age

sixty-three, his disability finally forced him to give up operating—
after he had removed his two-thousandth brain tumor. At his death
on October 7, 1939, Cushing himself was discovered to have a small
brain tumor.

Dr. Young and Diamond Jim

A short time before Cushing came to Baltimore in 1896, another
physician destined to make a significant contribution to surgery
joined Halsted's staff. This man, Hugh Hampton Young, revolutionized the treatment of prostate disease and is universally regarded
as the founder of modern urology.

The prostate is a chestnut-shaped gland that encircles the base of
the bladder and produces the seminal fluid. Enlargement of this
gland has been a burden to elderly men since the beginning of time,
prompting physicians through the ages to attempt to relieve the resultant obstruction to the free flow of urine. Because eunuchs are
known not to develop prostatic enlargement, Dr. J. William White in
1893 tried castration to restore normal urination. But the benefits
were only temporary, and the method soon fell into disuse.

Hugh Young was a surgical resident when he treated his first prostate case, an elderly black man brought to the hospital in kidney failure secondary to severe prostatic enlargement. Since a catheter could
not be passed through the penis into the bladder, an incision was
made into the lower abdomen to allow urine to drain. In a few days,
a remarkable improvement had taken place: The kidney failure disappeared and the patient regained consciousness.

Realizing that a cure could be effected by restoring free bladder
drainage, Young stuck his finger into the bladder and shelled out the
enormous prostate, becoming first to perform an effective suprapubic
prostatectomy. The excellent results obtained in this initial case stimulated him to use the same method in additional patients. Young had
succeeded where others had failed because he had thought to provide
counterpressure against the prostate from below by inserting his
gloved finger in the rectum, then pushing the prostate up so that it
could be removed by the finger in the bladder above.

Unfortunately, bleeding during suprapubic prostatectomy is often profuse and poorly tolerated by the elderly men in need of the operation. To combat this problem, Young perfected a new technique—perineal prostatectomy—by dissecting scores of cadavers. His first opportunity to try the method occurred when a Mr. Samuel Alexander came from Hawaii to Baltimore with his doctor, daughter, and nurse.

"Doctor," said Mr. Alexander to Dr. Young, "I've read everything I could get hold of on the prostate. I like what you have written and have come to you for relief, but I honestly think you have not yet got the perfect method. Could you give me something better?"

Young could and did, performing the first perineal prostatectomy on October 2, 1902. Over the next fourteen months he operated on fifty cases without a death, when mortality from suprapubic prostatectomy was still 20 per cent. Two years later, he perfected a more radical technique and became first to remove prostate cancer successfully.

One day in 1912 Young received a very fat gentleman with a huge head and double chin—James Buchanan Brady. The neatly dressed "Diamond Jim" well deserved his famous nickname: Diamonds sparkled from his vest, watch chain, cufflinks, and the head of his cane. Even his tie was transfixed by a huge diamond stickpin.

Brady presented quite a complicated case. Chronic inflammation of the prostate had caused a bar to form at the neck of the bladder, obstructing the outflow of urine. This condition was aggravated by diabetes, heart disease, high blood pressure, and generalized urinary tract infection.

Diamond Jim had been to surgeons in Boston and New York. All refused to operate, and he had come to Baltimore as a last resort—a wise move, for Dr. Young had recently devised an instrument with which the entire procedure could be done through the urethra. Since no external cut was necessary, the general anesthesia considered so dangerous in such a case was not needed.

Dr. Young showed Brady the instrument—a tube with a short, curved inner end. On the under surface of the tube was a large hole or window into which the obstructing prostatic bar would fall as the tube was withdrawn. An inner cutting cylinder was then pushed in, severing and removing the entrapped bar. This simple device, called a prostatic punch, had already been used by Young in many cases.

In his autobiography, Young described the operation on Brady in great detail to refute fabricated press accounts. Some newspapers claimed that Brady's overworked stomach had been cut out and a new one installed; other stories held that the gall bladder had been removed. Though the actual procedure was much simpler and required only a few minutes to complete, the convalescence was stormy on account of the infection present. Diamond Jim had chills and fever, with increasing temperature every day.

Before the operation, Young had explained that he would leave in four days to deliver a paper to a London medical congress; Brady was quite willing to be left in the hands of other staff members. On the day of Young's departure, the patient looked worse than ever.

Young arrived in New York full of misgivings and uncertain of ever seeing Brady alive again. Much to the surgeon's surprise, he and his family were met at the Vanderbilt Hotel by the manager and his assistants, who conducted them to the enormous royal suite, specially staffed by maids and even a matron to arrange their clothing. Brady's secretary was there, too, with a fistful of expensive theater tickets.

"All this," Young marveled, "from a man I had known only a few days and who was in Baltimore so sick that I was not sure he would recover."

The next day brought more surprises. On board ship Young's staterooms were filled with presents: champagne, Scotch, rye, Irish whisky, red and white vintage wines, various liqueurs, Havana cigars —small, medium, and large—cartons of cigarettes, most of the month's magazines, and the New York newspapers.

Who was this lavish spender covered with diamonds? Brady, born on the Bowery of a drunken father and barmaid mother, was the most famous railroad-equipment salesman who ever lived. With the first money he could save, he bought himself a diamond pin, and then continued to buy diamonds and elegant clothes. He entertained his clients on a princely scale, and won new customers with a raffish charm. Once, for example, after persisting a week, he was finally admitted to see an arrogant railroad president named Baer.

"I understand your name is Brady," the president said. "Don't you know I never see salesmen? Why the hell have you been waiting this entire week in my office?"

With a broad smile, Brady replied, "I have been waiting to tell you, Mr. Baer, that you can go straight to hell." Brady left the office an hour later with a signed contract for five million dollars' worth of steel freight cars.

And despite Dr. Young's misgivings, Diamond Jim left Johns Hopkins Hospital in equally good shape. During the remaining five years of his life he was troubled no further by urinary obstruction. Immensely grateful, he built Young a urological institute, but apparently on account of the machinations of an evasive secretary, he left insufficient funds in his will for maintenance.

Diamond Jim Brady may have been Young's richest patient, but the most eminent one was Woodrow Wilson, who became ill at a pivotal point in his presidency.

Wilson had returned from Europe in 1919 to obtain ratification for the Treaty of Versailles and the League of Nations. In France he had been hailed as a great hero—a reception never before accorded an American head of state. But in the United States he was hated and suspected by many members of Congress. Their views were succinctly stated by one senator, Hiram Johnson, who thundered to large crowds, "He is asking us to hand American destiny over to the secret councils of Europe. It is the duty of the senators of this nation to keep America American."

To triumph over his opposition, Wilson headed west in a special train, speaking at almost every station. By the time he had reached the Pacific Coast, he was so overwrought that he could hardly sleep. Signs of cerebral vascular insufficiency began to plague him. At Seattle, where he addressed a crowd of ten thousand, his head ached so severely and his vision was so impaired that he was unable to see even the first row. Though his speech lasted only an hour, the headache continued night and day. Tortured by pain and insomnia, he managed to deliver one more address in Denver.

At five in the morning, as the presidential train sped toward the next engagement in Kansas, Admiral Grayson, the White House physician, was summoned. Entering the President's car, he found Wilson slumped in his chair, pale, dribbling saliva from the drooping left corner of his mouth. The stricken President was put to bed, and the darkened train rushed toward Washington. During the remainder of the trip, Wilson improved enough to walk to a waiting car at the station in Washington. A few nights later he was able to play a game of billiards.

But at 8:00 A.M. on October 2, 1919, Mrs. Wilson was awakened by the sound of a thump in the adjoining bedroom. She hurried in to find the President sprawled face down on the bathroom floor. Admiral Grayson was summoned, and his examination revealed that Wilson had suffered a severe stroke, paralyzing his left arm, his left leg, and the left side of his face.

This time the President's condition did not improve. Control over urination was lost and bladder distension ensued. Grayson and a urologist, Dr. A. H. Fowler, successfully emptied the bladder by catheterization on two successive days. But their third catheterization attempt failed. On October 17, after Wilson had gone thirty hours without urinating, Grayson summoned Dr. Hugh Young.

Young found President Wilson a desperately ill man. His abdomen was hugely distended, his mouth was drawn on one side, and the left side of his body was paralyzed. Many urologic instruments had been tried in vain, and the other doctors in attendance believed that the only recourse was a median line abdominal incision into the bladder to relieve the distension.

Dr. Young, however, knew otherwise. In France during World War I he had treated many soldiers with similarly severe bladder distension resulting from spinal cord injuries and had found that the bladder neck would relax spontaneously, allowing recovery without surgical intervention. The British, who usually made an opening to drain the bladder, later learned that most patients who were operated on died of infection.

Advising nonintervention, Young went with Dr. Fowler to buy a few instruments that had not yet been tried. When the two returned, there was a large wet spot on the sheet beneath the President that had not been there before. The sheet was changed, and within fifteen minutes the new sheet was wet.

"Procrastination and 'masterly inactivity' saved the patient," Young wrote in his autobiography. "Had I attempted to pass instruments, failure would have been almost certain, and an operation to relieve the distension would probably have ended fatally."

After a few weeks, natural urination was re-established. A few months later Wilson regained use of his limbs and was able to walk with a cane. But this recovery did not save the Versailles Treaty or the League of Nations.

"Talking to Wilson is something like talking to Jesus Christ," remarked Georges Clemenceau, the French Premier. After his stroke, the President became even more self-righteous and intransigent than before, refusing to accept even the slightest modifications of the treaty offered by the Senate.

"Better a thousand times to go down fighting than to dip your colors to dishonorable compromise," the President told his wife. And so on November 19, 1919, the Senate rejected the treaty.

Young continued to visit Wilson during the recovery period, and was often delighted by the President's charm. Once, noting the President's need of a shave, Young suggested, "Why don't you let Admiral Grayson shave you? You know, originally the surgeons were all barbers."

"Yes," Wilson replied, "they are still barbarous."

Dr. Kelly and God

While Hugh Young worked on the urologic problems of men, his colleague Dr. Howard A. Kelly made innovations relating to the female urinary tract. Kelly, an Osler protégé, graduated from the University of Pennsylvania Medical School in 1882 and rose rapidly to become its professor of obstetrics. In 1889 he was appointed the first obstetrician and gynecologist in chief at Johns Hopkins.

Kelly's interest in the female urinary tract began in 1892, when he began viewing the water-distended bladder through a cystoscope of his own invention, with the patient in the knee-chest posture. The instrument had a special glass partition to prevent the water from running out, permitting the bladder to be inspected by direct vision with a head mirror. When patients were in knee-chest position, Kelly noted that the bladder spontaneously filled with air. Now able to observe the ureteral openings in the bladder, Kelly could pass catheters into them in order to study kidney outflow. Quite a scientific dispute later erupted over priority for this technique, since a Czech physician named Pawlik had previously devised a blind catheterization method in a water-filled bladder.

A lifelong fascination with snakes and an obsession with religious fundamentalism made Kelly one of the odder figures at Johns Hopkins. Before operating, he always conducted a prayer meeting for nurses, surgeons, and observers. Always eager to foist his beliefs on others, he wore a lapel button with a question mark, and would ask its meaning of people he met—"The most important question in life," he called it. After the victim was stumped, he would joyfully blurt out, "The most important question is, What think ye of Christ? Whose Son is He?"

Equally obnoxious was Kelly's love of preaching at taxi drivers stopped at red lights. "Cabby," he would say, "I hope when you and I come to the gates of heaven, the light will be green."

As an editor of the *Christian Citizen,* Kelly's meddlesome attempts at "religious oriented civic uplift" managed to provoke the formidable H. L. Mencken. During one train ride with Kelly between Baltimore and Washington, Mencken became so furious that a fellow passenger and acquaintance, Dr. Laurence E. Karp, wrote that "three separate times I was on the point of jumping out of the train window."

To Kelly's advocacy of prohibition, Mencken retorted in the Baltimore *Evening Sun,* "[Kelly] happens to be a man I have long known, and in every respect save the theological, greatly respected. But in that theological aspect . . . he is so plainly a menace to the peace and dignity of this town that what he believes should be made known to everyone, that the people may be alert to his aberrations and keep a curb on his public influence. If he had his way . . . life here would be almost impossible to civilized men. He is against practically everything that such men esteem, at least in the way of relaxation and recreation, and he is moved by a perfect frenzy to put his prejudices into harsh and unintelligent laws."

Mencken habitually referred to his pious adversary as "Dr. Evangelicus," but Kelly payed little attention, running—unsuccessfully—for the Maryland Assembly in 1921. His platform: "No liquor, no race-track gambling, no unnecessary paid labor on Sunday." Mencken rejoiced that the voters were not taken in by Kelly's "whole scheme of sanctification by force," adding, "How long are the people of Baltimore going to stand this nuisance?"

A long time, as Mencken learned to his dismay. Yet, surprisingly, the two were never deeply antagonistic toward each other. "Dear Brother Mencken," Kelly once said, "I am a friend of his and hope someday to win him."

"More than once," Mencken wrote on Kelly's seventy-fifth birthday, "[Kelly and I] have been on opposite sides of some public matter, but every contact with him . . . has only increased my admiration for his immense energy, his unbreakable resolution, and his complete honesty. Baltimore owes him a lot."

CHAPTER SIX

The Search for Microbes

The revolution in the field of surgery during the last quarter of the nineteenth century astounded both the scientific community and the society around it. Lives that would have been lost a few years earlier were being saved by the newly devised operative techniques.

The success of these techniques was a source of wonder, based as it was only on a scientific theory—the germ theory of disease. Was the success pure luck? Was the new antiseptic surgery simply a method that worked without being understood?

Pasteur, the man most responsible for the germ theory, thought not, even in spite of one disturbing fact: No one had been able to prove that a single germ caused a particular disease. A German physician, Johann Lucas Schönlein, had come close, however.

Schönlein, the son of a Bamberg ropemaker, was one of the first outstanding clinicians—a physician able to make a correct diagnosis on the basis of a physical examination. Listening to the fine tinkling sounds made by the lungs, he was able to differentiate pneumonia from lung collapse. The rushing sound of a murmur that came through his stethoscope when placed over the femoral artery allowed him to identify a faulty aortic valve.

In 1839, suspecting that some skin inflammations were of a "vegetable nature," Schönlein carefully studied a group of patients with favus, a scalp condition. Within the pustules he found a fungus, *Achorion,* and correctly identified it as the cause of favus. But the report of this investigation—only twenty-three lines long—had negligible impact at the time, and Schönlein died in 1864 with little notion of the immense implications of his discovery.

The deficiency in Schölein's report was an obvious one: *Achorion* had not been proved to cause favus. Perhaps it was merely an incidental finding in all of the cases examined. Schönlein should have pursued his line of investigation, but he chose not to.

An identical problem soon cropped up during study of a much more serious disease—anthrax. Small farmers were often ruined by the anthrax epidemics that swept through pastures. Most stock was affected, including cattle, horses, and sheep, and the malady sometimes spread to humans. Superstition held that certain areas of soil— often quite fertile—were cursed with anthrax by evil spirits. This belief was validated by the observation that animals consistently became sick on certain fields.

The symptoms of anthrax were so characteristic that it could hardly be confused with anything else. First there was a rise in the animal's temperature, quickly followed by trembling, gasping for breath, and convulsions. In the acute form, death ensued within a few days. The thick black blood that emerged through any scratch in the skin had suggested to early observers the name anthrax, from the Greek word for coal.

In 1850 two French scientists, Pierre François Olive Rayer and Casimir Joseph Davaine, found that the blood of sheep that died of anthrax could cause the disease when inoculated into healthy sheep. Within the diseased blood, Davaine identified "threadlike corpuscles of about double the length of the blood corpuscles" that did not show any spontaneous movement.

But the work of Rayer and Davaine suffered from the same deficiency as the work of Schönlein, since the two Frenchmen were unable to prove that the blood-borne bacteria observed in sick sheep were the cause of anthrax—not just an incidental finding. The elegant solution to the anthrax problem and the first rigorous proof of the germ theory of disease finally came from an unlikely source: an obscure, young German doctor, Robert Koch, working alone in an isolated Prussian border town.

Robert Koch and Anthrax

Both Koch and Pasteur had similar origins—poor country families with intellectual aspirations. Koch, one of thirteen children of a mining engineer, was born in 1843 in the German town of Klausthal. As a child, young Robert was pale and myopic, tortured by sexual guilt. At age fifteen he wrote, "I became, about the age of four or five, weak and sickly; I fell behind many contemporaries, as far as my body was concerned; how could that be otherwise when I squandered the noblest sap of my body, without knowing or even realizing it. Only when I was twelve did I learn, quite by chance, what consequences sexual sins have." These ruminations over masturbation were soon displaced by a deep passion for women. Much later in life, Koch's undiminished sex drive was to cause him considerable difficulty and embarrassment.

The elder Koch had determined that young Robert learn the shoemaker's trade, but a sudden upswing in family fortunes allowed the boy to pursue an academic career instead. At Easter in 1862, at the age of nineteen, he entered the University of Göttingen as a medical student.

Just at this time, Germany was emerging as the pre-eminent world center of medicine. The beginning of the nineteenth century found the German schools filled mainly with romantic philosophers, but while these men ruminated over *Sturm und Drang,* the romantic agony, their students were slipping off to Paris. There, the foggy speculations of old academics were being cut through by dissections, experiments, and statistics. When the students returned to their homeland to teach, they entered an educational system unparalleled in Europe. While in France the sciences centered around Paris, each of the German petty states had excellent universities. As the old philosophers died off, the young French-trained scientists moved into their chairs, converting many schools into research centers. Within a few decades, German chemists were dazzling the scientific world with their discoveries. In the meantime, other German scientists were borrowing the experimental techniques from the chemistry laboratories and applying them to problems in physiology and pathology.

The most eminent of the German physiologists was Johannes Müller, a shoemaker's son, who studied medicine before turning to physiology. After numerous animal experiments, Müller solidified understanding of the functioning of the nervous system. Among his many other contributions to physiology was a magnificent textbook, the *Handbook of Human Physiology*.

Müller trained many of the men who shaped German medicine in the last half of the nineteenth century: Emil Heinrich Du Bois-Reymond, the founder of electrophysiology; Hermann von Helmholtz, who made many contributions to both physiology and physics; and Jacob Henle, famous for his studies of the kidney and his theory that living carriers spread disease.

Henle was professor at Göttingen when Robert Koch arrived in 1862. Henle's dictum, "Before microscopic forms can be regarded as the cause of contagion in man they must be found constantly in the contagious material, they must be isolated from it and their strength tested," produced a deep impression on the young Koch, who later made it famous in a slightly modified form.

Even as a medical student, Koch showed great scientific promise. His essay—dedicated to his father—on the occurrence of ganglion cells in the nerves of the uterus won a school prize. He also tried to determine the origin of succinic acid in man, becoming on one occasion quite sick to his stomach after a series of self-experiments.

In 1866, at the age of twenty-two, Koch took his first medical job —an internship in Hamburg. His academic career appeared to have come to an end because of his marriage to a cousin, Emmy Fraatz. Emmy was a strong, nagging woman, who dominated the household. Her husband had dreams of emigrating to the United States, but Emmy would not hear of it, and pushed him instead into a general practice in the little German town of Rachwitz.

Koch's career did not prosper, however, and he moved his family several times. He was a kind, patient, responsible man, but apparently just not suited to be a private practitioner. The Franco-Prussian War provided him with a break from this life, and also allowed him some time away from Emmy. As a military surgeon, he saw in a few weeks a range of injuries never to be seen in a lifetime of ordinary practice.

At the end of the war he was able to secure a much more stable, better-paid job: district medical officer in Wollstein, an east German town, in what is now part of Poland, with a large Polish-Jewish population. Satisfied with this new position, Emmy gave her husband a microscope for his twenty-ninth birthday.

Koch was delighted with this gift. Already quite interested in photography and biology, he believed that the microscope could be used to photograph bacteria. So Emmy divided his consultation room with a brown curtain. In the back half, behind the curtain, he rigged up a laboratory, put in his newly acquired equipment—his plates, slides, white mice—and went to work. In this tiny, cluttered space, one of the most important discoveries in the whole science of healing was made.

Earning his living as he did in a country practice in a farming community, it was natural that Koch should pick anthrax—the scourge of farmers—for study. He knew that the French had demonstrated bacteria in the blood of infected animals, but was also aware that these micro-organisms might be incidental rather than causative.

Miles away from the nearest university laboratory, Koch began experimenting with the primitive tools he had. Animal inoculation was carried out with a splinter of wood smeared with infected tissue; autopsies were performed on the tiled surface of a stove. The anthrax bacillus was not a particularly safe one to work with, since infections at that time were incurable.

In Sinclair Lewis's novel *Arrowsmith,* a German bacteriology professor, Max Gottlieb, warns his students, ca. 1900, of the dangers involved: " 'This, gentlemen, iss a twenty-four-hour culture of *Bacillus anthracis.* You will note, I am sure you will have noted already, that in the bottom of the tumbler there was cotton to keep the tube from being broken. I cannot advise breaking tubes of anthrax germs and afterwards getting the hands into the culture. You might merely get anthrax boils—.' " The class shuddered. Gottlieb infected guinea pigs, then prepared slides of the blood for the students to examine after the animals' deaths. "But [the students] were uneasy, for Gottlieb remained with them that day, stalking behind them, saying nothing, watching them always, watching the disposal of the remains of the guinea pigs, and along the benches ran nervous rumors about a bygone student who had died from anthrax infection in the laboratory."

Despite the hazards, in three years of spare-time work Koch achieved the triumph that would soon revolutionize bacteriology, and wholly through ingenious and elegant techniques of his own design. First he made a small trough in a glass slide, into which he put aqueous humor from the eye of a dead ox along with infected matter.

Then he covered the trough with a second slide and sealed the edges to protect the mixture from the surrounding air. In this simple but brilliant manner he was able to study through his microscope the life cycle of the tiny anthrax organisms trapped between the slides, as they fed on the nutritive fluid of the eye. While he watched, the bacilli grew into long cylindrical rods covering the whole slide. Shortly afterward, Koch could see spots forming—the thick-walled spores or seeds of anthrax.

Now certain that he had found the germ of anthrax, Koch injected the bacteria he had grown into mice. Sure enough, the mice developed the disease. By 1876 he had worked out the life cycle of the anthrax bacillus and had demonstrated conclusively that anthrax spores from pure cultures could infect and kill inoculated animals. For the first time, a germ grown outside the body was proved to be directly responsible for a disease. A specific germ caused a specific disease. In the case of one disease—anthrax—Koch had succeeded in proving this essential postulate of the germ theory.

To obtain help in getting his work published, Koch wrote to Ferdinand Cohn, director of the Botanical Institute in nearby Breslau. Cohn had been approached frequently by bungling amateur scientists and later wrote how he assumed Koch was just another one of these. But the director was a polite, kindly man, not given to snubs. He invited Koch to come and demonstrate.

The pale, bearded young country doctor arrived at the institute in Breslau a few days later, loaded down with samples and equipment. After a few moments, Cohn stood transfixed by this amateur able to produce the proof that had eluded the greatest scientists in Europe. Thoroughly excited, Cohn sent a messenger to the Breslau Pathological Institute for its director, Julius Cohnheim, one of the outstanding German pathologists. Cohnheim came, saw, and hurried back to his institute, ordering his assistants, "Drop everything and go at once to Koch. This man has made a splendid discovery which is all the more astonishing because Koch has had no scientific connections and has worked entirely on his own initiative and has produced something absolutely complete. There is nothing more to be done. I consider this the greatest discovery in the field of bacteriology and believe that Koch will again astonish and shame us with still further discoveries."

Within three months, Koch had written up his results and published them in Cohn's *Journal of Plant Biology*. Yet even then the anthrax problem was not settled. So unbelievable and revolutionary were Koch's findings that many scientists remained unconvinced.

To gain support for his work, Koch decided to approach Rudolf Virchow, the most famous of all contemporary medical scientists. Virchow, the chief pathologist at the Berlin Charité Hospital, had an enormous reputation. He was a formidable politician and leader of the Opposition in the Reichstag; he was an archaeologist, who had dug with Schliemann at Troy; but above all he was distinguished for his cell theory and pathologic studies of disease. Koch knew that a benediction from Virchow could make his career. Unfortunately, the extremely busy and peppery Virchow had also been known to ruin careers. A former student, anxious to finish his examination, once caught Virchow dressed in tails, about to rush off to a session of the Berlin City Council. The candidate was invited to join him in his coach, where Virchow proceeded to quiz him. After a ride along Unter den Linden, they reached the famous Brandenburg Gate. Here Virchow served the student an abrupt notice: "Please get out, you failed."

Koch did no better. He arrived in Berlin on an unbearably hot day. Virchow was in a bad temper, though even in the best of humors he was highly skeptical of bacteriologic claims. As Koch waited in suspense, the great pathologist turned over a few pages of the anthrax manuscript, then muttered, "The whole thing seems highly improbable."

Though brutalized by Virchow, Koch managed to recover. He spent the evening in a music hall before returning to his laboratory in Wollstein. There, using organic dyes as stains, he was able to photograph previously unrecognized bacteria with a new tool: a Zeiss microscope.

This instrument was designed by a German physicist, Ernst Abbe, the son of a spinning-mill foreman from the little town of Eisenach in the grand duchy of Saxe-Weimar. Abbe, educated at the universities of Jena and Göttingen, taught first at Frankfurt, then at Jena, and in 1866 was invited by the industrialist Carl Zeiss to be optical consultant at the Zeiss Instrument Works at Jena—the most famous consultant in the history of the microscope. Abbe discarded all preconceived ideas about microscope-making, working out in their place exact mathematical formulae for achieving optimal performance. The Abbe sine condition, the Abbe number, the Abbe refractometer, the Abbe condenser, and the oil immersion lens soon made Zeiss optics the finest in the world and allowed Robert Koch to make another significant discovery.

Since Lister had introduced antisepsis in 1865, there had been no proof of why the method was effective. But, using his new microscope, Koch was able to stain with methyl violet the blood of animals with sepsis and see tiny bacteria among the blood cells. After exceptionally skillful experiments he was able to pass a mixed bacterial infection from an original fluid to a chain of animals, so that by the time the infection reached the last animal only one type of bacteria remained and there could be no doubt that the disease from which the animal was suffering had been caused by this bacterium. Thus Koch was able to identify for the first time the organisms responsible for the common forms of septicemia, gangrene, abscess, and erysipelas.

By this time, Koch's scientific success had reached the point that his supporters Cohn and Cohnheim tried to secure for him a professorship at the University of Breslau. Though the attempt failed, the post of town medical officer in Breslau became available in 1879. Seizing this opportunity to escape the anonymity and isolation of Wollstein—even though he would not have a university appointment—Koch moved Emmy and their daughter to a new house in Breslau.

Unfortunately, Koch did not do well. He had intended to supplement his small municipal salary with income from private practice. Two months after he arrived, with no private practice in sight, he was forced to return to Wollstein and his laboratory behind the brown curtain. But in 1880, because of the influence of Cohn and Cohnheim, he was offered a job in the Imperial Health Office, which he eagerly accepted. Three days after the cable confirming the appointment arrived, Koch and his family packed and hurried to Berlin, leaving half their belongings behind.

In Berlin, Koch was given not only a laboratory and money for equipment; he was given two assistants as well—Friedrich Löffler and Georg Gaffky. These two men, the first of an entire school of bacteriologists that he trained, marveled at the techniques this isolated genius had devised in the back of his Wollstein consulting room.

The elegant simplicity of Koch's methods is best illustrated by his procedure for separating a mixture of micro-organisms into its component parts. Taking a drop of the mixture, he would smear it on a sterile slice of boiled potato, where each individual bacterium would proceed to grow into a small, pure colony. Before the invention of this method, pure cultures could be obtained only if a single bacterium could be isolated from a hanging drop of mixture—an uncertain task at best.

Another of Koch's remarkable innovations was the use of agar jelly as a solid culture medium. This medium—still in use today—is so advantageous because any nutrients required to grow the organism in question may be mixed in with the jelly before it solidifies. The source of Koch's inspiration for both the potato and the jelly was the same: Emmy's kitchen.

In 1881 Koch was invited to address the Seventh International Medical Congress in London. With a magic lantern and his photographic slides he demonstrated his technique for obtaining pure cultures on solid media. Louis Pasteur and Joseph Lister were among the members of the audience, and the gentle, friendly Lister decided to introduce Pasteur to Koch.

This was not a simple task. The mutual antagonism between the Germans and the French was so deep that Lister could not have both to dinner at his home on the same day. And there was no more rabid anti-German than Pasteur, who wrote during the Franco-Prussian War, "I want to see France resisting to the last man and the last defense work, I want to see the War prolonged into the depths of winter, so that, with the elements rallying to our side, all those vandals confronting us shall perish of cold and hunger and disease. All my work, to my dying day, will bear as an inscription, 'Hatred towards Prussia! Revenge! Revenge!' "

Somehow, Lister managed to get the two scientists together. Pasteur gritted his teeth, took Koch's hand, and mumbled with suppressed jealousy, "That's great progress, Monsieur." These were the last civil words that the Frenchman ever spoke to his German colleague. Pasteur by this time had repeated and embellished Koch's anthrax work, and in addition had developed an effective anthrax vaccine. Koch's haughty response: Pasteur really hadn't accomplished what he claimed and had added nothing new.

Certainly Koch could have afforded to be more charitable, for he had long since finished with anthrax. In strictest secrecy, not telling even some of his closest friends, he had begun work on an even more formidable disease—tuberculosis. His celebrated studies of this fierce epidemic illness were to bring him both fame and a certain measure of disgrace.

Koch and the White Plague

Tuberculosis, the "white plague," is one of the diseases that is as old as the human race. Stone Age and Egyptian Old Kingdom skeletons have been diagnosed as exhibiting signs of tubercular damage. The earliest written record appears in the Laws of Manu of India, composed thirteen hundred years before the birth of Christ. No doubt some of the maladies of the Old Testament, which the prophets so kindly and charitably wished on their enemies, were forms of tuberculosis.

Remedies for tuberculosis are also quite ancient. Because of the dreaded emaciation that occurs, the Greeks named the disorder *pthisis* ("wasting") and described the frequently fatal outcome in the Hippocratic corpus. Their treatment: a milk diet, with goat or ass milk preferred to cow's milk. The Roman physician Galen wrote extensively on pthisis and also recommended a milk diet, though preferring breast milk to other forms. Since tuberculosis was frequently spread by contaminated milk before the advent of pasteurization, the wisdom of the ancients in this case is open to question.

By medieval times a particularly repugnant form of the disease had become quite prevalent. Scrofula, or the king's evil, as it came to be known, occurred with tuberculous involvement of the lymph nodes—especially in the neck—and produced ugly, smelly, continuously draining abscesses. One famous sufferer was Dr. Samuel Johnson, who went to Queen Anne to be touched by the royal hand in order that he might be cured.

He wasn't, but the king's touch remained a popular remedy. One of the most ancient forms of healing, it had begun with the Merovingian kings in the sixth century, reaching even greater prominence under Philip I of France in the eleventh century. The custom traveled to England with the Norman Conquest, where it remained for many years thereafter. Charles II is alleged to have touched 100,000 persons—almost half the entire population. The king not only laid on hands but presented the sufferer with a gold piece or "angel," perhaps the only instance in the history of medicine in which a patient got paid by a doctor for being cured.

Yet in some tuberculous patients not afflicted by scrofula, cure was not always fashionable or desired. During the nineteenth century the pale, gentle, weak appearance of the consumptive was part of the romantic mystique and was thought to be an intrinsic part of the charm of such figures as Keats, Byron, Shelley, Goethe, and Chopin. The existence of one whole family of tuberculous romantics, the Brontës, even suggested that the disease might be hereditary.

Most physicians, however, were not favorably disposed to tuberculosis, an illness that caused millions of deaths in no way romantic. Whole books were written on the subject of cause and cure. One of the earliest—by a Dutchman, Franz de le Boë (his name was Latinized as Franciscus Sylvius), who taught at Leyden between 1648 and 1672—is noteworthy for its clinical descriptions. A few years later Richard Morton of London wrote a detailed study, *Phthisiologia,* in which he asserted that consumption was caused by blood spitting—a perfect mirror image of the correct notion.

There was no less confusion over treatment. The most irrational method was the famous cowhouse therapy of Dr. Thomas Beddoes, the English pneumatologist and one-time employer of Sir Humphry Davy. Beddoes put his patients to bed in cow barns because he considered the exhalations of such surroundings to exert a beneficial influence over the course of the disease.

The first real step toward an understanding of the true nature of tuberculosis was made by a French physician, Jean Antoine Villemin. In a series of experiments carried out from 1865 to 1869 Villemin demonstrated conclusively that tuberculosis is a specific infection, due to an invisible, inoculable agent, and succeeded in passing the disease from man to rabbit.

Many contemporaries disagreed violently with these results. One who did not, however, was Julius Cohnheim, the brilliant chief pathologist at Breslau. Cohnheim discovered that he could infect rabbits with tuberculosis by inserting tuberculous lung tissue into the anterior chamber of the eye. By means of this clever experiment, Cohnheim was able to observe through the cornea the spread of disease within the eye.

After studying Cohnheim's experiments closely, Koch was convinced that tuberculosis was caused by a microbe. And the experiments had shown that if this microbe could be isolated and grown in pure culture, its identity as the tubercle bacillus could be proven by using it to infect an experimental animal.

So Koch set to work. His first tuberculous tissue was obtained from the body of a powerful thirty-six-year-old laborer. This man had been in perfect health until three weeks before his death, when he developed a cough, chest pains, and severe emaciation. Four days after entering the hospital he was dead, his body riddled with yellowish tubercles.

Koch ground up the tuberculous material between two heated knives and injected it into the eyes of rabbits and under the skins of guinea pigs. While waiting for infection to appear, he smeared the laborer's infected tissue on glass slides and peered at it through his microscope.

For days he saw nothing. The tubercle bacillus is extremely small —approximately a third the size of the anthrax bacillus—and is difficult to see because it congregates in small numbers. For this reason, other microscopists had failed to find it. But after hours of soaking in various dyes, the bacteria finally were persuaded to take up sufficient color to stand out from their surroundings. Among the diseased lung cells, Koch could see them—tiny blue-colored rods.

In the meantime, the infected animals began to die one by one. Koch pinned them down, soaked their hair with bichloride of mercury disinfectant, and cut them open. Inside were yellowish tubercles identical to those in the body of the laborer. Microscopic examination revealed the same tiny blue-colored rods.

Now certain that he had identified the tubercle bacillus, Koch went to hospitals everywhere in Berlin to obtain infected tissue from the bodies of patients who had died of tuberculosis. He injected this tissue into guinea pigs, rabbits, three dogs, thirteen cats, ten chickens, and twelve pigeons, as well as white mice, field mice, rats, and two marmots. Only when animal or man developed the disease could Koch find the blue-stained rods; never could the bacteria be found in healthy animals.

Yet the most difficult part of the study still remained: the organism had to be grown in pure culture and then used to produce the infection. Koch began by inoculating his regular solid media with diseased tissue. Nothing grew out. Then, reasoning that the bacillus must be a very fastidious one, he prepared a blood serum agar from heat-sterilized animal blood, which he inoculated with tissue from the lung of a diseased guinea pig.

One day passed. Two days passed. Still nothing appeared, though every other microbe he had worked with grew into large colonies within this period of time. Long after other investigators probably would have thrown the cultures away and started over, Koch waited with infinite patience, repeatedly inspecting the material in his incubator. Finally, on the morning of the fifteenth day, he was able to see through his pocket lens tiny glistening colonies on the surface of the agar. After making serial cultures with these organisms to exclude any residual animal matter, he was able to infect and kill guinea pigs with them.

On March 24, 1882, Koch presented his findings to the Berlin Physiological Society in one of its small reading rooms. On a table he spread out two hundred of his preparations—"like a cold buffet," remarked one observer. Then, in a halting, droning style he delivered the address that was to shake the scientific world. The first causative bacteria of an infectious disease in man had been isolated.

After Koch finished speaking, a long hush fell over the distinguished audience crowded into the room. Virchow, the doyen of German science, was there; he left without saying a word. Another young scientist present, Paul Ehrlich, dashed out to try the techniques for himself. The next day the discovery was front-page news throughout the world.

Soon Koch was inundated with aspiring microbe hunters: Japanese struggling to speak German, Americans such as pathologist William H. Welch. When not teaching—an activity he loathed—he helped his student Löffler to identify the diphtheria bacillus and Gaffky to find the typhoid bacillus. As Gaffky later remarked, Koch had shaken the tree, and discoveries were raining into his lap.

One man not delighted by this string of sudden triumphs was Louis Pasteur. He met Koch again at the International Congress of Hygiene in Geneva in 1882, and the antagonism between the two was intense. After Koch asserted that Pasteur had contributed nothing new to science, Pasteur furiously demanded a face-to-face confrontation, a debate. When Koch refused, Pasteur spent Christmas Day 1882 writing a biting letter to his German adversary. Thus the two most famous bacteriologists had shown themselves to be small, petty, jealous men.

And, like other scientists, they worked for the sheer joy of problem solving. Fine human motives were conspicuously absent, only created after the event by wide-eyed admirers. The discoveries themselves have since been employed like other scientific discoveries, for good—the prevention and treatment of disease—and for evil—germ warfare. But Pasteur and Koch seem to have given little thought to the ethical responsibilities of the scientist that receive so much attention today. Their only interest was in the bitter race to make more discoveries, a race in which Robert Koch won the next lap by identifying the organism responsible for another devastating human scourge—cholera.

Koch and the Vibrio of Cholera

Unlike tuberculosis, cholera was unfamiliar to Western civilization until the early nineteenth century. It has, however, long been endemic in Bengal, and it occasionally spread to other parts of India and adjacent regions.

The signs of cholera are violent and dramatic: diarrhea, vomiting, fever, and death, often within a few hours of the onset of illness. The rapidity with which cholera kills is profoundly alarming. In the days before adequate therapy, perfectly healthy people could never feel safe from sudden death when the infection was in the neighborhood. And the appearance of the victim is horrible. The severe dehydration causes the sufferer to shrink into a wizened caricature of his former self within a few hours, while ruptured capillaries discolor his skin, turning it black and blue. No illness more strongly reminds all who see it of death's ugly horror and utter inevitability.

Death from cholera was not only gruesome; it was sometimes widespread as well. In 1831, when the disease first struck Cairo, 13 per cent of the total population succumbed. Though such devastation was unusual in later European outbreaks, the psychological impact of cholera's approach was not diminished. It seemed capable of penetrating any quarantine, of bypassing any man-made obstacle. Victims appeared to be chosen erratically, mainly but not exclusively from the lower classes in European towns.

Europe first became strongly aware of cholera in 1817, when an unusually severe outbreak developed around Calcutta. From there it spread across India along the new British-imposed patterns of trade and military movement, finally overleaping its customary boundaries and extending into unfamiliar territory, where human resistance to it was totally lacking.

Before this outbreak, dissemination occurred mainly during Hindu pilgrimages and times of festival, when large crowds were drawn to the lower Ganges, a region in which cholera was endemic. Those celebrants who picked up cholera but did not die on the spot were likely to bring the disease back home, though well-defined custom usually kept it confined to India. It was sometimes carried as far as China by ship, but apparently nowhere else.

The 1817 epidemic broke all the old rules. English ships and troops on the scene carried the infection to new territory along two routes. One, the overland route, was limited. British soldiers fighting a series of campaigns along India's northern frontiers between 1816 and 1818 carried cholera from their base in Bengal to their Nepalese and Afghan foes.

But the second route, the sea route, led to wider dissemination. Ships brought cholera to Ceylon, Indonesia, the southeastern Asian mainland, China, and Japan between 1820 and 1822. In 1821 a British expeditionary force, intent on suppressing the slave trade, brought the disease to Muscat, in southern Arabia; and from there it passed south along the east coast of Africa, following the slave traders. The infection also turned up in the Persian Gulf area, Mesopotamia, Iran, Syria, Anatolia, and the Caspian shores. The Russians seem to have been spared because of the unusually harsh winter of 1823–24; the Chinese and Japanese were not, however, and in China the epidemic was particularly persistent.

This large outbreak was only a preview of what was to come in the 1830s. A new Bengal cholera epidemic in 1826 spread along its previous path into southern Russia. Then, troop movements resulting from Russia's wars against Persia and Turkey and the Polish revolt of 1830–31 carried cholera to the Baltic. (Karl von Clausewitz, author of *On War*, a famous treatise on military strategy died of cholera while observing the Polish campaign.) After spreading by ship to England, it appeared in Ireland. Irish immigrants carried it to Canada, from where it traveled into the United States and Mexico.

Besides invading Europe and the United States, cholera established itself at Mecca during the Moslem pilgrimage of 1831. This situation was potentially more disastrous than the Indian one because the followers of Mohammed came from as far away as Mindanao in the Philippines. Until Koch's work was accepted and the disease understood, no fewer than forty epidemics accompanied the Moslem pilgrims between 1831 and 1912.

World cholera deaths soon rose into the millions with no relief in sight. The long-standing quarantine regulations of Mediterranean ports did not seem particularly effective in halting spread of the disease, prompting British liberals to agitate for revocation on the basis that the laws infringed on the free-trade principle. To many, the proper explanation for cholera was the miasma theory, which held that sudden outbreaks of the disease were caused by an evil vapor, emerging perhaps from dead corpses or other rotting matter in the earth. When the miasma encountered appropriately weakened conditions, disease resulted.

One man who did not agree with this theory was an English physician, John Snow. A prudish, withdrawn celibate, Snow spent his life crusading against alcohol, perhaps in order that he might seem as pure as his name. Yet in spite of this eccentricity he was an outstanding medical scientist, who contributed to our understanding of the anesthetic properties of ether and chloroform. But he is best known for his perceptive observation of an English cholera epidemic, after which he was able to provide the first epidemiologic data verifying the infectious nature of cholera and its transmission by water.

Snow drew his now-famous conclusions after an 1854 outbreak of cholera occurring near the intersection of Cambridge and Broad Streets, Golden Square, London. In a period of ten days more than five hundred fatal cases were reported—a number that would have been considerably greater had not a large percentage of the population fled the city. Suspecting a much-frequented water pump in Broad Street, Snow investigated the case distribution carefully and found no increased cholera incidence in that part of London except in those people using the Broad Street pump. After convincing the city authorities, Snow had the handle of the pump removed, thus terminating the epidemic.

Surprisingly, this neat piece of medical detection failed to convince the scientific community, since Snow's argument was merely circumstantial. Europe's medical experts were so confident of the miasma theory that Snow's interpretation of his data commanded little attention.

By 1883, however, the situation had changed. Both Pasteur and Koch were convinced that cholera was an infectious disease caused by a micro-organism. Their opportunity to verify this theory arose with the outbreak of a severe cholera epidemic in Damietta, Egypt. Soon their field research had turned into an unseemly race.

The French gained a head start by managing to arrive first on the scene. Pasteur, fully occupied in Paris trying to cure rabies, had sent his two assistants, Emile Roux and Louis Thuillier. In August Koch came himself and brought along Georg Gaffky, miscroscopes, and experimental animals from Berlin. But shortly after the two Germans began work, news came that the French were packing their bags. Roux and Thuillier believed they had identified the germ of cholera.

Crestfallen, Koch approached the two Frenchmen to examine what they had found; his disappointment, however, was short-lived when he took one look at his competitors' specimens. They had mistaken blood platelets—a normal blood constituent necessary for coagulation—for the cholera bacillus.

Suddenly the epidemic began to wane. While the two French scientists relaxed and cooled themselves with swims in the sea, Koch and Gaffky sweated and dripped over their microscopes as they examined the last obtainable infected material.

At three A.M. on September 15 a messenger awakened Koch with the news that Thuillier was seriously ill with cholera. Koch hurried to the bedside where the twenty-seven-year-old Frenchman lay dying.

"Have we found the cholera bacillus?" Thuillier asked.

As Roux had requested, Koch lied and answered yes. Within a few hours, Thuillier was dead. Koch was one of the pallbearers and laid wreaths on the coffin.

Now the epidemic was over. Koch rushed back to Berlin with specimens containing the organism he had identified—a little vibrating bacterium, or vibrio, shaped like a comma. But to be certain that this vibrio was indeed the right bug, Koch went to India to study the regions where the disease had been endemic for so long.

The trip from Berlin to Calcutta was long, and Koch became quite seasick. But he was rewarded for his pains by finding the cholera bacillus in the dead bodies of forty Indian cholera victims. This same germ was not to be found in the feces of any healthy individuals, nor was it present in any animal.

The cholera vibrio, Koch found, could be easily grown on beef broth agar. Though it was quickly killed by drying, the organism readily infected healthy persons handling the soiled linen of cholera victims. And the germ could often be found in the dirty water tanks around the native huts. Only in this highly polluted water or in the human intestine could it survive.

When Koch returned to Berlin, he was feted as a conquering hero.

No lesser Prussian than Kaiser Wilhelm himself presented the famous microbe hunter with the Order of the Crown with Star. Yet not all scientists were convinced. One asked Koch to send over a vial of cholera bacilli, then publicly swallowed the contents, remarkably without ill effect.

The controversy continued to rage until 1892, when a final outbreak settled the matter. Hamburg, an old free city, had remained self-governing within the German Reich and drew its water from the Elbe without special treatment. Just adjacent was the Prussian town of Altona, where the imperial government had installed a water purification plant. When cholera broke out in Hamburg, it ran down one side of the street dividing the two cities, sparing Altona completely. No more graphic demonstration of the importance of the water supply could have been intentionally devised, and the miasmatists were silenced completely.

The Tuberculin Fiasco

After the discovery of the cholera bacillus, Koch's meteoric rise appeared to have halted. For six years he was able to produce nothing that matched the caliber of his early work. Increasingly, he became more nervous, secretive, and suspicious.

Additionally, his domestic life was not happy. Twenty years of marriage to the domineering Emmy had not improved the relationship, and at the age of forty-five the bespectacled, bearded, balding Koch began looking around. One day, while he was sitting in an artist's studio for an official portrait, his glance fell upon a finished canvas—the portrait of a seventeen-year-old girl, a beauty. Inquiry revealed that she was the illegitimate daughter of a Berlin workman. She played bit parts at the Schiller Theater in Berlin and was also the artist's student. A meeting was arranged; soon the girl, Hedwig Freiburg, was Koch's mistress and the center of his life.

These manifestations of the male mid-life crisis could not have occurred at a worse time in Koch's career. He was known to be studying tuberculosis, and high officials within the German government had heard rumors that he was on the verge of some dramatic new breakthrough. If so, what better occasion to reveal it than the Tenth

International Medical Congress, to be held in the summer of 1890 in Berlin? Gustav von Gossler, the minister of culture, even let Koch know that the Kaiser himself was awaiting the announcement of some sensational discovery.

As the day of the congress drew nearer, Koch agonized over the trap into which he had fallen. He had no announcement ready to make. Scientific research cannot be made to fit into a timetable, and the usually cautious Koch strongly considered abandoning his address altogether. No one today can say how much his crumbling marriage, his new mistress, and his need for more money influenced his decision.

In front of seven thousand conference delegates, Koch stood and made his address amidst a cardboard and plaster temple guarded by a statue of Aesculapius, a piece of kitsch the Ministry of Culture had deemed necessary for the occasion. He began by reviewing the latest developments in bacteriology, then arrived at the keynote of his speech.

"I have tested a large number of substances to see what influence they would exert on tubercle bacilli," Koch said as expectant silence enveloped the hall. After carefully mentioning numerous trials and failures, he added, "I have at last hit upon a substance that has the power of preventing the growth of tubercle bacilli not only in the test tube but in the body of an animal."

The hall erupted with excitement, and only a fraction of the audience seemed to be listening as Koch carefully began to qualify his remarks. His work was not yet complete. Thus far he had studied only laboratory animals.

The following day Robert Koch was again front-page news throughout the world. None save the scientists in the audience seem to have noted the fact that details of the nature of the new substance and its manufacture were not revealed. Only Koch's spectacular past triumphs lent credibility to this new wonder drug, which he named tuberculin.

Within a short time the great public expectation forced Koch to begin human trials. His first experimental subject: himself. After several hours of pain in the limbs, fever, and respiratory difficulty following the injection, he recovered. In November 1890 he published the results of his experiments with a small series of tuberculous patients, and though his success had been limited, the public went wild.

Consumptive patients and their families flooded into Berlin for treatment. Not enough tuberculin could be manufactured to satisfy the enormous demand, leading to a thriving black market and enormously inflated prices. The most well-known physicians in the city were using the new wonder drug to treat every conceivable tuberculous condition.

At first, treated patients showed a marked improvement. But then, a rapid decline and death would often ensue. This sequence of events occurred after Joseph Lister brought his sick niece to be personally treated by Koch. The girl worsened, as did so many others, and finally died.

Yet such setbacks did not seem to reduce the enormous demand for tuberculin. Hotels and hospitals in Berlin filled to overflowing with desperate sufferers. The cost of treatment became so enormous that Gossler, the minister of culture, was obliged to fix the price of the drug. And tuberculin that reached America was going for a thousand dollars per gram.

Koch had been awarded the Order of the Red Eagle by the Kaiser before the bad news was broken. In January 1891 Rudolf Virchow—always skeptical of Koch's discoveries—published the results of autopsies on twenty-one consumptives treated with tuberculin. All of the bodies had been riddled with miliary tuberculosis, the most advanced and dreaded form of the disease, worse than the famous pathologist had ever seen before. The uproar produced by this report forced Koch to reveal the exact nature of tuberculin.

To produce his wonder drug, Koch had grown tubercle bacilli on a glycerin broth for several weeks, then killed the bacteria with heat and filtered off the nutritive medium. This simple method had been employed earlier by Emile Roux to isolate diphtheria toxin, but why Koch believed that his filtrate would cure tuberculosis is unknown.

In fact, a valuable medical tool did emerge from the tuberculin disaster, though it was obscured by the terrible outcry at the time. Koch noted that tuberculin injected into the skin of tuberculous patients produced a reddish allergic reaction at the spot within forty-eight hours. This reaction, the Koch phenomenon, allows doctors today to determine whether an individual has been infected with tubercle bacilli, even before symptoms develop.

But discovery of the tuberculin skin test was of little immediate consolation. Koch had too many deaths on his conscience. The secrecy surrounding tuberculin, established to protect priority, was seen by detractors as Koch's way of assuring a fortune from the discovery—and they may have been right.

To escape the furor and enjoy a few weeks of peace, Koch left Berlin in the spring of 1891 for a vacation in Egypt. Thoroughly dispirited, he wrote to Hedwig, "As long as you love me, I cannot be beaten down by the vicissitudes of fate. Do not abandon me now, for your love is my comfort and the star to which I upward gaze."

Hedwig did not abandon her lover, and in a few weeks after his divorce from Emmy she married him. The German government was displeased. So were fellow townsmen from Klausthal, who unceremoniously ripped a commemorative tablet from Koch's birthplace. Remarked one American observer, "You couldn't blame Koch, but what on earth did she see in him?"

Fortunately, the Prussian Parliament was not deterred from offering state support for medical research, and by the autumn of 1891 Koch had his Institute for Infectious Diseases. There, he continued to work on tuberculosis, and he also traveled widely to study other infections: bubonic plague in India, cattle plague in South Africa, tsetse disease in West Africa, and malaria in the East Indies. Even after receiving the 1905 Nobel Prize, he remained as obsessive as ever about his work. Once during a research trip to Africa, Koch shook awake his assistant, Friedrich Kleine, at five A.M. for help dissecting an infected horse that had just died. Kleine, completely exhausted by Koch's demands, answered that he was too tired and had dreamed of horses all night long. "How can you hope to make any progress," the astonished Koch asked, "if you don't dream about horses?"

Pasteur and the Bacteria of Animal Disease

While Koch was at work on his sensational proofs that microbes cause animal disease, Pasteur was also pursuing investigations along the same line. Koch, it may be recalled, began by scrutinizing an infection of cattle and sheep. But Pasteur launched his investigations in this area with a study of disease in a lower animal form—the silkworm.

In 1865 Jean Baptiste Dumas, the minister of agriculture, asked Pasteur to determine the cause of maladies which were then destroying the silk industry of France. In 1853, before the silkworm epidemic, France produced no less than twenty-six million kilograms of silk at an average price of five francs, or sixty cents, per kilogram. As a result of the disease devastation, however, the French were soon losing a hundred million francs, or twelve million dollars, per year. At first the silkworm breeders were able to buy eggs from abroad, but as the epidemic spread to other countries, only the Japanese were left with eggs to sell.

"I have never even touched a silkworm," the surprised Pasteur protested to the minister of agriculture's request. And he further verified his ignorance when shown a handful of cocoons by an entomologist.

"Why, there is something inside," said Pasteur as he shook a cocoon.

"The chrysalis," answered the entomologist.

"What is a chrysalis?" asked Pasteur.

But he learned quickly, and within five years he had found out everything. The worms, he discovered, were actually suffering from two diseases, not one. Both diseases were caused by micro-organisms and though contagious could be prevented by keeping the animals away from infected matter on clothes, on hands, and in the air.

This foray into the fight against infectious diseases of animals was terminated by another commission. Pasteur was to look into the problems in the manufacture and preservation of beer, so that after the disastrous defeat suffered in the Franco-Prussian War of 1870, France might manage to fight on—at least on the brewing front. Just as in the case of wine, micro-organisms were found to be disordering fermentation, and again Pasteur was able to devise a brilliantly simple, effective solution to the problem.

In 1877 Pasteur again began to investigate animal disease. Though partially incapacitated by a weak, dangling arm and dragging foot, the residua of his paralytic stroke in 1868, he seemed even more perceptive than before. Probably inspired by Koch's publication, he chose to study anthrax.

And with good reason. So revolutionary was Koch's recent proof of the germ theory that some French biologists still claimed that the organism present in the blood of anthrax-infected animals was incidental and that the disease could be passed on without it. As this controversy raged on, anthrax continued to decimate French agriculture.

Pasteur began his study at Chartres, where the incidence of anthrax had been particularly high. At a local slaughterhouse, he obtained anthrax-infected blood from the carcasses of a horse, a sheep, and a cow. He found that under sterile conditions the blood did not putrefy, since it contained only the anthrax bacillus.

This characteristic of the disease allowed Pasteur to obtain pure cultures of anthrax bacilli in flasks of urine. After sowing a drop of infected liquid from one urine flask to a sterile urine sample, then sowing a drop from this sample into another, and so on for a hundred transfers, Pasteur could still produce anthrax in an animal with material from the last transfer.

Just at the time of these experiments, the Eure-et-Loir district of France was especially hard hit with anthrax, and Pasteur was requested by the minister of agriculture to investigate the problem. On arriving, the famous scientist was greeted with great excitement and expectation by the local farmers. They were not disappointed.

During his studies at Eure-et-Loir, Pasteur was able to make a number of crucial observations. The most important: An animal which recovered from an attack of anthrax was henceforward immune to the disease. This key finding immediately suggested the possibility of an anthrax vaccine.

Pasteur also noted that anthrax bacilli and their spores could live and multiply within the soil. These bacilli infected an animal through wounds in its mouth, a fact demonstrated in a clever manner. When animals were fed alfalfa mixed with anthrax spores, they remained well; only when sharp-pointed thistles were added to the mixture did the disease occur.

But how could anthrax be kept from blighting a field? Careful observation revealed that bacilli from the carcasses of infected animals, even when buried deep in the earth, were brought to the surface by earthworms in the casts which they produced. Dust from worm casts scattered the spores of the bacteria onto plants, and in this way the disease was passed to domestic animals. Pasteur therefore recommended burning the bodies of animals that had died of anthrax or burying them very deeply in specially prepared trenches far from any cultivated land and well away from flocks and herds.

Pasteur continued his anthrax studies in Paris. By means of a cold-water bath he was able to lower the body temperature of a hen from

42° to 38° C and then successfully infect the animal with anthrax. Ordinarily, fowl are not susceptible to this disease because the bacilli do not thrive at the bird's normal body temperature, which is higher than that of most mammals.

These results Pasteur announced in a particularly lively manner. A professor at the Alfort School of Anatomy named Colin had claimed that for twelve years he had carried out more than five hundred experiments on anthrax and had successfully infected birds. Doubting this claim, Pasteur sent Colin a culture of anthrax bacilli and publicly challenged the anatomist to produce an anthrax-infected hen. In March 1878, after no such hen was forthcoming, Pasteur described the situation at a full meeting of the Academy of Medicine, which the luckless Colin happened to attend.

"I saw Monsieur Colin coming into my laboratory," Pasteur told his audience, "and even before I shook hands with him, I said to him, 'Why have you not brought that diseased hen?' 'Trust me,' answered Colin, 'you shall have it next week.'"

Of course, Colin had never brought the hen. Pasteur was merely playing the situation for laughs. When poor Colin stood up to announce that he had attempted the experiment but had closed the hens' cage improperly so that the birds were mauled by a dog, the Academy burst into peals of mirth. A few days later Pasteur brought before the members one of his own hens dead from anthrax.

While Pasteur was at work making chickens susceptible to anthrax, a real epidemic—chicken cholera—was sweeping through the French poultry industry. Soon the industrial troubleshooter *par excellence* was at work trying to conquer this new economic threat.

Chicken cholera, like human cholera, is a particularly repulsive disease. An affected bird totters on its legs with drooping wings, while its feathers stand on end, giving it the form of a ball. It staggers along until it can go no further, flutters its wings, falls, and dies.

At the time Pasteur began his studies, little was known about the malady. An Alsatian veterinary surgeon named Moritz identified a micro-organism in infected animals, and this finding was confirmed by Eduardo Perroncito, an Italian professor of veterinary medicine at Turin. H. Toussaint, a Toulouse veterinary surgeon, had carried out a pathologic study of the blood of infected cases, and it was he who had consulted Pasteur, sending the head of an affected cock to Paris for examination.

From this head, Pasteur was able to grow the organism in a

chicken broth. If a bit of the infected broth was fed to an unsuspecting chicken, the animal would rapidly develop the disease, which then spread via droppings to the remainder of the flock.

Perhaps Pasteur's knowledge of chicken cholera might have stopped here but for an accident. During the summer of 1880, just before leaving on vacation, Pasteur instructed his assistant, Charles Chamberland, to inoculate a few hens with the cholera bacillus. But Chamberland did not carry out this order before leaving on his own holiday; only a few weeks later did he pick up where he had left off. Now the month-old bacterial culture made the chickens ill, but they soon recovered.

Chamberland naturally assumed that some error had been made, and was in the act of tossing the faulty culture out when Pasteur stopped him. In a flash of intuitive genius, Pasteur in some way had guessed that the recovered animals now might be immune, as were the animals at Eure-et-Loir that had recovered from anthrax.

And he was right. When infected with a new culture of chicken cholera bacilli, the hens did not turn a feather. But a new group of chickens bought from the local market quickly succumbed to the same bacteria. Chamberland had stumbled over the greatest discovery of his life, and would have kicked it out of his path had not Pasteur been watching. For the first time, a vaccine against chicken cholera could be made.

The presentation of these remarkable results at a meeting of the Academy of Medicine provoked one of the most discomfiting scenes of Pasteur's long career. When the address was completed, Dr. Jules Guérin, an eminent, elderly Paris surgeon, made a few particularly sarcastic remarks about so much fussing with mere chickens. Thoroughly enraged, Pasteur stood up and began to taunt Guérin about the stupidity of one of the surgeon's pet operations. The eighty-year-old Guérin furiously rushed at the sixty-year-old, partially paralyzed scientist, and the two men were kept from blows only by frantic Academy members who jumped in to intervene.

The next day Guérin, demanding satisfaction, sent his seconds to Pasteur with a challenge to a duel. But Pasteur had no desire to die from a gunshot wound. He sent a note to the Academy offering to temper his criticism and defense of the day before, thus backing out of the fight in as graceful a manner as was possible under the circumstances.

Unfortunately Pasteur soon became as emotional about his new chicken cholera vaccine as he had been about Guérin. Deciding that he might have discovered a universal protector, he injected inoculated hens with anthrax bacilli—and the animals survived. Quickly he dashed off a letter to the Academy of Sciences, which was then duly published in its *Reports*. Though he never made a formal retraction, Pasteur soon discovered that he had erred, and with this discovery he began his search for a real anthrax vaccine.

But anthrax proved to be much less tractable than chicken cholera. Anthrax bacilli cultures—unlike those of cholera bacilli—were not attenuated after standing for a month. In fact, the exposure to air allowed the anthrax organisms to continue forming spores, and the disease could be caused as readily by these spores as by the bacilli themselves.

After further study, however, Pasteur and his assistants found that spores did not form at a temperature of 42–43° C, though the bacteria would continue to multiply. Maintaining the bacilli between 42° and 43° C for eight days yielded organisms of attenuated virulence and also free of new spores. Vaccination of guinea pigs, rabbits, and sheep with these attenuated organisms protected the animals against anthrax.

In March 1881 Pasteur reported his discovery of the anthrax vaccine to the Academy of Sciences—he had avoided the Academy of Medicine after the dispute with Guérin. But many scientists remained skeptical, since two previous investigators, Toussaint and Louvrier, both veterinarians, had devised methods of anthrax protection that proved to be failures.

One especially important skeptic was a Monsieur Rossignol, an editor of *The Veterinary Press*. Rossignol had recently written a parody of the germ theory in which a Pasteur-like figure was wont to announce pontifically, "I have spoken." Now, doubting that Pasteur had done any better than Toussaint or Louvrier, Rossignol proposed that funds be subscribed so that the new anthrax vaccine could be given a thorough public test. The money would be used to pay for facilities and a large number of experimental animals.

Pasteur was well aware of the risk that he was taking, but he accepted the challenge nonetheless. Rossignol designated his farm at Pouilly le Fort, near Melun, as the site for the test. The skillfully promoted event drew correspondents from the most prominent Parisian newspapers, and even the London *Times* sent its famous Paris correspondent Henri de Blowitz, nicknamed Blowitz-own-Tromp by *Punch*.

The rules were simple. Rossignol had designed them to lay to rest the fiction that bacterial vaccination could protect against disease, and to humiliate Pasteur deeply in the process. Sixty sheep had been purchased with the proceeds of the public subscription. Twenty-five were to be inoculated with Pasteur's anthrax vaccine—two doses at twelve- to fifteen-day intervals. A few days after the last dose had been given, the inoculated sheep and twenty-five uninoculated sheep were to be infected with live, virulent anthrax bacilli. The remaining ten sheep would serve for comparison with the surviving animals—if there were any. Old Baron de la Rochette, the chairman of the Melun Agricultural Society, asked Pasteur if ten cows might also be included in the test. Though he had not experimented with cattle, Pasteur—showman that he was—agreed.

But Pasteur's two assistants, Charles Chamberland and Emile Roux, were not so blithe to risk a public humiliation as was their boss. The vaccine intended for use was a new one, attenuated with potassium dichromate rather than heat, and more easily prepared in open conditions. Moreover, it had not been extensively tested. Yet Pasteur was still confident, and when Chamberland and Roux complained, he roared back, "What worked with fourteen sheep in our laboratory will work with fifty at Melun!"

The day arrived to begin the test, May 5, 1881. All bottles and syringes had been made ready. The flasks of virulent and attenuated material had been carefully labeled.

"Be sure not to mix up the first and second vaccine, boys," Pasteur teasingly admonished his two helpers as they left for the train to Melun.

A huge crowd had assembled at Rossignol's farm to greet the three scientists from Paris. Present were senators of the republic, veterinarians, dignitaries, hundreds of farmers, and other scientists. Present, too, was a local veterinarian, a friend of Pasteur's old enemy Colin. Apparently believing that the tubes of virulent bacilli had been rigged to contain two layers, the top inert and the bottom active, Colin had sent his friend to give the tubes a thorough shake in public, which he did.

Pasteur, however, was far above petty chicanery and looked on with amused interest as the veterinarian vigorously jiggled the tubes Then, to heighten the drama and further confound his critics,

Pasteur announced that, when the time came to administer the virulent bacilli, he would administer triple doses to all the animals, and that vaccinated and unvaccinated animals would be injected alternately.

As the flock of newspapermen looked on, the sheep to be vaccinated were herded together and injected with a weak vaccine that would kill mice but not guinea pigs. Twelve days later the show was repeated. This time a stronger vaccine, capable of killing guinea pigs but not rabbits, was used.

The day of reckoning arrived May 31, when all the animals, vaccinated and unvaccinated, received a fatal dose of virulent anthrax bacilli. That night, realizing that his whole scientific reputation hung in the balance, Pasteur could not sleep. And a few days later his nightmares seemed to be coming true.

Chamberland and Roux, who had gone back to Pouilly le Fort to examine the infected sheep, now returned to Paris with bad news. Both vaccinated and unvaccinated animals were ill—weak, breathless, and feverish. Upon hearing this, Pasteur turned on Roux in a rage, blaming his hapless assistant for the foul-up. Roux, he declared imperiously, must be the one to face the humiliation at Pouilly le Fort. Fortunately, next morning a telegram arrived stating that all the vaccinated sheep were well.

On June 2, 1881, the day set for public assessment of the experimental results, the crowd was even larger and more distinguished than before. General Councilors as well as senators were present. And all of the newspaper reporters were clustered around Blowitz, the gentleman from the *Times*.

As Pasteur triumphantly entered the farm yard at two P.M., the audience applauded and cheered. Not a single vaccinated sheep had a trace of illness. But twenty-two carcasses of the unprotected animals had been laid out in a row—dead and stiff. Two more unvaccinated sheep staggered on the point of demise, and obligingly expired as everyone looked on.

Suddenly the gathering turned almost into a revival meeting. One veterinarian and former critic came forward and cried, "Inoculate me with your vaccines, Monsieur Pasteur—just as you have done to those sheep you have saved so wonderfully. Then I will submit to the injection of the murderous virus. All men must be convinced of this marvelous discovery!"

"It's true," said another erstwhile foe, "that I have made jokes about microbes, but I am a repentant sinner!"

"Well, allow me to remind you of the words of the Gospel," answered Pasteur. "Joy shall be in heaven over one sinner that repenteth, more than over ninety and nine just persons that need no repentance."

The almost unbelievable outcome was also not lost on the newspapermen. Blowitz cheered before racing off to wire his report to the London *Times* and the world press: "The experiment at Pouilly le Fort is a perfect, an unprecedented success." In response to the news, the French went wild. Pasteur was called the country's greatest son and received the Grand Cordon of the Legion of Honor. Letters and telegrams began pouring in, begging Pasteur for vials of his lifesaving vaccine.

In his great elation of the moment, Pasteur made one of the more serious misjudgments of his career: to begin mass-producing anthrax vaccine in his Paris laboratory on the rue d'Ulm immediately. Roux and Chamberland worked frantically at this task with crude, improvised, improperly sterilized equipment. Then, dead tired, they took the vaccine to the countryside to perform the inoculations. All the while, demands for more vaccine arrived.

Soon Pasteur began to be inundated with a different sort of mail. Angry farmers from a dozen towns in France and as far away as Hungary wrote that their sheep were dying of anthrax and other infections brought on by the faulty, hastily concocted vaccine. Pasteur began to hate opening his letters.

The worst blow fell when Robert Koch in Berlin managed to obtain a sample of vaccine. Koch not only verified that the material killed the animals it was supposed to protect, but also identified within the liquid numerous harmful contaminant bacilli. After accusing Pasteur to his face at a scientific meeting of withholding reports of the unfavorable results, Koch added disdainfully, "Such goings-on are perhaps suitable for the advertising of a business house, but science should reject them vigorously."

Pasteur may have been thrown into a rage by such invective, but France was not. What could one expect from a German, anyway? The Académie Française elected Pasteur a member, the ultimate honor that could be bestowed on a Frenchman. Ernest Renan, the French author famed for his life of Jesus, praised Pasteur as a ge-

nius, one of the greatest men who ever lived, and administered only
this mild reproof:

"Truth, Sir, is a great coquette; she will not be sought with too
much passion, but often is most amenable to indifference. She es-
capes when apparently caught, but gives herself up if patiently waited
for; revealing herself after farewells have been said, but inexorable
when loved with too much fervor."

Toxin, Antitoxin, and Money

Pasteur's discovery that anthrax and chicken cholera could be prevented by an attenuated bacterial vaccine stimulated great interest in
an attempt to produce other vaccines. But simple attenuation techniques were soon found inapplicable to many infectious diseases, especially those in which the causative bacteria produce a toxin responsible for the illness itself. For such maladies, other methods of treatment and prevention remained to be devised. Diphtheria is a case
in point.

Unlike tuberculosis, diphtheria was not identified as a distinct disease until the early nineteenth century. Before this time it seems to
have been confused with a number of other conditions affecting the
throat, the mouth, and adjacent tissues. Yet despite this confusion,
the mention of certain symptoms uniquely characteristic of diphtheria indicates that this infection is indeed an old one. For example, the
paralysis of the soft palate with resultant regurgitation of fluid
through the nose during the attempt to swallow, a particularly
distressing manifestation, was described in a sixth-century text,
though undoubtedly recognized hundreds of years before.

Epidemics of diphtheria are no doubt also quite old. During the
years 1735 to 1740 New England and the Middle Atlantic states
were ravaged by a "throat distemper"—almost certainly diphtheria
from its description—which may well have killed more than 20 per
cent of the entire population under fifteen years of age. Medical historians speculate that diphtheria might even have caused the death of
George Washington during another outbreak.

In 1826 a French physician, Pierre Bretonneau, was the first to
recognize the infectious nature of diphtheria and also to describe the

characteristic symptoms. The throat pain and the slimy gray pseudo-membrane in the throat are still sometimes called Bretonneau's angina or Bretonneau's disease. As the condition progresses, the patient, usually a child, develops a peculiar gurgling cough and paralysis, then turns blue while gasping for breath—as though being strangled to death slowly by a powerful, unseen hand.

This unseen hand was identified as belonging to tiny, Indian-club-shaped bacteria in 1883 by a German pathologist, Edwin Klebs. From the pseudomembranes in the throats of patients with "laryngeal croup" Klebs managed to isolate *Corynebacterium diphtheriae* and grow it in pure culture.

In his original bacteriologic studies Robert Koch had established a set of rules or postulates to prove that a particular organism caused a disease. Klebs had fulfilled two of these in his diphtheria studies by isolating and growing the correct germ. But he did not fulfill the third postulate by using the cultured organism to produce the disease in an animal. This was accomplished by Koch's student Friedrich Löffler.

Well, sort of. Löffler isolated the organism from the throats of children dead of diphtheria and, using an alkaline solution of highly concentrated methylene blue dye, identified it microscopically as the Indian-club-shaped bacillus that Klebs had previously seen. Then, after growing it on Koch's nutritive jelly medium, Löffler injected the bacillus into various animal species. Rats and mice were immune, he found, though guinea pigs, rabbits, and small birds were readily infected.

But Löffler was puzzled by what he observed. Susceptible animals would die in two or three days—like a child, or even more rapidly. Yet at post-mortem the organisms could only be found at the injection site, quite unlike the anthrax or tubercle bacilli, which are widely disseminated. Also, the animals did not manifest the paralysis that frequently occurred in human cases. To explain these anomalies, Löffler postulated a diphtheria toxin, a diffusable poison, which inflicted the widespread damage that could not be attributed to the bacteria alone.

Four years later, Löffler's prophecy was validated by Pasteur's colleague, Emile Roux. Roux was a hawk-faced consumptive, who liked to work wearing a small black cap, perhaps in imitation of his mentor, Pasteur. Yet members of the opposite sex were quite attracted to the precise, collected Roux, once leading him to remark, "Women are like drugs. When they no longer act, one must change."

Roux began his work on diphtheria with another of Pasteur's pupils, Alexandre Yersin. Yersin had visited for a short time at Koch's institute in Berlin, where he was able to observe Löffler's results at first hand. A few years after the studies on diphtheria, Yersin was to identify the organism responsible for the black death, *Pasteurella pestis*.

During a severe outbreak of diphtheria in Paris, Roux and Yersin went to the Hospital for Sick Children and there isolated the same bacillus Löffler and Klebs had found. After culturing the organism in broth, the two Frenchmen injected large volumes of the liquid into rabbits, successfully producing the paralysis which Löffler had failed to observe. For Löffler had grown his *Corynebacterium diphtheriae* on solid jelly and was unable to introduce a sufficient amount of toxin during his experiments to paralyze animals.

Performing autopsies on the rabbits, Roux observed, as had Löffler in children, that despite widespread tissue destruction few diphtheria bacilli were to be found. Immediately Roux realized that Löffler's guess was correct, that the organisms did indeed produce a toxin. Attempting a proof, the two French scientists used high air pressure to force infected broth through a Rube Goldberg porcelain filter, thereby excluding the bacteria; the resultant thin, amber-colored fluid was then injected into guinea pigs. Nothing happened.

The same experiment was performed again, but with a larger dose of fluid. Still there was no effect. Finally the exasperated Roux injected an enormous amount of the amber fluid, almost inundating the guinea pig in the process. After forty-eight hours the animal began to breathe in little hiccups. In five days it had died with signs of diphtheria.

Now a reason for the previous failures could be postulated. The bacilli had been incubated in the broth only four days—not enough time to produce a lethal concentration of toxin. So bacteria were left to incubate in another broth sample for forty-two days.

This time, minute amounts of the fluid were incredibly toxic. Enormous dilution was necessary for inactivation. Roux dried the toxin, tried to analyze it chemically, and failed. Only in 1958, with techniques far more sophisticated than those available in the late nineteenth century, was diphtheria toxin successfully crystallized and shown to be a high-molecular-weight protein. But Roux was able to make a striking estimate of toxicity: One ounce, he calculated, was sufficient to kill six hundred thousand guinea pigs or seventy-five thousand large dogs.

Here Roux's research took a turn in the wrong direction. Apparently, he correctly hypothesized that the toxin could be used to prepare a diphtheria vaccine. But then, instead of testing his hypothesis, he turned to showing doctors how to take pure throat cultures at the bedside, and tried suggesting useful gargles. The discovery of diphtheria toxin, however, did not go unnoticed by the scientists at Koch's institute in Berlin. And one, Emil Behring, was able to use it successfully in treating children with diphtheria—not directly, but by means of a specially prepared antitoxin.

Behring, like Koch, was born to a poor family with thirteen children. Like Mendel, he prepared for the priesthood to obtain a free university education, but then transferred into the army medical school. As a medical officer, Behring was something of a swashbuckling type and ran up sufficient gambling debts to provoke a minor scandal before resigning his commission.

In 1889, at the age of thirty-five, Behring joined Koch's Institute of Hygiene and soon began to study diphtheria. At first he tried to treat the disease in animals by administering various inorganic and organic compounds: gold salts, naphthylamine, and others. His rationale—one that was to trip up many future scientists seeking drugs to cure infection—was deceptively simple: Chemicals capable of killing bacteria in a test tube ("in vitro") should be useful for combating infections in an animal ("in vivo"). Behring killed a large number of guinea pigs before he finally grasped how innocent this assumption really was.

But during the chemical tests Behring made the fortuitous observation that some iodine compounds tended to attenuate the virulence of *Corynebacterium diphtheriae*. When injected into guinea pigs, these attenuated organisms would produce immunity to diphtheria. But they sometimes killed the guinea pig first, indicating that they would be too dangerous for human immunization.

Behring circumvented this problem in a highly ingenious manner. First he withdrew blood with a syringe from an immunized guinea pig, then allowed the blood to stand until a straw-colored serum rose to the top of the container while the clotted cells sank to the bottom. The serum, he found, when injected into another guinea pig, would protect against diphtheria and even sometimes cure an infected animal. This effect resulted from a substance within the serum—antitoxin—which inactivated the diphtheria toxin. For the first time, immunity to disease had been passively transferred from one animal to another via serum; before Behring's discovery, active immunity, conferred by inoculation, was the only preventive measure known.

Almost immediately, Behring applied transfer of passive immunity to the treatment of another disease: tetanus. A Japanese working in Koch's laboratory, Shibasaburo Kitasato, had identified the germ of tetanus, *Clostridium tetani,* and showed that it too killed by means of a toxin. Together, Kitasato and Behring were able to immunize a rabbit passively against tetanus. During World War I Behring was decorated by the German government in recognition of the many soldiers' lives that his tetanus antitoxin had saved. And even earlier, in 1901, he was awarded the Nobel Prize in Medicine for discovering the phenomenon of passive immunity.

But these honors were far in the future on Christmas night 1891, almost a year after his paper on diphtheria antitoxin had been published, when Behring made the first human trials on children in the Bergmann Clinic on Brick Street in Berlin. In some of the children the results were astounding, but others died. One, the son of an eminent Berlin physician, expired just after the injection had been made. Only later did physicians come to understand the hazards of introducing animal serum into a human being.

The reports of Behring's qualified success encouraged Emile Roux in the Pasteur Institute to begin treating French children with diphtheria antitoxin produced in horses. Roux was under some pressure to test the effectiveness of treatment by dividing the children into two groups: a treated group, and a control group which would receive no treatment. Only by comparison of the two groups could a valid proof of the worth of diphtheria antitoxin be made.

The humane Roux, however, chose to give antitoxin to all of the sick children under his care. The result: a great reduction in mortality during a four-month period in 1894. Meanwhile in a nearby hospital where the serum was not being used children were dying at a significantly higher rate.

Unfortunately, Roux's humanity left some continuing doubt as to the value of antitoxin, for diphtheria and other infectious diseases tend to wax and wane in virulence. During some decades 60 per cent of those affected will die, during others only 10 per cent. Skeptics examining Roux's results pointed to a hospital in England, where during 1894 the death rate from diphtheria had spontaneously plummeted from 40 per cent to 29 per cent, no antitoxin having been used.

This terrible problem in medical therapeutics—the necessity of denying a possibly lifesaving remedy to those needing it in order to prove its efficacy—was not lost on the public. During a climactic episode in *Arrowsmith,* Dr. Martin Arrowsmith must deny a potentially effective plague vaccine to half the population of an island, St. Hubert, ravaged by plague. Only after the death of his own wife from plague does Dr. Arrowsmith reject the demands of science and—like Roux—give the vaccine to everyone.

The fictional Dr. Arrowsmith and the real Dr. Roux may have been sorely troubled by this ethical problem, but Emil Behring was not. The now-famous German scientist had a considerably more important matter on his mind: money. Roux had fastidiously followed the French scientific tradition and refused any personal financial recompense for antitoxin. Behring, troubled by no such scruples and eager to earn a quick mark, had immediately patented his new treatment for diphtheria. But one obstacle, in the person of Paul Ehrlich, still stood in his way.

Ehrlich was an untidy man of dazzling brilliance, an eccentric Jew who had spent several years in Koch's laboratory. His suits were eternally soiled by the huge Havana cigars that he delighted in smoking, while he defaced set after set of detachable cuffs with his copious laboratory notes. Though possessed of a mature, sophisticated scientific insight, Ehrlich was almost childlike in his interpersonal relations and was given to periodic infantile outbursts when disturbed.

During the early diphtheria work, Behring had approached Ehrlich because of the latter's special knowledge of immunity. Ehrlich was immediately able to suggest modifications that vastly increased the strength and yield of antitoxin; then, after a large number of careful experiments, he devised a way to quantitate blood antitoxin levels and calculate a safe curative dose for humans. These fundamental improvements, which made commercial antitoxin production possible, gave him a legitimate claim on a portion of any royalties. But the childlike Ehrlich proved to be no match for a man as slick, shrewd, and money-hungry as Behring.

Through his useful contacts in the Ministry of Culture, Behring promised to arrange a salaried government post for Ehrlich in exchange for Ehrlich's renunciation of all patent claims. The naïve, trusting Ehrlich readily agreed when reassured that the job would be one most commensurate with his great abilities. Behring, however, treated this promise as he had his army gambling debts. Ehrlich never got his job.

After discovering that he had been duped, Ehrlich hid his anger from no one. His fury continued to intensify as he watched the commercial production of antitoxin become increasingly profitable. Bitterly, he carried his grievance to the highest levels of the Prussian government, always disparaging Behring's scientific abilities. Behring "wanted to be a superman," he once wrote, "but—thank God—he did not have the necessary superbrain."

As Ehrlich fumed, Behring prospered. His antitoxin patents brought him a large fortune—and for a time, a fame that exceeded Koch's. The once poor boy was made a professor and ennobled; with great pride he proceeded to call himself *"von* Behring." At the Monte Carlo gambling tables, his luck proved considerably better than it had in the army; on one occasion he won enough to buy a villa on Capri. He also constructed a castle overlooking the town of Marburg, where he lived and entertained in baronial splendor. In one wing of the building he built his own laboratory, in another a mausoleum. Not far away he established his own chemical company, the Behring Works. And in early middle age he married the twenty-year-old daughter of the Berlin Charité Hospital's director.

Though Ehrlich adamantly refused to speak to his erstwhile collaborator, Behring, perhaps pricked by guilt, was never vindictive. As an elderly cripple leaning heavily on a cane, Behring walked behind Ehrlich's coffin to the grave. "If we have hurt you," he said, "forgive us."

Behring took a final step toward preventing deaths in children by discovering that toxin neutralized by antitoxin could confer a long-lasting, active immunity against diphtheria, as opposed to the short-lived, passive immunity produced by antitoxin injection. And in 1923, six years after Behring's death, Gaston Ramon, a French bacteriologist, found that the preparation's effectiveness could be increased after formalin inactivation. Today, Ramon's vaccine, called diphtheria toxoid, has almost eliminated diphtheria as a disease of childhood.

Microbes and Vectors

The infectious diseases mentioned so far—anthrax, cholera, tuberculosis, diphtheria, tetanus—proved relatively easy to understand because their transmission was direct. Early microbe hunters had no trouble showing that they were passed from subject to subject by direct contact or by contact with an infected substance—water, food, clothing.

But another series of infectious diseases was initially much more difficult to comprehend. In these diseases, an organism might be identified, but often it could neither be grown nor used to infect an experimental animal. Further, the means of spread from victim to victim was completely mysterious. Examples are filariasis, Texas cattle fever, typhus, African sleeping sickness, and—most important of all—malaria, a condition as widespread as the common cold, yet deadly and disabling beyond belief. The first step toward prevention and eradication of these maladies was the discovery that they spread in an unusual manner—via an insect carrier, or vector.

Filariasis

Filariasis, the first insect-borne disease to be understood, is also the most deforming. One of its disturbing manifestations is elephantiasis, the tremendous enlargement of the victims' body tissues, particularly in the legs and scrotum. The scrotum in some cases can attain a weight of fifty pounds and a size so great that a wheelbarrow is needed to carry it around.

A Scottish surgeon, Sir Patrick Manson, proved that filariasis was transmitted by a mosquito. Manson's discovery earned him the title Father of Tropical Medicine and the distinction of being the first to show that insects transmit disease.

One of the truly eminent microbe hunters, Manson became a physician only by accident. He was born near Aberdeen, Scotland, October 3, 1844, the second son in a family of nine children. At fifteen he was apprenticed to a firm of ironmakers preparatory to the study of engineering. But not long at work, he developed spinal curvature and a weakness in his right arm. On the advice of a physician, he quit his job and for six months led the life of a semi-invalid, studying natural history for a short time each day at the Marischal College of Aberdeen.

When he resumed normal activity, Manson discovered that natural history was not applicable to an engineering degree. But further inquiry revealed that this subject was acceptable as part of the medical curriculum. Thereupon, Manson switched from engineering to the study of medicine.

His first post after graduation was a dreary one—assistant medical officer of an insane asylum. To escape this job, he accepted the more adventurous assignment as medical officer for Formosa in the service of the Chinese Imperial Maritime Customs. In June 1866 he began his official duties at the port of Takao on the southwest coast of Formosa, inspecting each ship in port and treating crew members. During his free time he did some private practice among the Europeans and Chinese, and also made frequent trips to the interior of the island. It was here that he was first able to observe elephantiasis, a common disease in that part of the world.

In 1870 Manson was transferred to Amoy, where he spent the next thirteen years. Few Europeans lived in this port city, and since his official duties for the customs service were light, Manson was able to spend considerable time treating and observing the native Chinese.

At first, few of the natives trusted him. Looking about, he soon discovered the reason. Chinese doctors practiced in the open street to prove that there was no trickery involved in their work. So Manson moved his consulting and operating rooms to the ground floor, where passersby could observe everything through the windows. Within a short time he was widely recognized as one of the most skillful surgeons on the China coast, and his practice flourished.

Of the common diseases to be seen in Amoy, elephantiasis, about which very little was known, interested Manson most. After some experimentation he was able to devise an effective surgical procedure for removal of the enormously enlarged scrotum. As word spread, his surgery was crowded with elephantiasis victims seeking relief.

Manson's first insight into the cause of elephantiasis was gained during a trip to London in 1875. There he learned that Timothy Lewis, an officer in the Army Medical Service in Calcutta, had discovered a microscopic worm, which he named *Filaria sanguinis hominis,* in the blood and urine of an elephantiasis patient. This parasite was identical to one first seen by a French surgeon in Havana, Jean Nicholas Demarquay, in 1863. But neither Lewis nor Demarquay was able to explain how this organism entered the body, nor how it spread from one person to another. Manson, blessed with extraordinary insight, persistence, and luck, was to succeed where his predecessors had failed.

After returning to Amoy with a new wife and a new microscope, Manson set out to discover how many in the native population were infected with filariae. To his amazement he found that the worms were almost as common as chopsticks and could be found in one city dweller in ten. An even higher proportion of old people were infected—one in three—implying that the probability of the disease increased with age. Yet in some individuals he knew to be heavily infected, Manson could find no parasites at all. Only by an extraordinary piece of good fortune did he discover why.

In order to search for filariae methodically, Manson had hired and trained two Chinese students, who took blood specimens and prepared them for study. One of these boys had an invalid mother to care for during the daytime and so could work only at night. The other student did his job during the day. To his great amazement, Manson discovered that the slides made by the night student always showed the most parasites. Thinking that perhaps the night student might just be more efficient, he put both boys to work on the same infected patient. The difference between day and night specimens persisted, seeming to confirm his suspicion.

Now, however, Manson began to note just what time the specimens were taken. The parasites could rarely be located in specimens taken early in the day. But when Manson and his assistants were so busy with routine duties that specimens could not be obtained until evening, the worms were present in abundance. The blood of two infected patients, examined every four hours during four days and nights, illustrated the time discrepancy even more clearly. Worms began to appear in the blood around sunset, increasing in number until midnight, then decreasing until nine or ten in the morning, when they practically disappeared. This temporal fluctuation occurred day after day.

When these remarkable findings were first presented at a London scientific meeting, Manson was laughed at and ridiculed. One member of the audience even rose to ask whether Manson had seen the filariae carrying watches. But the laughter quickly died out after the same experiment was repeated by many observers and found to be correct. Twenty years were to pass, however, before Manson could locate the daytime haunt of the parasites, again by pure luck. During an autopsy on a filariasis patient who had committed suicide with prussic acid at the convenient hour of eight-thirty A.M., Manson found that the parasites had migrated to the lungs and large arteries.

"It is the discrepancy that teaches, if you would learn," Manson once remarked. And it was the time discrepancy in filariasis that allowed him to recognize the mode of transmission.

At first, the periodicity of the parasite's appearance seemed to depend on meteorologic fluctuation, so Manson studied temperature changes and swings in barometric pressure. When these proved unrelated, he investigated the effect of sunlight by keeping a patient in a darkened room. The periodicity was unaffected.

Manson hit upon the correct explanation for the spread of the parasite while vainly trying to find the cause for the periodicity. In a flash he concluded that the immature worms must be removed from the blood by a blood-sucking insect. And of all such insects only one —the mosquito—altered its biting habits according to time of day. At twilight and early darkness, the exact time that the parasites appeared in the blood, the mosquitoes did most of their feeding. Manson's happy inspiration allowed him immediately to exclude fleas, ticks, and lice.

In his initial attempt to verify that the mosquito was indeed the vector of filariasis, Manson was again quite lucky, this time on account of a bit of ignorance. Charting the worldwide incidence of the disease, he found that it coincided quite closely with the known habitats of the mosquito: warm climates. A few years later, the mosquito was discovered to thrive all over the world, and had Manson been unfortunate enough to learn this during his work, he might have gone off in the wrong direction entirely.

To test his hypothesis, Manson collected a few mosquitoes, which he allowed to feed on the blood of a filariasis patient. Here is his description of what the insects revealed:

"I shall not easily forget the first mosquito I dissected. I tore off its abdomen and succeeded in expressing the blood the stomach contained. Placing this under the microscope, I was gratified to find that, so far from killing the filaria, the digestive juices of the mosquito seemed to have stimulated it to fresh activity.

"I followed it up as best I could with the meager appliances at my disposal, and after many months of work, often following up false scents, I ultimately succeeded in tracing the filaria through the stomach wall into the abdominal cavity and then into the thoracic muscles of the mosquito. I ascertained that during this passage the little parasite increased enormously in size. It developed a mouth, an alimentary canal, and other organs. . . . Manifestly it was on the road to a new human host."

After observing the growing worm until "it was equipped for independent life and ready to quit its nurse, the mosquito," Manson saw the parasite develop what appeared to be a boring or piercing device at one end. Because he erroneously believed that the mosquito died in the water where it laid its eggs, Manson theorized that the filaria escaped the dead mosquito and remained in the water until swallowed by a human, then bored through the bowel into the blood stream. Only fifteen years later, after Ronald Ross had shown that malaria resulted from a mosquito bite, did others prove that filariasis was also transmitted in this way.

Yet despite this error, Manson's positive identification of an insect vector ranks as one of the most important discoveries in the history of infectious disease. It stimulated the search for other insect-borne diseases and eventually led to the control of these great threats to human health.

But for a while, Manson was regarded as nothing more than a crackpot. Once, during a walk in a London street, he encountered two prominent physicians and nodded a greeting. After the two doctors had passed, the one who recognized Manson was queried by his companion as to who this florid gentleman might be. "Mosquito Manson," the man replied, pointedly tapping his temple with his forefinger.

Despite such slurs, Manson continued to study the mosquito and found that only one of the four species indigenous to Amoy—*Culex fatigans*—could harbor the filaria. In an 1883 publication he described the appearance and habits of this particular insect in detail, then added a final caveat for his critics: "All the principle facts I have stated are true. I have verified them over and over again."

In addition to his studies of filariasis, Manson made many other important contributions to medical science. These included a description of the fungus *Trichophyton mansoni;* identification of the eggs of *Schistosoma mansoni,* a parasite causing a widespread tropical disease; and discovery of the lung fluke, *Paragonimus westermani.* This fluke was encountered quite by chance in 1880, and Manson's account has the quaint, Kiplingesque flavor of the white Victorian among the natives:

"On one occasion I was consulted by a Chinaman, a petty mandarin, about an eruption between his fingers, to wit, the itch. While I was engaged in examining his hands my patient began to cough. He hawked up, and, after the manner of his race, incontinentally expectorated the result of his efforts onto my study carpet. I observed that the expectorated material was red and viscid; and so, instead of reproaching him for spitting on my carpet, requested him to repeat the cough and this time to deposit the sputum in a watchglass. He very obligingly did so. My forbearance was rewarded. On placing a little of the rusty sputum under the microscope I found it to be loaded with little brown operculated bodies, manifestly the ova of a parasite."

Besides his other accomplishments, Manson came exceedingly close to making three especially significant discoveries, yet in one way or another managed to let them slip through his grasp. Two eventually led to Nobel prizes for others.

In February 1879 Manson began to experiment with a liquid he called "leper juice," obtained from lesions of patients with leprosy. Microscopic examination revealed minute rodlike bodies, which Manson tried but failed to cultivate in a hen's egg. Only years later were these lepra bacilli successfully grown by others in the foot pads of mice. Before Manson was ready to publish his work, Armauer Hansen identified and reported the same organisms, which are now known as Hansen's bacilli.

Manson's failure to investigate closely an effective remedy resulted in his losing credit for an even more well-known discovery. He encountered this remedy when a Chinese woman dying of profound anemia was brought to him. After having given the case up for hopeless, he happened to see the apparently doomed woman again months later—alive and in excellent health. Hearing this remarkable cure attributed to some mysterious pills prescribed by a native doctor, Manson immediately sought the doctor out and plied him with strong wine until the secret was revealed. The magic substance proved to be dried crow's liver, a venerable Chinese drug.

So impressed was Manson with the results that he started treating other anemia patients with liver. Because many benefited, he continued to administer liver soup routinely in all cases of anemia. In 1926, four years after his death, George Minot and William Murphy discovered liver therapy independently, and found that only one form of anemia—pernicious anemia—was helped. The Nobel Prize that went to Minot and Murphy could have been Manson's had he only tried to determine which type of anemia was improved by liver. Perhaps he was lucky that he did not live long enough to learn what he had so nearly missed.

But after having come tantalizingly close to solving the riddle of another disease, malaria, he was not so fortunate.

The Fever of Bad Air

Malaria is the oldest and most widespread disease known to man, the disease that has killed more human beings than any other. True, the bulk of malaria occurs in tropical and semitropical regions, but it is by no means confined to these areas. It has been reported north of the Arctic Circle and as far south as the extreme tip of South America. Only recently have new insecticides and drugs eradicated malaria from North America. In the 1940s the disease was especially prevalent in the southern United States, and it still appears in small, sporadic epidemics when brought back by visitors from malarious areas and armed forces personnel.

In countries still affected, malaria brings economic and social ruin. Characteristically beginning in childhood, the infection debilitates when it does not kill, making chronic invalids of young adults and precluding all productivity. As former Surgeon General Hugh S. Cumming once remarked, "Malaria has the disastrous effect of permitting human existence while precluding the possibility of human health and happiness."

The history of malaria and its terrible effects is as ancient as the history of civilization. The disease has been responsible for the decline of nations and crushing military defeats, often having caused more casualties than the weapons themselves. For centuries it prevented any economic development in vast regions of the earth.

Because of its ubiquitous nature, malaria is familiar to almost everyone, and its symptoms are well known: the chill with its violent shivering, the chattering teeth and goose flesh, the high fever accompanied by headache and torturing thirst, followed by a drenching sweat as the fever departs.

One American physician, Dr. Victor Vaughan, recalled an attack which occurred during his early childhood in the summer of 1865: "On a hot August morning, as I sat on my horse in the treeless prairie, I felt cold chills playing hide and seek up and down my spine. As the sun's rays became more vertical, the chilly sensations grew in strength. Soon my teeth were chattering. . . . As the God of Day heralded his coming by flaming banners in the east, my fever left me, and was followed by the sweating stage. As fast as the sun dried my clothes on the outside, the flowing pores of my skin wet them within. . . . This was my first and last personal experience with malaria."

Most sufferers, unluckier than Dr. Vaughan, have multiple attacks, often consistently separated in time. Noting this phenomenon, the ancient Romans named the disease by measuring the elapsed time from the beginning of the first episode to the end of the second. Thus, fever recurring on Tuesday and Thursday was called a *tertian* or "every third day" fever, although only forty-eight hours separated the two attacks. A fever appearing on Tuesday and Friday would be called *quartan*.

Today, malaria is classified according to the type of parasite responsible for the infection. Of the four species affecting man, *Plasmodium vivax,* a one-celled protozoan, is most commonly responsible for tertian fever. Since a vivax infection is rarely fatal, it has been called "benign tertian fever"—something of a misnomer when one considers that the victim may suffer eight to ten relapses, each with its long series of chills and fever, followed by a profound prostration and debility.

But *P. vivax* may sometimes seem benign when compared to its brother, *P. falciparum,* the parasite of malignant tertian fever. Surpassing all of the other plasmodia in virulence, this organism is responsible for the most severe forms of malaria, including cerebral malaria and blackwater fever, the latter being a condition in which hemoglobin from dissolving red cells is suddenly discharged into the urine, imparting the characteristic color.

The two remaining human malarial parasites, *P. malariae* and *P. ovale,* generally produce the mildest infections. *P. ovale* infection may be recognized by the propensity of the chills and fever to recur at regularly spaced intervals. *P. malariae* infection, like vivax malaria, has the tendency to relapse.

Sometimes a single infection may be caused by two or more types of plasmodia. Ancient physicians recognized such an infection by virtue of its *quotidian* or daily fever. When a quotidian fever is treated with drugs, the more susceptible type of plasmodium often is destroyed first, causing the fever to change from quotidian to the type characteristic of the survivor.

Early man, confronting the manifestations of malaria, attributed the fevers to supernatural influences—evil spirits, angered deities, or the black magic of sorcerers. The ancient Chinese believed the frightening symptoms and signs to be the work of three demons—one with a hammer, one with a pail of cold water, and a third with a stove. A fever goddess—three demons rolled into one—was worshiped by the ancient Romans.

Because the connection between malaria and swamps was evident even in antiquity, the evil spirits or malaria gods were believed to live within the marshes. This belief is likely the origin of the Greek fable of Hercules and Hydra. Hercules set out to destroy this monster, so the story goes, a nine-headed beast that resided in the swamps around Lake Lerna. But the task proved to be a difficult one, since as each head was struck off, two new ones appeared. Hercules finally triumphed by ordering his servant Iolaus to burn the wound after each head was severed. Some historians feel that this legend resulted from an attempt to reclaim a formerly uninhabitable swamp.

The impact of malaria on Greek history, however, is anything but fictional. The disease struck Alexander the Great just at the height of his power. By force of arms, this Macedonian general had joined the Greek states in an unwilling alliance and led their armies against the Persians, successfully capturing the entire coastline of the eastern Mediterranean. Then he had conquered Syria, Phoenecia, Arabia, and Egypt before finally destroying the armies of Darius, the powerful Persian king. Alexander's momentum had carried him into northern India, where he had again been victorious in spite of fierce opposition from the hill tribes. Finally, after conquering the entire known world, he had set out to subjugate the earth. An enormous harbor holding a thousand ships had been dug, and a gigantic fleet assembled. Men had been trained, supplies obtained. But just as Alexander was to depart with his army in early June 323 B.C., he contracted a fever and the voyage was postponed.

At first the thirty-three-year-old general regarded his illness as nothing more than a temporary setback. Fevers were not uncommon throughout Greece and Asia Minor, and Alexander himself had had an attack ten years before from which he had quickly recovered. Some of the soldiers even attributed the present illness to an episode of carousing.

But Alexander continued to deteriorate until he lapsed into a deep coma, his blinded, glazed eyes fixed on the ceiling, his ears deaf, his body racked by fever. One by one, his loyal warriors were allowed to pass through his chamber and pause by his bedside to say good-bye. The next day he died.

Malaria, by striking Alexander, had altered the course of history. Had the great military leader survived, he might well have succeeded in uniting east and west, fusing Greeks and Orientals into a single nation. But in his absence, his empire crumbled, his army collapsed. Still later, historians believe, malaria was instrumental in the downfall of all Greek civilization by sapping the strength of the people and depopulating the countryside.

Naturally, the prevalence of malaria afforded Greek physicians ample opportunity for meticulous observation of signs and symptoms, all duly recorded in the Hippocratic corpus. This ancient medical text correctly distinguishes the intermittent malarial fever from the continuous fever more commonly observed in other infectious diseases, and also notes the daily, every-other-day, and every-third-day temperature rise that the Romans later named. Though it incorrectly attributes malaria to ingestion of stagnant water, the Hippocratic corpus was the first document to contain an important observation of splenic change: "Those who drink [stagnant water] have always large, stiff spleens and hard, thin, hot stomachs, while their shoulders, collarbones, and faces are emaciated; the fact is that their flesh dissolves to feed the spleen. . . ."

The combination of splenic enlargement and intermittent fever is so characteristic of malaria that it permits historic identification of the disease with a high degree of certainty. One particularly famous case with these signs was that of the artist Albrecht Dürer, who contracted malaria in 1520 during a trip to the province of Zeeland in Holland. Dürer sought medical advice by sending his physician a now-famous drawing. The sketch shows the upper half of the artist's body, with an index finger pointing to a yellow spot over the spleen. Above the self-portrait Dürer wrote, "Do der gelb fleck ist und mit dem finger drawff dent, do ist mir we," or, freely translated, "The yellow spot to which the finger points is where I hurt."

In the first century A.D., Marcus Terentius Varro, the Roman scholar whom Caesar named director of the imperial library, suggested the presence of the disease in his book on agriculture, *De Rerum Rusticarum*. Swamps, Varro wrote, breed "certain animalcula which cannot be seen with the eyes and which we breathe through the nose and mouth into the body, where they cause grave maladies." Shortly thereafter, Celsus described malaria in detail and apparently agreed with Varro about the cause.

But Galen, a much more important and influential physician in Rome, did not. Galen believed that malaria was due to a disorder in the four humors of the body. Tertian fever, for example, was the result of an imbalance of yellow bile; quartan was caused by too much black bile, and quotidian by an excess of phlegm. A blood abnormality was the cause of continuous fever. So to set matters right again, Galen wrote, the physician must restore the normal humoral balance by bleeding, purging, or, even better, by both. These tenets were accepted without question for the next fifteen hundred years.

Perhaps the Romans were fortunate to have embraced Galen's incorrect theory and totally worthless therapeutic measures, for unchecked malaria served to protect Rome from repeated Hun invasions. In the swamps of the Campagna that surrounded the city, in the Pontine Marshes, hordes of malaria-infected mosquitoes thrived. On numerous occasions invading barbarians were forced to withdraw, their ranks decimated by malaria, their surviving troops too ill to fight.

Even the most formidable Teuton of all, Alaric, king of the Goths, was thwarted by the disease. After successfully plundering Greece in the fourth century A.D., Alaric turned his attention to Rome. But his plans were received with horror by his old warriors, who desperately attempted to dissuade him. The Roman poet Claudian recorded one as warning grimly, "If the tradition of our fathers is true, then none return who wantonly attack this town."

All to no avail. Rome, the Big Apple of its day, had a charismatic attraction. Alaric knew that he could not be counted a major-league barbarian until he had plundered the Eternal City. After much bloodshed, his wish was granted. But his triumph was short lived. Hardly had he arrived in town when he sickened with malaria and died. His soldiers built a dam to deflect the Busento River and buried their leader in the river bed with some of his spoils. Then the dam was taken down, the river directed again into its usual channel, and the laborers who had accomplished the task killed so that no one might learn the last resting place of the king of the Goths.

A century later, another warrior, Belisarius, didn't get as far as Alaric had. In 536 Belisarius, leading the army of the Eastern Empire, surrounded Rome, planning to starve the city into submission. To facilitate their plan, the soldiers ravaged the farms producing food and destroyed aqueducts to cut off the Roman water supply. But they made a fatal error by digging their entrenchments in the Campagna. With summer came malaria, which quickly decimated the ranks. Belisarius himself was severely stricken with fever but survived, a beaten man.

Throughout the Middle Ages the Roman malaria continued to subdue would-be conquerors from the north. The Emperor Otto I attacked the city in 964 to suppress a revolt there but "was overcome by a fate more unhappy than he could have ever looked for, for in his army there broke out so great and deadly a pestilence that almost all died, and those who still kept their health only dared to hope to live from one evening to the next morning," wrote a contemporary historian, Otto's second son. Some years later the eldest son, Otto II, perished miserably in spite of medical intervention: "Greedy for health, he took too much of the remedy composed of aloes, which had been prescribed for him, and died at the age of twenty-eight years."

Frederick I, called Barbarossa, did no better in his attempt to conquer Rome than had Otto the First, but the lessons learned were not lost on some of the later German kings. The army of Henry II was wiped out by malaria, but Henry IV managed to besiege Rome four times, always withdrawing the bulk of his soldiers during the summer months from the Campagna. The tiny force left behind was invariably annihilated by fever.

"Nor do hot fevers sooner quit the body if you toss about on a pictured tapestry and blushing purple than if you must lie on a poor man's blanket," wrote the Roman poet Lucretius. The princes of the

Church were well aware of this fact. One pope after another succumbed to malaria, just as the military leaders had. Pontiffs from the
north were especially vulnerable—so vulnerable, in fact, that sometimes candidates for the papacy were difficult to find. The cardinals,
too, were not immune, and consistently lost members to fever when
gathering to choose a new pope. Finally, in the fourteenth century,
foreign popes were no longer permitted to live in Rome, a regulation,
according to the poet Petrarch's letters, wholly due to fear of "Roman
fever." Malaria even inspired one cleric to express the universal dread
in verse:

Rome, voracious of men, breaks down the strongest human nature—
Rome, hotbed of fevers, is an ample giver of the fruits of death.
The Roman fevers are faithful according to an imprescriptable
    right:
Whom once they have touched, they do not abandon as long as he
    lives.

A few years after these lines were written, the nefarious Cesare
Borgia plotted to dominate all Italy. But shortly after the death of his
father, Pope Alexander VI, Cesare contracted an especially severe
case of malaria. Only the resourcefulness of the kindly family doctor saved the day, so the story goes. The desperately ill patient was
given the largest poultice in the history of medicine by being secreted
within the carcass of a recently disemboweled mule. By the time
Cesare Borgia grew well enough to crawl out of the mule, his moment
of opportunity had passed.

But malaria did not confine its attentions to Italians and Goths
alone. Sir Walter Raleigh, sentenced to die on the gallows, pleaded
with his executioners to arrange the event at a certain time of day so
he would not be seized by a malarial chill that could be construed by
the audience as a sign of fear. Lord Byron, James I, and Lord Nelson
also suffered from malaria.

And in 1493 malaria appeared in North America. On his second
voyage to the New World, Columbus dropped anchor at the site of
an old Indian village on Hispaniola to build a fort and colony. After
a month, an epidemic of terrible fever afflicted the entire party, including Columbus himself. Where did the fever come from? Medical
historians generally agree that malaria did not exist in America until
it was brought by Europeans. The Hispaniola settlement was at the

mouth of a river, an ideal breeding place for mosquitoes. No doubt the malarial parasites that eventually infested the whole settlement were carried by one or more infected Spaniards.

Further evidence of the European origin of American malaria is provided by the experiences of the two earliest English settlements, Roanoke Island, Virginia, and Jamestown. Sir Walter Raleigh recruited the Roanoke colonists from his native Devon, a region of England then free of malaria. Though Roanoke eventually proved an ideal spot for malaria, Raleigh's Devon settlers appear not to have incurred a single case of the disease.

The Jamestown colonists were not so fortunate. Recruited mostly from London, which was plagued at the time by malaria, the settlers remained in good health until two months after their arrival. Then in July 1607 a fever epidemic occurred, killing almost half the population by September and severely debilitating the rest. Malaria continued to haunt the settlement until the founding fathers were forced to move the capital of the colony from Jamestown to Williamsburg in 1699.

Settlers in the Carolinas and Georgia also found malaria to be a problem, indeed one so annoying that the region might have remained entirely unsettled but for the discovery that the marshy flatlands were perfectly adapted for cultivation of rice. Enormous, profitable plantations spread out over the area, producing so much rice that by 1700 not enough ships were at hand to transport all of it.

But the amount of rice and the amount of malaria grew apace. Only the Negro field hands seemed relatively impervious to the fever, an immunity now known to be conferred by sickle-cell hemoglobin, the abnormal blood protein that evolved after millennia of exposure to the African malarial parasites. The white overseers and masters, having no such hereditary protection, fled the marshes for more healthy higher ground during the summer months.

Just at the time that rice-growing began to boom, physicians started to suspect strongly that the cause of malaria might lie in the environment rather than in the four humors of the body as Galen had postulated. In 1717 an Italian doctor, Giovanni Maria Lancisi, echoed the old theories of Varro and Celsus by speculating that malaria was due to minute "bugs" or "worms" which entered the blood. But others were not so sure, and many attributed the disease to the noxious vapors or marsh air of swamps, *mal'aria*—"bad air"—in Ital-

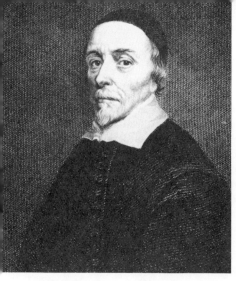

William Harvey In 1628 Harvey published the results of his experiments proving that the blood circulates — the single most important discovery in the science of physiology. His report of this work, a book entitled *De Motu Cordis,* was printed on thin, cheap paper that quickly deteriorated. It teemed with typographical errors, suggesting that Harvey did not even take the trouble to proofread it.

Edward Jenner (bottom left)   Two experimenters before Jenner had successfully used cowpox to inoculate against smallpox. But these two men did not bother to publish their results, and one of them, Benjamin Jesty, lived to rue his mistake. Jenner, who published in June 1798, is now credited for the discovery.

William Withering (bottom right)   In 1785 Withering published a detailed, systematic account of the use of digitalis in the treatment of heart failure. This drug, contained in the foxglove plant, had been a component of folk remedies since ancient times, but Withering was the first to recognize its indications and limitations.

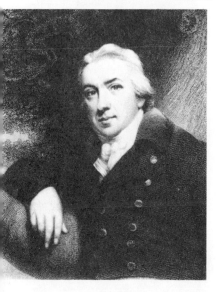

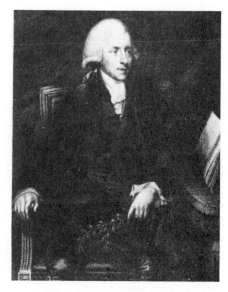

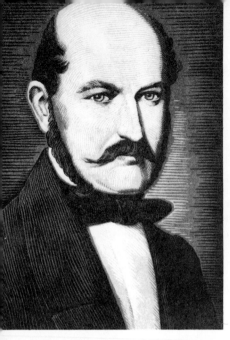

Ignaz Semmelweis This Hungarian physician realized in 1847 that puerperal sepsis, a severe disease occurring in women after childbirth, was infectious and caused by minute organic particles. But because of his unpleasant, tactless manner, he was unable to convince many of his colleagues. Before he could be recognized as correct, Semmelweis died tragically, infected by the same bacteria that cause puerpal sepsis.

Louis Pasteur The greatest medical scientist of all time, Pasteur made many discoveries forming the basis for bacteriology, virology, and immunology.

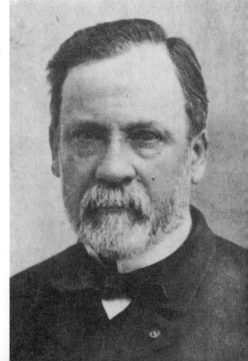

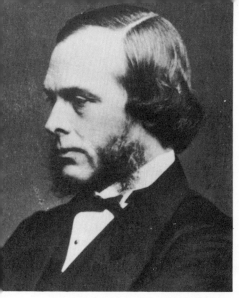

Joseph Lister Influenced by the work of Pasteur, Lister learned how to prevent infection in a surgical wound—the finding that made possible all modern surgical techniques. But Lister was not above a little capitalizing on his fame, and permitted his name to be used on a patented concoction in exchange for a royalty—which is still being paid. As a consequence, he is an integral part of the Listerine ads and the battle against halitosis.

Robert Koch (bottom left) While district health officer in an isolated Prussian border town, Koch demonstrated that anthrax, a disease of live-stock, is caused by a bacillus. This first rigorous proof of the germ theory of disease catapulted Koch to fame. He subsequently discovered the germs of cholera and tuberculosis but was shamed by tuberculin, a worthless cure for tuberculosis that he had devised.

Antoine Lavoisier and his wife (bottom right) The eighteenth-century French scientist who correctly described the process of chemical combination, Lavoisier also showed that animal respiration involves oxidation of carbon. This brilliant investigator was guillontined at the peak of his scientific career, during the French Revolution, by a judge who declared that the republic had no need for scientists. "This probably saves me from the inconveniences of old age," Lavoisier calmly remarked of his sentence.

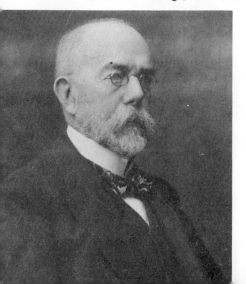

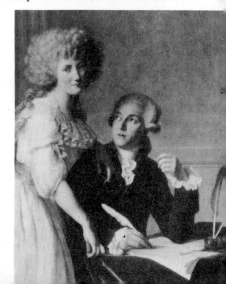

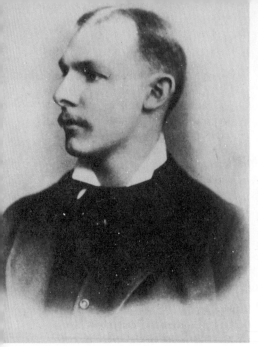

William Stewart Halsted The most innovative of all American surgeons, Halsted introduced a successful method of hernia repair, the radical mastectomy, and rubber surgical gloves. But his life was blighted by a long addiction to morphine, which he was never able to overcome.

Harvey Cushing The techniques of neurosurgery were perfected by this American surgeon, who had been trained by Halsted. During his lifetime, Cushing was as famous for his bad temper and difficult personality as for his scientific accomplishments.

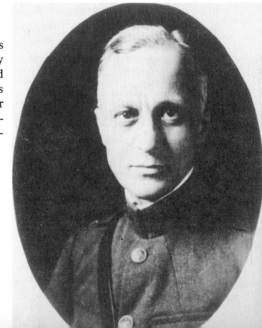

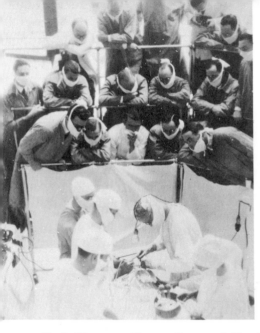

Cushing operating By the time that age and infirmity had forced him to abandon surgery, Cushing had removed more than two thousand brain tumors.

Hugh Hampton Young (bottom left) Another of Halsted's residents, Young vastly improved surgery of the urinary tract. Among his famous patients were the *bon vivant* Diamond Jim Brady and President Woodrow Wilson.

Alphonse Laveran (bottom right) This French military surgeon was awarded the 1907 Nobel Prize for his identification of the malarial parasite. But, try as he might, Laveran was unable to determine how the disease was transmitted.

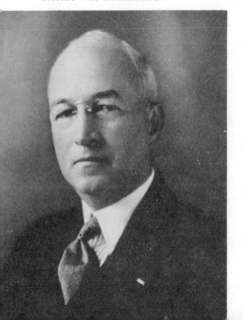

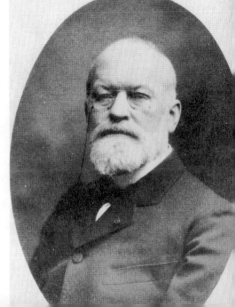

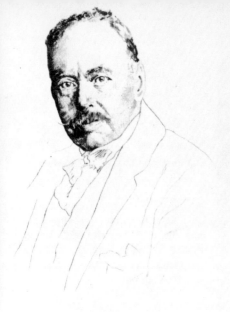

Ronald Ross Ross was a contentious, dissatisfied physician in the British Indian Medical Service when he proved that the malarial parasite is transmitted by the anopheles mosquito. The priority for this discovery, one of the most important in the science of infectious disease, was later bitterly contested, since Ross had done his work on bird malaria and was blocked by superiors before he could repeat his experiments in humans.

Marie Curie This French scientist, who discovered the elements radium and polonium, made valuable contributions to physics, chemistry, and medicine. Regettably, she suffered intensely in her last years from radiation burns incurred during her research.

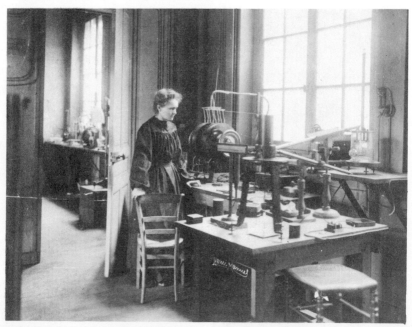

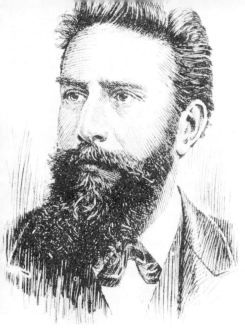

Wilhelm Roentgen When he discovered X rays in 1895, Roentgen was an obscure German physics professor. So simple were the rays to produce that he said nothing of his discovery to anyone until after it had been published, obviously fearful that a competitor might repeat the procedure and get into print first.

Paul Ehrlich (bottom left) "Dr. Fantasy," colleagues named Ehrlich for his belief that chemical "magic bullets" could be used to kill germs within the body and cure disease. But their snickering stopped when Ehrlich synthesized Salvarsan, the first effective drug against syphilis.

Frederick Grant Banting (bottom right) Banting was a young orthopedic surgeon when he set out to isolate the pancreatic hormone that prevents diabetes. Assisted by Charles Best, a fourth-year medical student, he succeeded spectacularly where the world's greatest physiologists had failed. A Rumanian physiologist, Nicolas Paulesco, who isolated insulin at the same time, is now largely forgotten, probably because his work was overlooked by the Nobel Committee when the Nobel Prize was awarded.

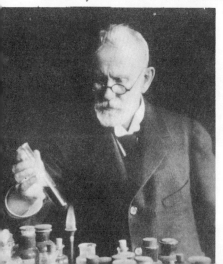

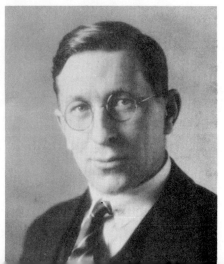

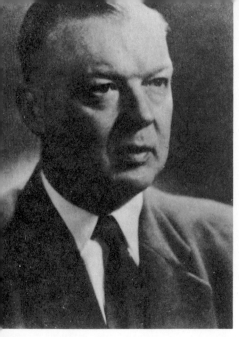

Werner Forssmann "People often ask me if I wasn't afraid," Forssmann remarked of his 1929 experiment in which he inserted a long tube through an arm vein into his own heart, then injected an iodine contrast medium to get an X-ray picture of the heart chambers. "I must confess that I was slightly nervous . . . and it took me a few days to make up my mind to carry out the injections." For this study that made possible the dramatic heart operations of today, Forssmann was awarded the 1956 Nobel Prize in Medicine.

Francis Crick, James Watson, and **Maurice Wilkins** These three scientists were awarded the 1962 Nobel Prize for their discovery of the structure of DNA, the most important finding in twentieth-century biology. Tragically, Rosalind Franklin, whose studies of the DNA molecule contributed to this discovery, was not cited by the Nobel Committee.

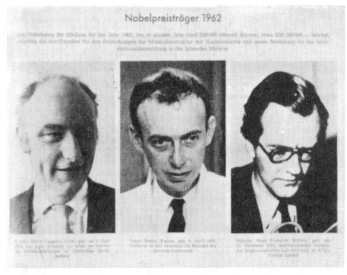

ian. The term *malaria* was first used in a French medical publication in 1743.

Malaria continued to spread throughout North America during the Revolutionary War. Whole British garrisons are recorded as having succumbed to the disease, and some historians even speculate that the eventual British surrender at Yorktown may have been partly due to a severe fever epidemic. But neither were the Americans spared; George Washington suffered several attacks. Washington was fortunate, however, because he was cured at least once by a remarkably effective malaria remedy—cinchona bark.

Cinchona, the Countess's Powder

For fifteen centuries after the death of Galen, countless malaria patients received the disastrous remedies that this ancient physician prescribed—bloodletting and purgation. The bleeding supposedly rid the body of "corrupt humors." The vomiting accompanying malaria was believed to be the body's attempt to expel poisons. What, therefore, could be better than a few good purges to help things along?

In fact, matters were not so simple. Each chill actually results from the destruction of thousands of red cells, and repeated bleedings only made the ensuing anemia that much worse. When compounded with the disability brought on by powerful purgatives (the gentle laxative did not exist in those days), the debilitating effects of the disease itself often finished off most sufferers in a short time. Lucky indeed were the country folk and townspeople too poor to afford the ministrations of the medical profession.

These common citizens turned to witchcraft, a form of treatment often less harmful than the orthodox methods. The Dominican scholar Albertus Magnus, teacher of St. Thomas Aquinas, may well have consulted a contemporary witchcraft text for this thirteenth-century remedy: "Take the urine of the patient and mix it with some flour to make a good dough thereof, of which seventy-seven small cakes are made. Proceed before sunrise to an anthill and throw the cakes therein. As soon as the insects devour the cakes the fever vanishes."

If the ants weren't hungry, Albertus had another potion: "The matron of a noble family cut the ear of a cat, let three drops of blood fall in some brandy, added a little pepper thereto, and gave it to the patient to drink."

Sound delicious? If not, there were other measures. The patient's body could be rubbed with chips from a gallows on which a criminal had been recently executed. At least the rationale here was not as complex as Galen's. Since the spirit causing malaria was an evil one, it could be warned off by a reminder of the penalty for heinous crimes.

In the mid-seventeenth century, from among the wealth of useless potions and incantations emerged cinchona bark. Its active principle, quinine, is the one naturally occurring substance effective against the malarial parasites.

Like another folk remedy, digitalis, cinchona has origins that remain shrouded in mystery. One story holds that the bark was first discovered by a member of a Peruvian Spanish garrison. This soldier, overcome by malaria, was left behind to die by his comrades. Tortured by thirst, he crawled to a shallow pond, where he drank deeply and fell asleep. On awakening he found that his fever had disappeared, and then he remembered that the water had a bitter taste. A large tree trunk, split by lightning, had fallen into the pool; the bark from this tree, the soldier soon discovered, had both the bitter taste and the remarkable power to cure malaria.

There are other stories. One famous tale attributes the identification of cinchona bark to South American Indians. These natives supposedly noted that sick mountain lions chewed on the bark of certain trees. Malaria patients were given the bark and found to be helped.

In 1630 the first written record of a malaria cure with cinchona bark appeared. Don Juan López de Canizares, the Spanish governor of Loxa, a flourishing Peruvian city, was relieved of fever by drinking a cinchona infusion. Three years later Antonio de la Calancha, an Augustinian monk, wrote, "A tree grows which they call the 'fever tree' in the country of Loxa, whose bark, of the color of cinnamon, made into powder amounting to the weight of two small silver coins and given as a beverage, cures the fevers and tertians; it has produced miraculous results in Lima."

At about the same time, the first cinchona bark appeared in Europe, probably as part of a shipment from the New World, but after years of controversy historians still don't know who first brought cinchona across the Atlantic.

The original candidate for this honor, the Countess of Chinchón, was designated in an account by an Italian, Sebastiano Bado, published in 1663. The fourth Count of Chinchón, Don Luis Gerónimo Fernández de Cabrera de Bobadilla Cerda y Mendoza, was appointed by Philip IV to rule the vast Spanish South American empire. The count and his wife, Señora Ana de Osorio, arrived in Lima in 1629. Shortly thereafter, according to Bado, the countess became severely ill with tertian fever, and news of her suffering soon spread throughout the colony. The governor of Loxa wrote the count, recommending that some of the same medicine by which he had been recently cured be given to Señora Ana. Don Juan was summoned to Lima, the remedy was given, and the countess was cured.

Soon the natives were swarming around the palace, both to express their joy at the recovery and to learn the secret of the remedy. Upon hearing the people's pleas, the generous Señora Ana ordered a large quantity of the bark and gave it personally to the sick. The grateful sufferers, all of whom were cured, named the new remedy *los polvos de la condeça,* "the countess's powder."

In 1639, according to Bado, the countess returned to Spain, bringing a large quantity of bark with her. She distributed her remedy among the peons on the Chinchón estate, and also sent some to an ailing theology professor at the University of Alcalá de Henares. At the same time, Juan de Vega, Señora Ana's physician, who had also returned to Spain with a supply of bark, sold part in Seville at an exorbitant price—one hundred reals per pound. This unscrupulous practice was to be repeated by many men in many places before the precious bark became readily available.

Bado's romantic tale was accepted without question by Carolus Linnaeus, the Swedish botanist, when he designated the genus of tree producing bhe bark as *Cinchona.* But, as is apparent, Linnaeus misspelled the name—or rather he spelled it as had Sebastiano Bado, who had partially Italianized the count's name, since *c* before *i* in Italian is pronounced like the Spanish (and English) *ch.* After Linnaeus's death the error was discovered, much too late to effect a change.

An even bigger mistake came to light in 1930, when the official diary of the Count of Chinchón was discovered. This diary was written by Don Antonio Suardo, the count's secretary, who recorded every minute of his boss's day with compulsive detail. A careful reading reveals multiple inconsistencies with Bado's account that suggest the latter is chimerical.

For example, the diary states that Ana de Osorio, the first Countess of Chinchón, died in Spain at least three years before Philip IV appointed the count viceroy of Peru. It was the second countess, Francisca Henríquez de Ribera, who accompanied her husband to South America. And while Doña Francisca continued to enjoy excellent health, the count had several episodes of fever, none of which was treated with bark.

Bado's story is totally demolished a few pages later, when Don Antonio records that even the second countess never returned to Spain; instead, she died in the port of Cartagena, Colombia, during the trip home. Juan de Vega, her supposed rascal of a physician, who, according to Bado, extorted enormous prices in Seville for the bark, never in fact left Peru because of an appointment as professor of medicine at the University of Lima. The count himself did return to Spain in 1641, and though he probably brought some bark with him, none reached the professor at the University of Alcalá de Henares, for this theologian had already been cured of his fever two years earlier.

In light of the evidence in Don Antonio's diary, historians have been forced to conclude that cinchona bark appeared in Europe entirely by accident. Another Peruvian bark, balsam, was a popular though worthless remedy for syphilis, and since the two barks could not be readily distinguished, greedy merchants substituted one for the other. Only later was cinchona seen to be of value in malarial fever, a condition which may have been mistaken for syphilis in some cases.

The first Europeans to appreciate the true value of cinchona were the Jesuits. Throughout the Spanish New World empire, Jesuit priests proselytized and cared for the natives and, in doing so, quickly ascertained the medicinal properties of the Peruvian bark. Large shipments were forwarded to the Jesuit pharmacy in Rome, where Juan Cardinal de Lugo ordered that the new medicine be given gratis to the ailing poor. While on a visit to Paris in 1649 the cardinal even used some of his cinchona to treat the young Louis XIV. After the king's recovery, the French eagerly embraced the new remedy.

But the English didn't. The Protestants were intensely suspicious of anything related to "popery," especially "Jesuit's bark," which was said to be nothing more than a Catholic plot to rid the world of heretics. Oliver Cromwell, who had ordered the execution of Charles I, steadfastly refused cinchona during a severe attack of malaria in 1658, and died as a result.

In other countries that initially accepted cinchona the drug was sometimes used improperly. For example, the Austrian governor general of the Netherlands, Archduke Leopold William, was given cinchona with excellent results by Chifflet, his physician. But when the malaria recurred a month later, the archduke blamed the cinchona and foolishly refused to take more. His subsequent demise gave the medicine a bad name throughout Europe, and even Chifflet somehow came to believe that cinchona "fixed the humors" while reducing the fever, making recurrence certain and death likely.

The widespread resistance to the use of cinchona was finally overcome by Robert Talbor, an English quack. Talbor was born in Cambridge in 1642, one year after the death of the Countess of Chinchón in Colombia. He entered St. John's College but dropped out at the age of twenty-one, becoming apprenticed to a Cambridge apothecary from whom he first learned of cinchona.

At this time, Thomas Sydenham, an eminent English physician, published a book called *Method for Curing the Fever*. A firm believer in the remedies of Hippocrates and Galen, Sydenham staunchly adhered to the old humoral theory of malaria. Grudgingly, though, he admitted that cinchona might be of some benefit if given after the fever had declined.

Yet just as Sydenham's halfhearted endorsement appeared, word came from the marshy, malaria-infested Essex coast that Talbor, a nonphysician, was curing malaria with a secret remedy. By 1668 Talbor had become so successful that he was able to establish a London practice which quickly came to include high government figures. The apogee was reached when he cured Charles II of malaria, an act which earned the former college dropout knighthood and an appointment as court physician. All the while, Talbor adamantly refused to reveal the contents of his remedy, skillfully disguising the bitter taste of the cinchona with opium and wine. Further to protect his secret, he made careful slurs against the Jesuit's bark.

The Royal College of Physicians was furious at Talbor's doings and advocated his prosecution for practicing medicine without a license. But the king would not hear of such a thing; in an angry, threatening letter, he warned the College members that any interference with Talbor would be certain to arouse the royal displeasure.

The king went even further to demonstrate faith in his new physician. When the dauphin, last living son of Louis XIV, became ill with fever, Charles II sent Talbor to the French court as a gesture of goodwill. Louis had sheltered the English monarch in his period of exile during the Protectorate of Cromwell. Now the favor was returned. Sir Robert cured the stricken dauphin.

Anxious to learn the secret of the marvelous remedy, Louis XIV asked Talbor to name his price. As a consequence, Louis got the secret with the proviso that it would not be made public until after Talbor's death. The king could have saved money had he only remembered his childhood cure by the same remedy. Sir Robert was made chevalier, given the enormous sum of three thousand gold crowns, and awarded a pension for life.

And he continued to effect miraculous cures: the Prince de Condé, the Duc de la Rochefoucauld. When the queen of Spain became ill with fever, Louis sent Sir Robert to treat her, too.

Forbidden to employ the new remedy, the jealous French physicians tried vainly to humiliate this foreign upstart. "What is fever?" they asked.

"I do not know," replied the wily Talbor. "You gentlemen may explain the nature of fever; but I can cure it, which you cannot."

After returning to England, Talbor, now rich and famous, tried to become even richer. Covertly he cornered the cinchona market by buying all the bark he could find. But he did not live long enough to enjoy his wealth. He died in 1681 at the age of thirty-nine, and was interred in Cambridge's Holy Trinity Church.

Fearing that in death his enemies in the medical profession would defame his memory, Talbor included a bit of professional advertising in his epitaph: "most honourable Robert Talbor, Knight and Singular Physician, unique in curing Fevers of which he had delivered Charles II King of England, Louis XIV King of France, the Most Serene Dauphin, Princes, many a Duke and a large number of lesser personages." In the same church, another imposing tablet hailed him even more eloquently as "Febrium Malleus," smasher of fevers.

In 1682, shortly after Sir Robert Talbor's death, Louis XIV ordered the secret of the fever remedy revealed. Nicholas de Blegny, physician-in-ordinary to the king, thereupon wrote a small book which was quickly translated into English: *The English Remedy: Or Talbor's Wonderful Secret for the Curing of Agues and Fevers—Sold by the Author, Sir Robert Talbor to the Most Christian King and since his Death ordered by His Majesty to be published in French, for the Benefit of his Subjects.* Cinchona had been included in the London Pharmacopoeia in 1677, but the new French book greatly increased the drug's popularity.

At the beginning of the eighteenth century, as the use of cinchona spread throughout Europe, apothecaries and chemists began to question what specific substance contained in the bark was active against malaria. The identification of an active principle was important for at least two reasons. First, since unscrupulous traders sometimes substituted medicinally worthless bark for the real thing, ability to identify the active principle chemically would prevent a pharmacologic flim-flam from being perpetrated on consumers. Second, even the real bark varied greatly in potency; only by extracting the active agent could dosage be standardized.

The first attempt to isolate the active principle in cinchona was made by Count Claude de la Garaye, a French pharmacist. In 1745 Garaye announced that he had successfully extracted the "essential salt." Unfortunately, Garaye's preparation was soon found to be no more effective against malaria than ordinary table salt.

A French chemist, Antoine François Fourcroy, confronted the problem next. Fourcroy, possessed of considerably more ego than chemical ability, was insanely jealous of his rival, Lavoisier, and conspired with the revolutionary terrorists to guillotine him. Though ultimately succeeding in this nefarious task, Fourcroy failed in his studies of cinchona. In 1790 he did extract a resinous substance with the characteristic color of the bark and for a time maintained that he had isolated the active principle. When the resin was later found medicinally worthless, he made a number of observations that brought him quite close to the discovery of quinine. But he gave up too soon, writing only that "these researches will no doubt lead to the discovery one day of an antiperiodic febrifuge, which, once known, may be extracted from various vegetables." And so today Fourcroy is mainly remembered for the glowing eulogy he delivered at a ceremony in Lavoisier's memory.

Armand Seguin, Fourcroy's student, did no better than his teacher. Somehow he came to the absurd conclusion that the active principle in cinchona was gelatin and published his findings despite inadequate experimental data. For years thereafter, many physicians reading Seguin's paper adopted clarified glue to treat their malaria patients.

This enormous error is all the more surprising because Seguin was actually quite a facile chemist. In 1804 he devised a method for extracting morphine from opium, and he read his results to a scientific meeting, though he did not publish them for ten years. Such hesitation was unfortunate because in 1806 Friederich Sertürner, a German chemist, published his technique for isolating morphine and so is now credited with this discovery. Besides being hesitant, Seguin was also a rather devious fellow, and was once punished by Napoleon for selling adulterated drugs to the French Army.

The first partially successful separation of the active principle from cinchona was achieved in 1811 by a Portuguese naval surgeon named B. A. Gomez. But the unlucky Gomez happened to choose a quinine-poor variety of cinchona known as the gray bark. The crystalline powder he isolated and named "cinchonine" was in reality a mixture of quinine and another chemical. Only good fortune permitted the eventual discoverers of quinine to recognize Gomez's mistake.

These two men were French pharmacists, Joseph Pelletier and Joseph Bienaimé Caventou. Both were exceptionally gifted scientists, especially Caventou, who at age twenty-two was appointed full professor of toxicology at the École de Pharmacie in Paris. The technique for isolating morphine had inspired their work, and they had previously used Sertürner's method to extract emetine from ipecac, strychnine and brucine from nux vomica, carmine from cochineal, and veratrine from sabadilla seeds. Some of these alkaline compounds, called alkaloids, were once widely employed in medical therapeutics: strychnine as a central nervous system stimulant, emetine as a treatment for amebiasis, and veratrine as a heart drug. Today most have been discarded, though carmine is still employed as a tissue stain and strychnine survives as a rat poison.

In 1817, learning of Gomez's work, Pelletier and Caventou correctly guessed that the active principle of cinchona was an alkaloid and therefore extractable by Sertürner's method. Like Gomez they began with the gray bark and so were able to isolate only a quinine-poor powder, medicinally worthless. But then they recalled that gray bark was sold very cheaply because of its questionable ability to cure malaria. Another substance, however, called yellow bark, was of great curative value. From yellow bark Pelletier and Caventou succeeded in isolating a sticky, pale yellow gum that could not be induced to crystallize. The gum was soluble in acid, alcohol, and ether and highly effective against malaria. The two men named the new chemical quinine after *quinquina,* an old Peruvian Indian name for the bark.

Pelletier and Caventou, like Pasteur a few years later, refused any profit from their discovery. Instead of patenting the extraction process, they published all the details so that anyone could manufacture quinine. They received many honors, the greatest of which was the Prix Monthyon of ten thousand francs awarded by the French Institute of Science.

Yet quinine remained difficult to obtain; a hundred years after it had been brought to Europe, Peru was still its only source. And early attempts to remove cinchona plants from the country were uniformly jinxed.

The first was made in 1735 by Charles de la Condamine, a French naturalist and explorer. Condamine was determined to bring the trees back to France and grow rich selling the bark. He collected a large number of seedlings, planted them in boxes of earth, and then braved swamps, jungles, hostile natives, dangerous animals, and wild river rapids to reach the coast. After a perilous eight-month journey, within sight of the ship for Paris, his small boat was swamped by a wave and his plants washed away.

One member of Condamine's expedition, Joseph de Jussieu, remained in the South American jungles for seventeen years to study cinchona. When he decided to return to France in 1761, he carried with him cinchona seeds packed into a wooden strongbox. But on the day of departure from Buenos Aires, a "trusted servant" made off with the box in the mistaken belief that it was filled with money. Jussieu returned to France ten years later, hopelessly insane.

Other endeavors also failed. A Jesuit expedition was able to transport cinchona seedlings to Algeria, but the plants died in their new home. Seeds carried to Paris and Java by French and Dutch expeditions failed to germinate. In 1860 an English government clerk, Clements Robert Markham, carried seedlings to England; shortly thereafter, a distinguished botanist, Dr. Richard Spruce, did the same. These plants supplied the London market for only six years before being destroyed by insects. Spruce had contracted severe rheumatism and intermittent paralysis in the South American jungles and spent the last twenty years of his life flat on his back, a hopeless, penniless invalid.

In the meantime, to protect their monopoly, Peruvian authorities had barred foreigners from the cinchona forests. But in 1865 Charles

Ledger, an Englishman living in Peru, obtained sixteen pounds of seed from a loyal native servant. A pound of this seed was sold to the Dutch in Java, and though apparently decayed on arrival, it germinated readily, giving birth to an enormous Dutch cinchona industry. Finally, the high price of quinine was driven down, and for the first time the drug was made available for large numbers of impoverished malaria sufferers.

The Parasite

Still, quinine could only suppress malaria, not prevent it. And the cause of the disease remained unknown. Far into the nineteenth century most medical men continued to believe the old ideas about bad air. In Robert Louis Stevenson's *Treasure Island,* for example, Jim Hawkins tells of Dr. Livesey's first impression of the island from aboard the ship *Hispaniola:*

> There was not a breath of air moving, nor a sound but that of the surf booming half a mile away along the beaches and against the rocks outside. A peculiar stagnant smell hung over the anchorage—a smell of sodden leaves and rotting tree trunks. I observed the doctor sniffing and sniffing, like someone tasting a bad egg.
> "I don't know about treasure," he said, "but I'll stake my wig there's fever here."

Where did the poisons in the swamp air come from? Some believed that they were given off by marsh vegetation; others held that they were elaborated by microscopic animals. One American physician, James K. Mitchell, wrote that malaria was due to certain spores present in marshy regions.

But in 1846 Giovanni Rasori, an Italian physician, guessed with remarkable accuracy the true cause of malaria. "For many years," he wrote, "I have held the opinion that the intermittent fevers are produced by parasites which renew the paroxysm by the act of their reproduction which recurs more or less rapidly according to the nature of the species."

Rasori's intuition was soon supported by a bit of experimental evidence. In 1867 a German pharmacologist, Karl Binz, discovered that quinine was highly toxic to the tiny organisms in impure water. This finding suggested that a similar type of microscopic animal might cause malaria. Binz went on to make other studies of the properties of quinine and devised a chemical procedure for detecting small amounts of the drug in urine.

Twelve years after Binz's work, malaria research suddenly took a wrong turn. The powerful influence of the germ theory of disease had convinced most scientists that all epidemic diseases were caused by bacteria. Thus a great deal of excitement and very little skepticism greeted the announcement that a malaria bacillus had been found.

The discoverers were Edwin Klebs, the German pathologist who had isolated the diphtheria bacillus, and Corrado Tommasi-Crudeli, an Italian bacteriologist. Working in the Roman Campagna, these two scientists isolated a microbe from the soil, a short rod that they named *"Bacillus malariae."* This organism, they wrote, could be found in damp soil and low-lying air in malarious regions, and would grow on fish gelatin. Soil infested with the bacteria, when injected into rabbits, was said to produce a malarial fever and enlargement of the spleen; soil from malaria-free regions caused a different sort of fever and splenic change. The two authors even asserted that humans receiving an injection of pure *"Bacillus malariae"* cultures would develop the symptoms of malaria. Probably no scientific article ever written has contained more wishful thinking than this one.

Klebs's reputation was so great that when others attempted to duplicate his findings and failed, many in the medical community were not dissuaded from believing in the existence of a *"Bacillus malariae."* In an 1879 editorial, one prestigious British medical journal declared that the malaria problem had been solved.

And in reality, the correct solution was at hand, though no one recognized it at first. For centuries, the victims of malaria were seen to have a characteristic black pigmentation of the brain and spleen, first described in 1716 by Giovanni Maria Lancisi. In 1847 a German physician, Heinrich Meckel, discovered the origin of this pigmentation. After a careful microscopic study of tissue from malaria victims, Meckel was able to identify round, ovoid, or spindle-shaped structures containing black pigment granules. Though Meckel's work was consistently confirmed by many others, the little black granular bodies were somehow never suspected to be the cause of malaria, despite the fact that their presence in the blood was soon noted in malaria victims.

So characteristic were the granular bodies in the blood of malaria patients that they proved crucial in a murder trial. In 1878 a Mississippi village storekeeper was robbed and savagely slain. His bloody body, its skull brutally fractured, was found in his blood-spattered store. Immediately, a riverman with a larcenous reputation was spied to have fresh bloodstains on his clothes and arrested by the ever-vigilant sheriff. But confronted with his evil deed, the thug staunchly proclaimed his innocence. The stains, he said, were paint from barrels he had loaded on a steamer.

In order to disprove this fishy alibi, the sheriff consulted Dr. Joseph Jones, a professor of chemistry in the medical department of the University of Louisiana, who was frequently called as an expert witness in forensic medicine. Obtaining specimens of the victim's blood, Jones found pigmented malaria bodies. An inquiry with the local physician revealed that the storekeeper had been afflicted with fever shortly before death.

Dr. Jones then examined stains from the riverman's clothing and found them to be human bloodstains, not paint stains, as the suspect had claimed. Jones also demonstrated that the bloodstains held the same malarial bodies discovered in the blood of the victim. A thoroughly convinced jury subsequently convicted the riverman.

Two years later another scientist, Alphonse Laveran, found that the pigmented malarial bodies were the cause, not the result, of malaria. But the scientific community proved to be much more difficult to sway than a Mississippi jury.

Laveran was born in Paris in 1845, the son and grandson of French military surgeons. After military training and medical school, he was assigned as surgeon to Paris's St. Martin Hospital. A few weeks later, when the Franco-Prussian War erupted, Laveran was shipped to the front. There he served with distinction in numerous campaigns before being taken prisoner at the Battle of Metz.

At the close of the war the young surgeon returned to the Paris hospital, where he took a particular interest in studying the infectious diseases of soldiers. So innovative was his work that he was appointed to the chair of epidemics and diseases of armies in 1874, the identical post his father had held for many years. But in his new job Laveran found that teaching and administration precluded most research. Finally in 1878 these burdens were removed when he was transferred to the military hospital at Constantine, Algeria.

In Constantine, Laveran was confronted with a particularly vexing problem—malaria. The hospitals were full of it. Whole platoons were decimated by it, and rarely could an entire squadron be assembled at once for active duty. New recruits succumbed with sickening regularity, always showing on autopsy the same graphite pigmentation of the brain and spleen, the same black granular microscopic bodies in the blood.

No more appropriate investigator could have been found to investigate this disease than the calm, reserved, unemotional Laveran. He was as slow and methodical in his speech as in his work, a stiff, aloof, quiet man; yet he was exceptionally astute both as physician and scientist.

For two years Laveran sweated under the burning Algerian sun as he pored over tissue specimens from malaria victims. All of his efforts revealed to him nothing more than the changes already described by Lancisi and Meckel. In desperation he decided to confine his search to the fresh blood of malaria patients—an extremely lucky choice.

Still not knowing what he was looking for, Laveran began taking blood specimens from pinpricks in the fingers of sick soldiers. After spreading a droplet into a thin film on a glass slide, he would peer at it for hours through a small, crude microscope.

Laveran had no difficulty locating the little malarial bodies filled with their tiny black granules. They had been seen many times before and accepted without question as the result of malarial infection. But on November 6, 1880, while examining a fresh blood specimen taken from a new hospital arrival, his eye was caught by a moving object on the slide. Under high power, this proved to be a tiny malarial body wriggling vigorously. Laveran watched amazed as the little crescent-shaped object lashed about so energetically that an entire red blood cell jiggled. Even the pigment granules appeared to be in frenzied motion. Why had this important observation—which was to win for Laveran the 1907 Nobel Prize in Medicine—never been made before? Probably because no previous investigator had used wet blood films.

Instantly, Laveran realized that he had found the cause of malaria —a tiny, living organism. He named the parasite *Oscillaria malariae* and identified it within the blood of 148 other patients out of a total of 192 examined. It developed, he observed, from a small, colorless structure one-sixth the size of a red cell, gradually growing as large as the cell and meanwhile forming pigment granules. The larger malarial parasites had a crescent shape with pigment granules arranged in a ring. These organisms, often quite active, would suddenly produce lashing, whiplike filaments.

From his observations, Laveran deduced that the large, crescent-shaped organism was the fully developed parasite or "perfect form," as he called it. After growing over a period of days, imbibing nourishment from the red cell, the parasite could survive independently in the blood. The appearance of filaments represented the climax of the process. Tertian, quartan, and quotidian malaria, he believed, occurred during different stages in the parasite's development. Laveran wrote a letter to the Academy of Medicine in Paris, communicating his discovery.

The observations were quickly confirmed. Laveran reported them to a friend, Dr. E. Richard, stationed at Philippeville, a French Mediterranean military base fifty miles from Constantine. After finding the fully developed, wriggling parasite, Richard identified an even younger form than Laveran had seen—merely a tiny, colorless spot in the red cell. Laveran believed that the organism lived on the surface of the cell, but Richard correctly observed that it developed within the cell, growing larger and larger until it finally burst out.

In the face of such apparently incontrovertible evidence, the European scientific community remained unconvinced. So powerful an influence was the new bacteriology that no one could believe the pigmented malarial bodies were the cause of malaria. The arguments presented by Klebs and Tommasi-Crudeli for their *"Bacillus malariae"* had been accepted almost without question, and an Italian pathologist, Ettore Marchiafava, even claimed to have found the bacillus in several dead malaria patients. Laveran traveled to Rome in 1882 to demonstrate the parasites to Marchiafava, but failed to shake the pathologist's belief in the bacillus.

The Americans, however, were more open minded about the matter, since patriotic considerations were not involved. To resolve the controversy, the Army sent Major George Sternberg to study malaria in New Orleans, where the incidence was particularly high. Sternberg, a graduate of New York's College of Physicians and Surgeons, had attained great standing as a bacteriologist. He had isolated *Diplococcus pneumoniae,* the germ of pneumonia, at the same time as Pasteur, and later developed an antityphoid vaccine. During the Spanish-American War he was appointed surgeon general.

On arriving in New Orleans, Sternberg assembled a laboratory and began making bacterial cultures from the air, from mud, and from nearby marshes. No organism he found was capable of producing malaria in an animal. By 1881 he had shown positively that the *"Bacillus malariae"* of Klebs and Tommasi-Crudeli was not responsible for malaria.

In 1884 Marchiafava, too, became convinced that a bacterium was not involved. Studying wet-blood smears with the new oil-immersion lens, he was able to perceive wriggling even in the earliest forms of the parasite. With Angelo Celli, another physician, he verified unequivocally Laveran's observations. *Plasmodium malariae,* the name chosen for the parasite by the two Italians, turned out to be an incorrect one, since the organism is not actually a plasmodium. But like the dropped *h* in *Cinchona,* the name stuck despite years of haggling.

The old ideas about bad air tended to persist as well. In 1886 Dr. William Osler, an authority on blood microscopy, stated that the malarial bodies were nothing more than incidental findings. When persuaded by a colleague, Dr. William T. Councilman, to reconsider, Osler spent many hours looking at wet-blood films. After convincing himself that there were indeed parasites present, Osler decreed that no patient in his clinic could be declared to have malaria without a positive demonstration of the malarial bodies in the blood. In this way, other diseases—typhoid, infectious hepatitis, dysentery—would no longer be confused with malaria.

Yet in the first edition of his textbook *The Principles and Practice of Medicine,* in 1892, Osler continued to maintain a peculiar ambivalence toward the cause of malaria, stating only that the work of Laveran and others pointed "strongly in favor" of a malarial parasite that produced the disease. Though devoting two pages of text to the parasite studies and the repudiated *"Bacillus malariae,"* Osler spent almost another whole page rehashing the old bad-air theory. "Many facts," he wrote, "are on record which seem to indicate that the poison may be carried to some distance by winds." A few lines later, he remarked, "That the distribution of the poison of malaria is influenced by gravity has long been conceded." He even intimated that susceptibility might be related to social stratum, a comfortably Victorian notion: ". . . the majority of cases admitted into hospital are of the poorer class, who have returned from picking cranberries and peaches in Delaware and New Jersey."

Despite Osler's reservations, evidence for the parasite theory continued to pile up. An especially important contribution was made by the Italian pathologist Camillo Golgi. Golgi showed that when the malarial chill occurred, the parasite could be seen to segment like a cut pie. This segmentation was different in cases of tertian and quartan malaria, implying that the two diseases were caused by two distinct parasites.

Many scientists accepted Golgi's findings, but others—including Laveran—did not. The dissenters pointed to the work of a Russian physiologist, Basil Danielewsky, who had shown that malaria could occur in birds; they also cited additional studies identifying bat malaria and monkey malaria. How could so many varieties of parasite cause essentially the same disease?

The argument was ultimately settled by better blood-staining methods, and Golgi was shown to be correct. Many parasite varieties did indeed exist, often developing in the blood at different rates of speed. In each species there was a segmented form that reproduced by division and an ovoid form that never segmented.

At first, the role of the ovoid form was unclear. Many scientists held that extrusion of flagella by the ovoids was a sort of death spasm. But in 1897 Dr. William G. McCallum of Johns Hopkins found the true function of this process. Under the microscope McCallum saw one flagellum break away from its ovum, dart across the microscopic field, and penetrate another ovoid without flagella. He correctly recognized the process as fertilization of a female germ cell by a male cell. More study suggested that only plasmodia outside the body behaved in this fashion.

Though McCallum had been working with the parasite of bird malaria, his observation raised an important question about the human form of the disease. Did sexual reproduction of the parasite occur within the human host or somewhere else?

To answer this question, a knowledge of the mechanism of transmission of the malarial parasite is required. Laveran, the discoverer of the parasite, tried to provide an answer. In 1896 he left the army to join the Pasteur Institute. Now world famous, he continued to study tropical diseases and eventually identified more than twenty new organisms. As the grand old man of French military and tropical medicine, he often would discomfit the generals by publicly warning of the dangers of malaria in a particular area. But the positive identification of the mosquito as vector of malaria—one of the most dramatic and influential discoveries in the science of healing—was not made by the calm, methodical, persistent Alphonse Laveran. The man responsible for this discovery turned out to be Ronald Ross, one of the most surprising, colorful, unlikely characters in the history of medicine.

The Vector of Malaria

The belief that mosquitoes transmit disease is a truly ancient one, which originated thousands of years before Patrick Manson proved that these insects carry filariasis. A red, swollen, painful mosquito bite has always been viewed as harmful, and references exist throughout recorded history to a connection between mosquitoes and fevers.

The oldest, written several thousand years ago in cuneiform script on clay tablets, attributes malaria to Nergal, the Babylonian god of destruction and pestilence, pictured as a double-winged, mosquito-like insect. A few centuries later, Philistines settling in Canaan, on the eastern shore of the Mediterranean, were told by the natives of the god Beelzebub, lord of the insects. The evil reputation of this deity increased through the ages until the early Jews named him "Prince of the Devils."

The ancient Hindus were no less conscious of the mosquito's harmful potential. In 800 B.C. the sage Dhandantari wrote, "Their bite is as painful as that of the serpents, and causes diseases. . . . [The wound] as if burnt with caustic or fire, is red, yellow, white, and pink color, accompanied by fever, pain of limbs, hair standing on end, pains, vomiting, diarrhea, thirst, heat, giddiness, yawning, shivering, hiccups, burning sensation, intense cold. . . ."

So conscious were the ancient Romans of the association between mosquitoes and malaria that city officials would routinely prohibit human habitation in mosquito-infested districts. To protect themselves from the notorious Campagna mosquitoes, shepherds returning from a summer in the Apennines furnished their small cabins with a few sheep to satisfy the ravenous insects, thereby hoping to avoid malaria. Such a tactic was encouraged by the first-century B.C. agriculturist Collumella, who wrote, "A marsh always throws up noxious and poisonous steams during the heats and breeds animals armed with mischievous stings which fly upon us in exceeding thick swarms . . . whereby hidden diseases are often contracted, the cause of which even the physicians themselves cannot thoroughly understand."

Collumella's excellent observation was subverted for fifteen hundred years by Galen's dogmatic, widely accepted medical theories that attributed malaria to internal causes. But early in the seventeenth century Giovanni Maria Lancisi revived the old idea that mosquitoes might play a role. This Italian physician is one of the most remarkable figures in the history of malaria, for by intuition alone he came close to divining the causative agent, "microscopic worms," and he guessed the means of spread.

Lancisi was born in Rome in 1654 to middle-class parents, and, like his countryman Spallanzani, studied theology for a time before turning to natural science. After mastering anatomy, chemistry, and botany at the Collegio de Sapienza, he was awarded his doctorate at age eighteen. By age thirty he had been appointed professor of anatomy at his alma mater, and at age forty-three he was named professor of the theory and practice of medicine, a position he held until his death in 1720.

The extraordinary powers of observation Lancisi demonstrated soon attracted the attention of Innocent XI, who appointed him a papal physician in 1688. The appointment was renewed by Innocent XII and his successor, Clement XI. When Clement commissioned Lancisi to investigate the cause of sudden death in Rome, the resulting study became a classic in the history of cardiology. A voluminous writer, Lancisi composed three other major treatises, including the important *Aneurysms of the Heart and Blood Vessels,* a work which lucidly describes the vascular changes in syphilis. But today he is best known for his two-volume monograph *Noxious Emanations of Swamps and Their Cure.*

In this monograph, written in 1717 at the height of his fame, Lancisi postulates two ways in which malaria might be spread by mosquitoes. In one, the insects deposit microscopic organisms in uncovered food and drink, and the human consumption of this contaminated material produces the disease. Though not applicable to malaria, this hypothesis suggests Lancisi was aware that disease could be spread by food. And, in fact, typhoid—which at the time was frequently confused with malaria—is transmitted in this fashion.

Lancisi's second postulated mechanism was the correct one for malaria. Mosquitoes, he writes, "always inject their salivary juices into the small wounds which are opened by the insects on the surface of the body." Because "all their viscera are filled with deleterious liquids . . . no controversy can arise among professional men concerning the harmful effect which the insects of the swamps, by mixing their injurious juices with the saliva . . . inflict upon us." But, lacking proof, Lancisi conceded that there might still be some validity in the old bad-air theory.

Almost a century after this monograph appeared, a physician living in America, John Crawford, wrote a series of essays contradicting the bad-air theory. Crawford, an Irishman, had worked as ship's doctor on East India Company vessels before accepting a Dutch position in Guiana on the east coast of South America. But when the colony shifted from Dutch to British hands in 1796 and Crawford found himself without a job, he was helped by a wealthy brother-in-law to establish a thriving practice in Baltimore. It was here that he began to write about malaria.

Crawford developed his ideas about this disease by observing the behavior of a particular species of fly. After the adult insect laid its eggs in the body of a host animal, Crawford noted that the host perished when the eggs hatched. Malaria, too, he asserted, was "occasioned by eggs insinuated, without our knowledge, into our bodies." These eggs, laid during a mosquito bite, hatched in the wound and migrated through the host's body, producing the manifestations of malaria.

So absurd were these notions considered by contemporaries that local medical journals summarily rejected all of Crawford's articles. Eventually these were published in a little weekly paper, *The Observer and Repertory of Original and Selected Essays in Verse and Prose, on Topics of Polite Literature,* founded by Crawford and edited by his daughter Eliza. Disillusioned with the publishing business, Eliza quit after a year to marry a prosperous Baltimore architect. But before the little paper folded, the theories on fever had gotten into print.

Crawford's newly expanded bibliography in no way helped his professional standing. "The wildest of philosophical vagaries,"

sniffed his contemptuous colleagues. Soon he was being disparaged
so loudly that his medical practice began to suffer. Fearing ruin, he
carried his ideas no further. Yet the old miasma theory was finally
beginning to crumble, and within a few years Crawford's ideas were
echoed by two other Americans, Josiah Clark Nott and Lewis Daniel
Beauperthy.

Nott, a South Carolinian by birth, was a prominent surgeon in
Mobile, Alabama. Since malaria and yellow fever were widespread in
the South, Nott had considerable opportunity to observe these two
maladies, and he became convinced that an insect was involved. In
his essay "Yellow Fever Contrasted with Bilious Fever," published in
1850, he dismissed the miasma theory as worthless, arguing that both
diseases were caused by microscopic "insects" somehow transmitted
through mosquitoes.

A much clearer statement of this notion was formulated by Lewis
Beauperthy, a "traveling naturalist" for the Paris Museum in Vene-
zuela. In 1854 Beauperthy wrote that malaria and yellow fever "are
produced by venomous fluid injected under the skin by mosquitoes
like poison injected by snakes." Marshes and swamps, he added,
were not made treacherous by their miasmic vapors but by the mosquitoes that proliferated within them.

While the speculations of Nott and Beauperthy caused little stir,
those of Albert Freeman Africanus King generated considerable public interest. King, a graduate of the National Medical College, now
George Washington University, received his third name because his
father was a great advocate of African colonization. After service
with the Confederate Army during the Civil War, the young surgeon
returned to Washington, D.C., just in time to attend a performance of
Our American Cousin in Ford's Theater, April 14, 1865. He was sitting in an orchestra seat when John Wilkes Booth fired his fatal bullet. Climbing into Lincoln's box, King rendered first aid, then helped
carry the dying President to a rooming house across the street.

Though he eventually became a gynecologist at George Washington University and author of a famous obstetrics textbook, King
could not help but spend much of his time treating and thinking
about malaria. Because of its warm, moist climate and slimy
marshes, Washington was as filled with this disease as with bureau-
crats. During the notoriously feverish summers, the demand for quinine to medicate the thousands of new cases was enormous.

On February 10, 1882, King presented his ideas on malaria to the

Philosophical Society of Washington, and in September 1883 this lecture was published in *Popular Science Monthly*. The characteristics, King said, "may be explicable by the supposition that the mosquito is the real source of the disease rather than the inhalation or cutaneous absorption of a marsh vapor." After listing nineteen sound reasons for implicating the mosquito as the vector, he added, "While the data to be presented cannot be held to prove the theory, they may go so far as to initiate and encourage experiment and observation by which the truth or fallacy of the views held may be demonstrated . . . which either way, will be a step in the line of progress. . . ."

King's article attracted enormous popular attention, but in the end his ideas came to naught. Almost two centuries earlier, Lancisi had proposed the draining of marshes to eradicate malaria. King, a much more grandiose and impractical man, had an even better idea. Washington could be ridded of malaria, he claimed, by surrounding the entire city with an enormous screen of fine mosquito netting as high as the Washington Monument.

This farfetched suggestion was greeted with an enormous guffaw. Even today no one is certain whether King was serious or whether he might have been attempting a joke. But his crackpot plan roundly discouraged anyone reading his paper from testing the highly sensible mosquito hypothesis.

Mosquito Manson's Inspiration

At the time that Albert Freeman Africanus King's article appeared, Patrick Manson in China was also speculating about the nature of malaria. The regularity of the chills and fever seemed to Manson quite analogous to the periodicity of parasite appearance in filariasis. Could malaria, he wondered, also be caused by a parasite transmitted by a mosquito?

In 1878 Manson had begun to study the blood of malaria patients, intending to see whether a blood-borne agent was responsible for the fever. Unable to detect any abnormality, he abandoned the effort until 1881, when he learned of the supposed discovery of the "*Ba-*

cillus malariae" by Klebs and Tommasi-Crudeli. But try as he might, Manson was never able to isolate the bacillus from the blood of a malaria victim.

Nevertheless, Manson was growing increasingly successful and famous as both a surgeon and scientist. In December 1883 he moved from Amoy to Hong Kong and soon built a thriving private practice. Besides caring for patients, he devoted himself to many matters of public interest: the organizing of a local medical society, the establishing of a dairy farm to provide milk for children and invalids, the founding of a new medical school. One of the first six students was Sun Yat-sen, the future Chinese political leader. Manson remembered Sun as an especially bright pupil and later came to his aid in London when the Chinese government began to harass the young man on account of his revolutionary proclivities.

In the meantime, Manson continued to search in vain for the "*Bacillus malariae*." Then in 1884 he learned of Laveran's discovery and immediately set out to identify the parasite for himself. The plasmodium, however, proved to be as elusive to Manson's eye as the bacillus had been.

But fortune was not nearly so slippery. Within a short time, Manson had accumulated so much money that in 1889 he left the Orient forever and retired to a country home in his native Scotland. Here he might have abandoned medical research and practice permanently, living the pleasant life of a landed English gentleman, except for a cruel quirk of fate.

Manson had imprudently left all of his holdings in the volatile Chinese currency. In 1890 a precipitous decline in the Chinese dollar wiped out his entire life's savings. Compelled once again to take up private practice, he established himself in London. He also took up the investigation of tropical disease by arranging with missionary societies to provide him with blood smears and other material from Africans and Orientals. Soon he acquired a post with the Seamen's Hospital Society, directing a London waterfront ward for sick sailors. The blood specimens of these men from all parts of the world finally revealed to him Laveran's malarial parasite.

After seeing the plasmodium, Manson studied the observations of Golgi, Laveran, and others. He then confirmed to his own satisfaction that there were indeed several species of parasite that could infect a human being, each having its own appearance and producing its own symptoms and signs. Especially intriguing to Manson was "exflagellation," the formation by the ovoid form of the tiny, whip-like appendages first reported by Laveran.

Other observers, noting that this phenomenon took place only in blood removed from the body, believed with Laveran that they were witnessing nothing more than a "death spasm." Such a notion fit in with the old Hippocratic idea that malaria might come from ingesting stagnant water, and it also conformed to the newer theory that the organism was transmitted by contaminated water—like cholera.

Manson, however, thought otherwise. To him, the exflagellation represented another phase in the parasite's development. "Since the flagella appear only when malarial blood gets outside the body," he reasoned, "their purpose must be to continue the life of the parasite in the outer world." This logic had stimulated him to seek an ex-tracorporeal form of the filaria of elephantiasis and had led directly to his discovery of the mosquito as the vector. In addition, two other parasitic diseases—Texas cattle fever and African sleeping sickness—had just been proved to be transmitted by insect vectors.

The work on Texas cattle fever had been done in 1893 by an American physician, Theobald Smith, and an epidemiologist, F. L. Kilborne. The two men had been assigned to study the disease as an epidemic threatened to bankrupt the American cattle industry. After meticulous, painstaking field work, Smith and Kilborne proved that Texas cattle fever was produced by a parasite that reproduced asex-ually in cow blood, but also went through a developmental phase within cattle ticks. Like the mosquitoes in filariasis, it was proved that the ticks transmitted the disease. Smith and Kilborne, however, went a step further than Manson by using the vector to infect healthy animals, thus furnishing the final link in the chain of evidence for the insect-transmission hypothesis.

One year later, in 1894, David Bruce, a British medical officer, identified the causative organism and vector of an African animal in-fection, called *nagana* by the natives. This disease had desolated great stretches of South Africa, making farming impossible. In blood specimens, Bruce located the tiny, rod-shaped parasite, called a try-panosome, as it darted from one red blood cell to another. Then, suspecting the tsetse fly, *Glossina morsitans,* to be the vector, Bruce was able to use the flies to infect healthy horses, concluding correctly that big-game animals served as a reservoir for the disease. These findings produced a storm of controversy, especially when Bruce later proved that the tsetse also carried the trypanosome responsible for two formidable human infections, Gambia fever and African sleeping sickness, and attributed all three diseases to the same organism. To refute Bruce, a German named Taute working in Portuguese East Africa injected himself with five cubic centimeters of blood from animals dying of nagana and allowed himself to be bitten with nagana-carrying tsetse flies—and lived. Mortified at being shown incorrect, Bruce vengefully commented, "It is a matter for some scientific regret that these experiments were not successful. . . . As it is, these negative experiments prove nothing."

Reasoning by analogy with the findings of Smith, Kilborne, and Bruce, Manson postulated a mechanism for the transmission of malaria. According to his schema, when a mosquito fed on the blood of a human with malaria, the flagellated form of the plasmodium ended up in the insect's stomach. From there it migrated into the tissues, where it grew into a form capable of infecting another human.

This part of Manson's hypothesis is correct. To be complete, it lacks only the finding that was to be made by McCallum in 1897: The flagellum from the male parasite form had to fertilize the female form before development within the mosquito could take place. But Manson tripped up when postulating how the parasite passed from the mosquito back to man because entomologists at the time believed that the insect died after depositing its eggs in water. The parasites, Manson theorized, escaped from the dead mosquito's body and were carried to the next victim by contaminated water. Thus he had neatly fitted in another piece of the puzzle, yet was still forced to fall back on the old Hippocratic notion that attributed malaria to the ingestion of stagnant water.

This new theory of malarial transmission was quickly published. To allow it to gain acceptance, Manson eagerly accepted invitations to lecture on it and discuss it. Unfortunately, the theory was considered far out by the scientific establishment, and Manson was not able to get hold of the malaria-carrying mosquitoes that would enable him to clinch his argument. He applied for a scientific grant so that he might travel to a malarious area abroad and collect the evidence he needed, but no money was forthcoming. Skeptical members of the Royal Society had refused to appoint him a delegate, effectively discouraging the official backing needed for work among colonial natives.

Manson, however, was an indefatigable teacher and demonstrator, whose reputation as a tropical-medicine expert continued to grow.

Invariably his medical advice was solicited by younger men returning from the far corners of the Empire. And one of these men, Surgeon Major Ronald Ross of the Indian Medical Service, was to solve the puzzle of malaria transmission—after considerable help from Manson. Unfortunately, generosity was not one of Ross's virtues, and when he was awarded the 1902 Nobel Prize in Medicine for his great achievement, he selfishly refused to share it with his former mentor. Still later, Ross's jealous dispute over priority with another malaria investigator, Giovanni Battista Grassi, grew into one of the most vitriolic feuds in the history of medicine.

Ross and the Birds

An old aphorism holds that only a person with intense devotion to a career can expect to become prominent in it. No piece of conventional wisdom could be less applicable to Ronald Ross, a man who never wanted to be a physician at all and who continually flaunted his distaste for the practice of medicine. Born in May 1857 in the Himalayan Mountains of India, only three days after the outbreak of the Indian mutiny, Ross effectively carried on the conflict for the remainder of his life by contemptuously rebelling against superiors and colleagues.

Ross's father, Campbell Claye Ross, a major in the Indian army, was as authentic-looking a soldier as Queen Victoria could have hoped for. He had a ferocious countenance framed by bellicose side whiskers. Ross's grandfather, Lieutenant Colonel Hugh Ross, had also been a fierce Indian border fighter.

At the age of eight, young Ronald was sent to England to continue his education. But, as he later wrote, he was told in no uncertain terms what career to pursue: "I wished to be an artist, but my father was opposed to this. I wished also to enter the Army or Navy; but my father had set his heart upon my joining the medical profession and, finally, the Indian Medical Service, which was then well paid and possessed many good appointments; and, as I was a dreamy boy not too well inclined towards uninteresting mental exertion, I resigned myself to this scheme. . . ."

Though not too willingly. Most of his time in medical school was spent composing music or writing poems and plays. Not surprisingly, he completed his medical studies "without distinction" and flunked the qualifying examinations for the Indian Medical Service. When his father threatened to cancel his allowance, he took a job as ship's surgeon on a vessel sailing between London and New York. In 1881 he repeated the qualifying examinations and this time ranked seventeenth of twenty-two successful candidates. After four months' indoctrination at the Army Medical School, Ronald Ross finally fulfilled his father's wish by entering the Indian Medical Service.

He had not been long in India before he encountered the mosquitoes that were to occupy him, in one way or another, for the rest of his life. Outside his bungalow quarters they bred in a barrel, swarming in to attack him through an open window. Ross solved the problem by simply tipping over the barrel, though not everyone approved of this solution.

"When I told the adjutant of this miracle," Ross wrote, "and pointed out that the mess house could be rid of mosquitoes in the same way (they were breeding in the garden tubs, in the tins under the dining table and even in the flower vases) much to my surprise he was very scornful and refused to allow men to deal with them, for he said it would be upsetting to the order of nature, and as mosquitoes were created for some purpose it was our duty to bear with them! I argued in vain that the same thesis would apply to bugs and fleas, and that according to him it was our duty to go about in a verminous condition." Then Ross added, with the contempt that was later to shower his enemies, "I did not know then that this type of fool is very common indeed."

Ross spent his first five years in India as a hostile, recalcitrant medical officer, doing all that was required of him but no more. Though he saw service in the Burma War and in the Andaman Islands, he was still denied the promotions that he felt he richly deserved. He spent his free time concocting equations he hoped would revolutionize mathematics and writing poetry, music, plays, and bad novels that he published at his own expense.

In addition, he developed an interest in the tropical diseases that were everywhere about him—especially malaria, which was estimated at the time to kill more than a million persons in India each year. Of his first impressions of malaria, characteristically, he composed some appropriate verse:

> In this, O Nature, yield I pray to me.
> I pace and pace, and think and think, and take
> The fever'd hands, and note down all I see,
> That some dim distant light may haply break.
>
> The painful faces ask, can we not cure?
> We answer, No, not yet; we seek the laws.
> O God, reveal thro' all this thing obscure
> The unseen, small, but million-murdering cause.

On his first furlough in 1888, a welcome respite from dull garrison life, Ross returned to London. During his busy stay, he wrote another bad novel, invented a new shorthand system, devised a phonetic spelling for the writing of verse, and was elected secretary of a local golf club. He also took up the study of the new science of bacteriology and was granted a diploma in public health. And during this busy year he found time to court and marry Miss Rosa Bloxam, with whom he returned to India.

Back at his post, Ross began to formulate theories of malaria. Initially ignorant of the existence of the parasite, he hypothesized that "the unseen, small, but million-murdering cause" might lie within the bowel, presumably some form of poisoning. But in 1892 he finally learned of Laveran's discovery when several papers describing the parasite were published in Indian medical journals. After reading these, Ross decided that the malarial bodies did not exist, and published numerous articles saying so.

Soon, however, doubts began to creep in, and Ross sent to England for Laveran's original publications. Then he spent hours peering through his microscope at blood smears, yet was unable to see the little wriggling crescents. Thoroughly exasperated, he strongly questioned the soundness of Laveran's observations and even wondered if the Frenchman might have falsified his data. This inability to confirm Laveran's work—a problem shared by many investigators—was apparently due to the crude microscopic techniques of the day and the inferior illustrations in the original articles.

When he took his second furlough to England in 1894, Ross believed he had accumulated overwhelming evidence that Laveran was incorrect.

"Everything I had tried had failed," he told his colleagues. But they quickly informed him that the parasites did indeed exist and sent him to Dr. Patrick Manson.

"Within a few minutes," Ross wrote, "he showed me the Laveran bodies which are technically called 'crescents' in a stained specimen of malaria blood, and I recognized at once that no such bodies could exist in healthy blood. My doubts were now removed. . . ."

Though Ross would not have agreed, medical historians today are certain that his Nobel Prize–winning discovery of the vector of malaria could not have been achieved without Manson's help. When Ross was thwarted by superiors, Manson came to his aid. There was a continuous exchange of ideas between the two men, first directly and then by letter. Manson continued to suggest new approaches and to encourage Ross when he became depressed.

But sharing credit for a scientific discovery is more difficult than sharing money. If to speak the name of the dead is to make them live again, as the ancient Egyptians believed, then whoever makes a great discovery truly achieves eternal life. Huge fortunes have been made and lost, with no more than the remark, "Well, it was only money." But no one losing part or all of the credit for a great scientific discovery has yet been known to remark, "Well, it was only a Nobel Prize." Especially not Ronald Ross.

During his 1894 furlough Ross spent many hours tagging along behind Manson—on ward rounds at the Seamen's Hospital and in Manson's private laboratory. There, for the first time, Ross was able to locate the tiny malarial parasites under the microscope. One November afternoon in 1894 Manson, impressed with this eager, capable student, began to expound upon his ideas about the plasmodia.

"Do you know," he remarked to Ross while the two were on the way to the hospital, "I have formed a theory that mosquitoes carry malaria just as they carry filaria."

Though this nicely rhymed observation might have been made into another new poem, Ross was initially unimpressed. The mosquito had been suggested as a carrier of malaria many times before, he responded.

But then the two men discussed the facts that favored this argument. As Ross began to be swayed, Manson brought in his own theories. The filaments in the crescents—believed by everyone to be evidence of a death spasm—were actually living bodies. The mosquito, feeding on the blood of a malaria patient, sucked the filamented crescents into its stomach. The filaments proceeded to travel through the stomach into the insect's tissues. After the mosquito died laying its eggs, the "flagellated spores" emerged into the water, ready to infect anyone who came to drink.

These theories—which had earned for Manson the titles "pathological Jules Verne" and "Mosquito Manson"—sent the young Ross into raptures of ecstasy. Suddenly the fame that had eluded him despite years writing poems, music, plays, novels, and equations seemed within his grasp. He had but to prove what Manson had presented to sound like gospel truth.

Overwhelmed by the conviction that Manson was entirely correct, Ross made only the most superficial attempt to familiarize himself with the life of the mosquito, despite Manson's entreaties. After having failed to examine books on the mosquito in the library of the British Museum—the only place in England at the time with such books—Ross later confessed that he was "very badly equipped for the fray."

His ignorance, however, was offset by an almost manic enthusiasm. On the ship to India, Ross rushed among passengers and crew members, frantically pricking fingers and examining blood. At the ship's ports of call, he besieged the local hospitals for blood specimens of malarious patients. He even tried to prepare himself for anatomical studies of Indian mosquitoes by dissecting the ship's cockroaches.

At his new post in Secunderabad, Ross continued to dart around like a frenzied mongoose looking for cases of malaria. His preoccupation quickly incurred the hostility of his colonel. Even the natives, their fingertips inflamed from his repeated pinpricks, would dash to hide from him. He was thought so mad by colleagues that authenticated malaria cases were kept from him.

But he refused to give up. Spurned in his garrison hospital, he haunted the municipal hospitals and the other regiment infirmaries looking for cases of malaria. The local doctors would often turn over these cases to him just to rid themselves of his annoying presence. He offered the malarious natives he discovered a rupee a prick; yet many still fled. After he finally managed to obtain the co-operation of one patient with a documented case, fellow doctors challenged him to demonstrate the parasite. But somehow, when the moment came, the plasmodia mysteriously vanished from the blood. Poor Ross had to endure gales of laughter.

At first his luck with mosquitoes was no better. Following Manson's instructions, he captured the ubiquitous insects and tried to induce them to bite malaria patients. But they obdurately refused to bite any one—even Ross.

The mosquitoes caught were probably too frightened to bite, Ross reasoned. So he raised new mosquitoes from grubs. Still no luck. He baked the patients in the hot sun "to bring their flavor out." Nothing happened.

Then, on May 13, 1895, Ross's birthday, a heavy rain soaked the bed and netting of a malaria patient. Made ravenous by the moisture, the mosquitoes attacked the patient with alacrity. Ross grabbed four of them, expressed their ingested blood on a glass slide, and peered at it with his microscope. Just as Manson had prophesied, there were the parasites.

To be certain of the results, Ross tried the same experiment with six more mosquitoes the next day. Abjuring food and sleep, he peered through the microscope so intently that his eye was blackened by repeated contact with the eyepiece.

"Every point that you predicted seems to come true," he wrote to Manson. "Certainly there is nothing contrary to the theory. The parasites are present in the blood of the mosquito, and what is even more, they appear to be there in greater numbers than in blood from the finger. Also, the development of the crescents, and the formation of the flagella, seem to be favored by conditions in the mosquito's stomach. Yes, the crescent–sphere–flagella metamorphosis does go on inside the mosquito to a much greater degree than in control specimens of finger blood."

At one point, Ross became so enthralled watching a white blood cell try to engulf a flagellum that in his letter he compared the battle to a swordfight. "I shall write a novel on it in the style of the *Three Musketeers*," he added joyously.

Manson immediately wrote back with more instructions. "Let mosquitoes bite people sick with malaria," he advised, "then put those mosquitoes in a bottle of water and let them lay eggs and hatch out grubs. Then give that mosquito-water to people to drink."

So Ross allowed four mosquitoes to feed on a patient named Abdul Kadir. These insects were then kept in a bottle full of water until they died. After the promise of a suitable emolument, Lutchman, Ross's native servant, was persuaded to swallow the liquid in the bottle.

Day after day for ten days, Ross waited anxiously for Lutchman to develop fever. On day eleven, Lutchman complained of a headache and was found to have a slight temperature elevation. Now thoroughly excited, Ross admitted his experimental subject to the hospital and impatiently sat by him, measuring his temperature every thirty minutes.

Lutchman, however, probably only had the flu. Not a parasite was to be seen in his blood. A few days later, he had recovered completely. Ross repeated the experiment with other volunteers, and these men were totally unaffected by the mosquito water.

The volatile Ross was plunged into deep despair. Nothing seemed to be going right. Careful dissection of the mosquitoes revealed that the flagella Manson believed to be spores remained active but a few moments in the insect's tissue. Perhaps, thought Ross, ingestion of the parasites by the mosquitoes was only incidental, unrelated to human disease. Thoroughly discouraged, he began writing poems again. Maybe this was a better way to become famous.

From England, Manson desperately tried to re-energize his slacking convert. "Above everything, don't give it up. Look upon it as a Holy Grail and yourself as Sir Galahad and never give up the search, for be assured that you are on the right track. The malaria germ does not go into the mosquito for nothing, for fun, or for the confusion of the pathologist. It has no notion of a practical joke. It is there for a purpose and that purpose, depend upon it, is its own interests—germs are selfish brutes."

Unfortunately, the Indian Medical Service did not share Manson's views. To them Ross's search seemed more of an unholy nuisance than a Holy Grail. Finally, during a cholera epidemic in Bangalore, the ersatz Sir Galahad was ordered to clean up the area. For the next eighteen months Ross had little time to do anything but visit cholera cases and fight with civilian and military authorities over sanitary reforms.

Manson was distressed. Perhaps his precious theory might be appropriated by someone else who would give him no credit. "The Frenchies and Italians will pooh-pooh it, then adopt it, and then claim it as their own," he warned Ross in one letter, "see if they don't. But push on with it, and don't let them forestall you. They won't have this autumn, and they will not have a chance to work seriously at the matter until next June or so. You have got a year ahead of them."

By this time, the repeated failures had prompted Ross to question Manson's theory. So he began to formulate his own theories.

"She always injects a small quantity of fluid with her bite," Ross noticed. "What if the parasites get into the system in this manner?"

To test this eminently reasonable idea, Ross allowed mosquitoes that had fed on a malaria patient to bite a healthy man. Nothing happened. The experiment was repeated again and again. No fever developed. Still enthusiastic, he communicated his new notion to Manson.

Manson, however, had quite an imperfect understanding of mosquito behavior. Believing that the insect bit only once during its life, he was convinced that Ross could not be correct. "Follow the flagella," he wrote back, and forget this crazy idea.

Ross obediently went back to dissecting mosquitoes and in February 1897 was able to observe the true fate of the flagella. Within a blood smear he saw two parasites near each other. The first was giving off flagella, while the second, which was spherical and unsegmented, had a single flagellum wiggling slowly inside.

Had Ross begun a moment earlier, he might have watched the flagellum emitted by the first parasite penetrate the second and so perceived the true nature of the process. But from his unlucky vantage point, he surmised that the single wiggling flagellum was trying to escape the sphere rather than fertilize it. When McCallum in Baltimore correctly interpreted the process a few weeks later, Ross was deeply humiliated, and "always felt disgraced as a man of science" for incorrectly interpreting his own observation.

"I was now forty years old," he wrote dejectedly, "but, though I was well known in India, both for my sanitary work at Bangalore and for my researches on malaria I received no advancement at all for my pains." Still convinced that the study of malaria was to be his path to fame and fortune, he pestered the military hierarchy incessantly to allow him time for research. But he had stepped on too many toes to expect any favors from his superiors. In June 1897 he was sent back to the steamy, depressing hospital in Secunderabad.

Yet he refused to give up. He wrote to England, begging Manson to intercede with high government figures on his behalf. Manson thereupon approached Lord George Hamilton, the secretary of state, and even petitioned Lord Elgin, the viceroy of India. But Elgin, whose grandfather had brazenly pried the magnificent marble frieze off the Parthenon, refused to pry Ross out of Secunderabad.

On two months' leave taken at his own expense, Ross tried to continue his malaria work. Again he was unlucky. Within a few days he himself contracted malaria and spent his vacation too ill to do anything. When he finally recovered, the weather had turned hot and dry. A stiff wind filled his laboratory with mounds of dust. The sweat-rusted microscope, its one remaining eyepiece cracked, sat idle as Ross sulked, brooded—and wrote poetry:

What ails the solitude?
　Is this the Judgement Day?
The sky is red as blood;
　The very rocks decay
And crack and crumble, and
　There is a flame of wind
Wherewith the burning sand
　Is ever mass'd and thin'd

The world is white with heat;
　The world is rent and riven;
The world and heavens meet;
　The lost stars cry in heav'n

As he was emerging from this bleak period of depression, Ross was struck by the inspiration that was to make him famous. Rereading Manson's original article on filariasis, he was reminded of the fact that only one species of mosquito among the four found in Amoy—*Culex fatigans*—was capable of carrying filariasis. Manson had also suggested that each form of the malarial plasmodia might require a particular mosquito species.

Suddenly Ross realized that perhaps his experimental attempts to transmit malaria by mosquito bite had failed simply because he had used the wrong species of mosquito. Most of his cases had been falciparum malaria, and he had consistently employed the common house mosquito, a gray insect with plain wings that sat with its tail pointing down. The larvae of these mosquitoes floated head downward in water, breathing by means of a long tube.

After a little searching, Ross was able to come up with another species of mosquito. This "brown mosquito," as he called it, had no breathing tube and floated parallel to the water surface in its larval form. The adult sat with its tail pointed upward.

A malaria patient named Husein Kahn was the first experimental subject. Ross let loose a dozen of the brown mosquitoes under the mosquito netting of Husein Kahn's bed, and trapped each one, after it had fed, in a separate bottle.

Two mosquitoes were then examined immediately. Two days later others were dissected. More of the insects died during the night and quickly decomposed. In all of them Ross found nothing. Worse, search as he might, no more of the same species of insect were to be procured.

On August 20, 1897, a tired, discouraged Ronald Ross dissected one of the two remaining brown mosquitoes. Just as he was about to give up, he noted a queer structure within the cells lining the insect's stomach: an almost perfectly circular cell containing a group of black pigment granules very similar to those seen in the malarial parasites found in blood smears. Nearby were identical circular cells. Ecstatic with joy, Ross wrote, "Those circles in the wall of the stomach of the mosquito—those circles with their dots of black pigment, they can't be anything else than the malarial parasite, growing there. . . ." On August 21 he dissected and examined the last brown mosquito, and again saw the pigment-filled circles. To commemorate his triumph, he wrote—what else?—a poem:

> This day designing God
>> Hath put into my hand
> A wondrous thing. And God
>> Be praised. At his command
>
> I have found thy secret deeds
>> Oh million-murdering Death.
>
> I know that this little thing
>> A million men will save—
> Oh death where is thy sting?
>> Thy victory, oh grave?

But would this little thing really save a million men? Ross was nagged by doubt. Perhaps, he worried, the granule-containing, circular cells might be totally unrelated to the malarial parasites.

"I really believe the problem is solved," he wrote to Manson, "although I don't like to say so. I look at them myself daily; those of the fifth day have grown bigger than those of the fourth day. . . . Pigment—it is almost proof already! What else can the thing be? . . . What are we to think: What do you think?"

As luck would have it, swarms of brown mosquitoes suddenly appeared. Now able to repeat his experiment, Ross confirmed that only those insects which had bitten malaria patients carried the circular cells. He submitted the results to the *British Medical Journal,* and in December 1897 his report, "On Some Peculiar Pigmented Cells Found in Two Mosquitoes Fed on Malarial Blood," was published.

Then, just at his moment of triumph, Ross was foiled by his superiors. On September 22, 1897, he had written Manson, "I shall be much disappointed if I don't get a practical proof in a week's time," and was attempting to transmit malaria with the brown mosquitoes. Two days later, the following wire arrived:

UNDER INSTRUCTIONS FROM COMMAND HEADQUARTERS, SURGEON MAJOR R. ROSS, I.M.S., WILL PROCEED IMMEDIATELY TO BOMBAY FOR MILITARY DUTY.

Ross bombarded the commanding officers with angry telegrams. He pleaded with Manson to intervene. Nothing helped. His new station, to his great dismay, was totally unsuited to his research.

"Alas for your hope," he wrote to Manson, "that I shall have a plentiful supply of mosquitoes and cases here! None of either (or very few); the cold weather is in, and the people here so savage and superstitious that they won't allow experiments to be made on them."

Yet the resourceful Ross did not quite languish. He knew of Danielewsky's studies of bird malaria, and verified for himself that some types of pigeons carried the disease. At the time, many biologists believed mosquitoes did not attack birds. After studies of pigeons, sparrows, and crows, Ross verified that birds were indeed bitten by mosquitoes, as well as by other insects.

In the meantime, Manson reached the right bureaucrat. On January 29, 1898, after weeks of futile pleading for a furlough or a change of station, Ross was notified by wire of his attractive new assignment:

GOVERNMENT INDIA SANCTIONS YOUR APPOINTMENT ON SPECIAL DUTY UNDER DIRECTOR GENERAL FOR SIX MONTHS.

Ross found no shortage of mosquitoes at his new station, Calcutta, a city notorious for its Black Hole, its shanghaied sailors, its poverty, filth, and disease. He was assigned the dilapidated laboratory of a recently retired physiologist. Because the two native "dieners" were too old to be of any use, Ross advertised for assistants who would be paid from his own pocket.

Of the twenty or so job applicants, Ross chose two. His capriciousness would delight a modern corporate personnel director. One, Mohammed Bux, was picked because "he looked the most rascally of the lot and was therefore likely to have considerable intelligence." The other, named Purboona, was apparently a random selection.

Purboona disappeared after the first payday. But Mohammed Bux proved a particularly fortuitous choice. He became quite devoted to Ross and was singularly adept at the work. He would even sleep on the laboratory floor at night to keep stray cats from killing the experimental animals. His only recorded failing was a lamentable fondness for strong Indian marihuana, which would send him on weekly binges.

Ross directed Mohammed Bux to capture mosquitoes, hoping again to find the circular, pigment-filled cells within the insects' stomachs. Bux climbed through the sewers, the drains, the stinking tanks which abounded in Calcutta and brought back all kinds of mosquitoes. He also had an almost miraculous ability to induce the insects to bite patients when Ross was unable to make them bite at all. Unfortunately, the work had begun between malaria seasons. All the human experiments were a failure.

For this reason, Ross turned to the study of bird malaria. His laboratory soon became filled with the live sparrows, larks, and crows that were snared by Mohammed Bux. Into the cages covered with mosquito netting went the mosquitoes. In almost no time Ross could demonstrate that the plasmodium passed from bird to mosquito, just as it did in humans. Moreover, the same pigmented, circular cells would form in the wall of the insect's stomach. Only one difference was noted. The common gray mosquito was the carrier of bird malaria. The brown, dapple-winged vector of human malaria could not be infected by the bird parasite.

These studies were carried on in desperate haste. Ross was forever haunted by the fear that hostile superiors would once again interrupt his work. He was forbidden to publish any of his results, though compelled to send long, meticulously detailed summaries to headquarters. The only outsider aware of the research was Manson, who often received whimsical accounts. Here, for example, is one with Ross taking the role of the pigmented circular cell:

"I find that I exist constantly in three out of four mosquitoes fed on bird malaria parasites, and that I increase regularly in size from about a seven-thousandth of an inch after about thirty hours to about one seven-hundredth of an inch after about eighty-five hours. . . . I find myself in large numbers in about one out of two mosquitoes fed on two crows with blood parasites . . ."

But how did the parasite pass from the mosquitoes to the birds? According to Manson's theory, the parasites were ingested with water in which the mosquitoes had died while laying eggs. Ross easily tested this theory by feeding infected mosquitoes to healthy sparrows. The result: The birds remained free of malaria.

The true answer finally emerged as Ross continued to study infected mosquitoes. As the circular cells within the mosquito's stomach enlarged, the pigmented granules grew into little rod-shaped bodies. And soon, Ross discovered, these rods appeared in the insect's thorax. Since the stomachs of some mosquitoes showed only ruptured capsules where circular cells had been, the implication was clear: The rods migrated.

On July 4, 1898, Ross discovered their destination. Examining the insect's head, he noted the salivary gland to be so loaded with rods that it literally quivered. Here then was the answer. Malaria was passed back to the birds in the mosquito's saliva during the act of biting.

This remarkable finding, Ross later wrote, "brought him up standing." As a final verification, he sent Mohammed Bux to capture a group of healthy sparrows. Mosquitoes that had fed on infected birds were allowed to bite these healthy ones. Within a few days the blood of the new birds was loaded with malarial parasites.

Ross communicated his results to Manson in a state of intense excitement. "I think I may now say Q.E.D.," he wrote, "and congratulate you on the mosquito theory indeed. The door is unlocked, and I am walking in and collecting the treasures." But in the same letter, he gave an intimation of his ultimate refusal to share his prize: "Well, I have become unbearable with conceit. . . . I brag openly about it!"

Manson received the news at a meeting of the new Tropical Diseases Section of the British Medical Association. When he read Ross's report to the assembled delegates, the excitement generated was intense.

"I am sure you will agree with me," Manson added, "that the

medical world, I might even say humanity, is extremely indebted to Surgeon Major Ross for what he has already done, and I am sure you will agree with me that every encouragement and assistance should be given to so hard-working, so intelligent, and so successful an investigator to continue his work."

The audience may have agreed with Manson, but the Indian Medical Service did not. For Ross's original assignment was also supposed to include the study of another tropical disease—kala azar. And so, just at the peak of his success, Ross received instructions to abandon the malaria work and report to a new post in Assam to do research on kala azar.

"Columbus having sighted America was ordered off to discover the North Pole," he remarked bitterly. "No, the man who can do is not allowed to do—because the man who cannot do is put in authority over him."

In a state of deep despondency, Ross was forced to close his small laboratory. The birds were set free from their cages and the jars of mosquitoes emptied. After sadly wishing Mohammed Bux good-bye, Ronald Ross left Calcutta. His only consolation lay in his belief that what remained to be done was a job for children.

Unpleasantness

In reality, the research still to be done was more complex than that. For, as Manson remarked in his address to the Tropical Diseases Section, "One can object that the facts determined for birds do not hold, necessarily, for men."

The Italian physician Giovanni Battista Grassi, working independently of Ross, was finally able to verify the mosquito theory of malaria in man. It seems now almost inevitable that an Italian should fit in the last piece of the puzzle. As we have seen, malaria was common and devastating in Italy, especially in the neighborhood of the Roman Campagna. By the mid-nineteenth century, any scientist wishing to study the disease could be assured of financial support from Italian industrialists and agriculturists. Tommasi-Crudeli, Klebs, Celli, and Marchiafava all received such support.

In 1896, a year before Ross verified the mosquito as the vector of bird malaria, Amico Bignami, an Italian scientist, had attempted to prove Manson's mosquito theory in man. Bignami had captured mosquitoes from regions with a high incidence of malaria and allowed them to bite healthy human beings. But like Ross in his early work, Bignami failed to appreciate that only one type of mosquito could transmit human malaria.

Bignami's failure threw the mosquito theory into disrepute, though only for a short time. For Robert Koch had also been interested in malaria and the role of the mosquito since his first contact with the disease during his Indian cholera research in 1883. After learning of Manson's hypothesis, his interest was reawakened, and in 1898 he organized an Italian expedition. His goal: to demonstrate that human malaria was caused by a mosquito bite.

Koch stumbled over the same problem that had tripped up Bignami and Ross. He simply could not believe that a particular species of mosquito was necessary to transmit human malaria. In addition, he was convinced that the infant mosquito inherited the parasite from its mother. Theobald Smith had demonstrated this type of transmission in the ticks of Texas cattle fever, and Koch was probably basing his assumption on Smith's work.

Giovanni Grassi, who succeeded where Koch, Bignami, and Ross had failed, received his medical education at Pavia, a school made famous by Lazzaro Spallanzani a hundred years earlier. Grassi had little affinity for the practice of medicine, however, and was wont to sniff arrogantly that he was a zoologist, not a physician. Unlike the mercurial, fumbling Ross, Grassi was as precise, unemotional, and meticulous as a watchmaker. His scientific papers were models of perfection—classics in their own time—that he would labor over for years before publishing. Though his eyesight was terrible, he had become famous for his studies of the microbes that parasitized white ants and of the behavior of eels. After his investigation of the *Chaetognatha,* a genus of small marine worms, Pavia made him full professor of zoology at the age of twenty-nine. A fanatical worker, he was highly contemptuous of those who were not. "Mankind," he once said, "is composed of those who work, those who pretend to work, and those who do neither."

Grassi readily accepted the mosquito theory. In addition, even before he began his research, he had cleverly guessed that only certain mosquitoes were involved. Since mosquitoes were numerous in some locations where malaria was rare, while in other places malaria was common and mosquitoes rare, he deduced that only a particular mosquito could carry the disease. And no one was better qualified to identify this insect than Grassi, a superb taxonomist capable of recognizing each of the more than thirty species indigenous to Italy.

In the summer of 1898 Grassi began his search. Using large test tubes, he trapped every variety of mosquito that he spotted. At the same time, he recorded in a notebook the incidence of malaria at the place where each insect had been captured. After a summer spent visiting most of the swamps in Italy, Grassi was able to exonerate all forms of the culex, or common gray house mosquito—the insect that caused Ross to throw away almost two years' work. The type that appeared to be responsible was called *zanzarone* by the peasants; it had dappled wings and a tail that pointed upward when it sat—Ross's "brown mosquito." In September 1898 Grassi was able to report that this insect, *Anopheles claviger,* was the carrier of human malaria.

The proof was obtained by means of a human experiment. The subject, a Mr. Sola, had been for six years a patient in the Hospital of the Holy Spirit, a building high atop one of the hills of Rome. Malaria had never been seen in this vicinity and neither had the anopheles mosquito. With Mr. Sola's permission, Grassi and Dr. Bastianelli, a hospital physician, shut Mr. Sola in a room with anopheles mosquitoes every night for ten nights. On the eleventh day, the patient developed a malarial chill. Examination of his blood revealed large numbers of plasmodia: "The rest of the history of Sola's case has no interest for us," Grassi wrote, "but it is now certain that mosquitoes can carry malaria, to a place where there are no mosquitoes in nature, to a place where no case of malaria has ever occurred, to a man who has never had malaria—Mr. Sola!"

Grassi's successful repetition of the experiment on a number of other patients somehow leaked out. The newspapers were incensed and implied that Grassi was ruthlessly endangering the lives of his human guinea pigs. He ignored them and continued with his work.

For there was still Robert Koch's assertion that the infant anopheles inherited the malarial infection from its mother. To refute this, Grassi raised anopheles mosquitoes from eggs. Then he allowed the mosquitoes to bite him and six other volunteers. All remained free of malaria.

In the course of his experiments, Grassi came to read Ronald Ross's articles on bird malaria. After dissecting the anopheles, Grassi was able to observe the same pigmented circular cells and the same rods within the salivary gland. But when he published, he failed to give Ross credit.

Needless to say, Ross was furious. Thoroughly convinced that Grassi was trying to steal his discovery from him, Ross sent angry letters to the journals that had published Grassi's papers, asserting that Grassi was a mountebank, a cheap crook, a parasite who survived on the ideas of others. Grassi replied in equally acrimonious terms. So vicious did the correspondence soon become that journal editors, fearful of libel, hesitated to publish the letters.

But Ross and Grassi did not stop feuding. Both enlisted the aid of the greatest authorities on tropical medicine. Ross was able to obtain letters from Dr. T. Edmundston Charles, an English observer of the Italian work in Rome. Using this evidence, Ross asserted that Grassi had been aware of the studies on bird malaria, though Grassi later denied such awareness. When Ross could not find a publisher for a book containing his case against his Italian adversary, he paid for the printing himself, carrying the work through two editions. This bitter conflict lasted for more than two decades.

In the meantime Grassi began a campaign against malaria, since opposition to the mosquito theory was still widespread. He warned against taking walks in the twilight, the prime mosquito feeding time. "Don't go out in the warm evenings," he announced, "unless you wear heavy cotton gloves and veils." Naturally he was laughed at.

To prove his point, Grassi set up an experiment to prevent malaria in the most heavily diseased region in Italy—the railroad line that ran through the plain of Capaccio. With funds from the queen of Italy and authority from the railroad, Grassi installed fine mesh screens on the doors and windows of ten station-masters' houses. One hundred twelve employees were paid to stay inside during the twilight. Another four hundred fifteen workers went out as usual. At the end of the summer, almost all the unprotected developed malaria. But of the hundred and twelve protected individuals, only five got sick.

"In the so much feared station of Albanella," wrote Grassi triumphantly, "from which for years so many coffins had been carried, one could live as healthily as in the healthiest spot in Italy!"

Grassi's experiment was repeated in an even more dramatic fashion by Patrick Manson. During one phase, Manson sent men from the staff of the London School of Tropical Medicine to live and work in the Roman Campagna. One hour before twilight they repaired to special mosquito-proof tents, where they stayed until an hour after sunrise. Though everyone around them contracted malaria, these men stayed healthy. This outcome was dramatized by the fate of a police detachment sent from Rome to capture a famous criminal in the Campagna while the Englishmen were there. Though they remained in the Campagna for only a day, all the policemen developed malaria shortly after returning to Rome.

The second phase of Manson's experiment was most chilling, though fortunately it ended happily. Manson managed to obtain live, malarious Italian mosquitoes, which he permitted to bite his own healthy son. In fourteen days, the boy was ill with malaria. Manson's laboratory assistant, George Warren, then allowed a few more of the infected mosquitoes to bite him, remarking that it would have been "a great pity to waste them." He too quickly contracted malaria. Both young men survived. After these results had been reported in newspapers and magazines throughout the world, the last resistance to the mosquito theory finally crumbled. Simultaneously, an era was coming to an end.

Two Tales of the Golden Age

The years 1875 to 1910 are often referred to as the golden age of microbiology. During this period almost all of the bacteria causing human disease were identified, along with many human parasites, and the science of virology was begun. No previous era in the history of medicine witnessed such a rapid succession of great discoveries.

Two books embody the spirit and sense of the golden age of microbiology. One, *Microbe Hunters* by Paul de Kruif, is nonfiction. The other is Sinclair Lewis's novel *Arrowsmith*.

No doubt de Kruif (pronounced "de krife") was able to capture the excitement of the new science so well because he had been educated as a bacteriologist. He was born March 2, 1890, in Zeeland, Michigan, the son of Dutch immigrants. His father wanted him to be a doctor or lawyer, and the dutiful son enrolled in the premedical course of the University of Michigan. But during his second year he was inspired to change his field by an article about Paul Ehrlich, the German scientist who discovered a cure for syphilis.

After receiving a bachelor of science degree in 1912, de Kruif was awarded a Rockefeller fellowship to do bacteriologic research at the University of Michigan. In 1916 he received his Ph.D. By this time, the First World War was raging in Europe, and the young scientist joined the Army's Sanitary Corps in France. While still in the service he discovered a quick and practical method to produce antitoxin for *Clostridium welchii,* the bacterium of gas gangrene.

After the war, de Kruif returned to Michigan to do research. He was already married, the father of two sons, and his inadequate university salary left him gasping for cash.

Because he had developed literary interests, de Kruif wrote to his idol, the irascible H. L. Mencken, asking advice. Mencken's suggestion—free-lance writing—proved to be a mixed blessing.

While at Michigan, de Kruif wrote an excellent scientific article on his studies of the blood-dissolving poison of the hemolytic streptococcus. This paper resulted in his appointment in 1920 as associate at the Rockefeller Institute for Medical Research in New York. Here he might have spent his life as a researcher but for his pronounced mischievous streak. He wrote a rakish book, *Our Medicine Men,* which was published in 1922 and which he described as "a spoof of the exaggerated pretensions of a part of the medical profession." Unfortunately, that part consisted of colleagues at the Rockefeller Institute, parodied in thinly disguised caricatures.

"It caused me to get fired," de Kruif said some years later. "Exiled from science, I grubbed for a living, writing about medical science for popular magazines." He was in Chicago in 1922, busily grubbing, when a friend, Dr. Morris Fishbein, introduced him to Sinclair Lewis.

At this time, the thirty-seven-year-old Lewis had reached a high point in his career, buoyed by the enormous popular and financial successes of two novels, *Main Street* and *Babbitt.* He was considering a Christlike labor leader as the hero of a third book, and had come to the Middle West to talk to Eugene Debs, on whom he intended to pattern his protagonist. But during a boisterous evening with de Kruif and Fishbein, Lewis was persuaded that he was not ready to write about labor. The hulking, ebullient de Kruif, a huge man who wore a size-eighteen collar, matched drinks that night with Lewis in one roadhouse after another. Nobody, however, could outdrink the famous novelist. De Kruif and Fishbein watched amazed as Lewis picked up a fifth, put it to his lips, and literally poured the entire contents down his throat. Finally, in the early hours of the morning, Lewis was convinced that he should write a novel about medical science.

This was not a surprising decision, since the medical profession formed a prominent backdrop for much of Lewis's early life. As a student at Yale he had considered it for himself. His much respected older brother, Claude, was a surgeon in St. Cloud, Minnesota. Even in 1922 his aging father, E. J. Lewis, was still practicing as a country doctor in Sinclair's birthplace, Sauk Centre, Minnesota. A grandfather had also been a physician, and an uncle was a doctor in Chicago.

Lewis quickly struck a bargain with de Kruif and the publisher Alfred Harcourt to produce a novel about the medical profession. De Kruif, who would provide the background information, was to receive 25 per cent of the royalties, a ten-thousand-dollar advance, and an acknowledgment in the book. Lewis was to receive the remaining 75 per cent. Together, the two men began work—after a last night of carousing—on a freighter cruise to the West Indies.

The purpose of the cruise at the outset of the collaboration was twofold. First, since a plague on a tropical island was planned to form the climax of the novel, travel was essential to assimilate the atmosphere of Caribbean life. But second and more important, the time at sea was needed to educate Lewis in bacteriology, epidemiology, and the method as well as the spirit of research.

By the time the two-month cruise was over, a great deal of the plot had already been worked out on paper. De Kruif had written complete professional histories of the main characters, Martin Arrowsmith and Max Gottlieb. He had also produced ideas for other characters who would appear in the developing plot. As Lewis wrote, de Kruif continued to stand by in order to assist whenever technical information was required.

No such information was needed for the opening of the novel— which portrayed a fourteen-year-old boy, Martin Arrowsmith, in a small-town doctor's office. The boy is obviously young Lewis himself in an office somewhat more disorderly than his father's. But the old alcoholic Doc Vickerson of Elk Mills probably bore little resemblance to the elder Dr. Lewis.

De Kruif's contributions to the story first appear when young Martin proceeds to the University of Winnemac. The technical experience of life in a medical school might have come partly from Lewis's brother Claude, though some undoubtedly came from de Kruif. And the character of Max Gottlieb—the most important figure in the book next to Martin Arrowsmith—derives principally from Jacques Loeb, for whom de Kruif had worked as research associate at the Rockefeller Institute.

Loeb was a German biologist who had become famous for his experimental studies of parthenogenesis (reproduction without fertilization). Popular interest and some controversy had attended the first announcement of this work in 1899, for Loeb had succeeded in bringing about the development of sea urchin larvae from unfertilized eggs merely by exposing them to controlled environmental changes. Loeb later extended the technique to the production of parthenogenetic frogs, which he raised to sexual maturity. He thereby demonstrated that the initiation of cell division in fertilization was controlled chemically and was separated from the transmission of hereditary traits. His studies of cellular chemistry led Loeb to espouse the belief that life phenomena can be explained in terms of physical and chemical laws. Before joining the Rockefeller Institute in 1910, Loeb had taught at Bryn Mawr, the University of Chicago, and the University of California.

Like Loeb, Max Gottlieb was a German Jew who had taught at a small American college before moving to the University of Winnemac Medical School. Also like Loeb, Gottlieb attempted to explain biologic phenomena in terms of physical chemistry and mathematics. Despite his love for pure science, however, Gottlieb is a worldly, sardonic man; yet a strangely childlike streak of innocence runs through the hardened exterior. He believes that the Winnemac Medical School should be converted into a pure research institute and communicates this conviction to the dean by letter along with the suggestion that the dean resign. When the dean politely replies that the school is supported by the people of the state in order to train physicians, Gottlieb damns the people of the state; in their present condition of nincompoopery, he adds, they are worth no attention at all. He then goes over the dean's head to the president of the university.

"Really, I'm too engrossed to consider chimerical schemes, however ingenious they may be," the president tells Gottlieb.

"You are too busy to consider anything but selling honorary degrees to millionaires for gymnasiums," Gottlieb replies. He is fired the next day.

During this tragically comic altercation, Martin Arrowsmith graduates from Winnemac Medical School and moves to the small town of Wheatsylvania, Dakota. Here he fails in medical practice by offending too many of the locals, who resemble the characters satirized in *Main Street*. From Wheatsylvania, Martin proceeds to the medium-sized city of Nautilus, Iowa, as a public health official. This world of small-time hucksterdom Lewis had also dealt with in another novel, *Babbitt*. Again Martin cannot compromise his principles and is soon driven out by the many people he has offended.

The real story of *Arrowsmith*—the conflict between the ideal of scientific research and the crass threat of commercial compromise—emerges after Martin's next move to the slick Rouncefield Clinic in Chicago. Rouncefield is a place motivated by the conviction "that any portions of the body without which people could conceivably get along should certainly be removed at once." Uncomfortable in this milieu, Martin begins spare-time research with the intelligent, assiduous technique that so impressed Max Gottlieb at Winnemac.

Soon, like Paul de Kruif, Martin writes a paper on streptolysin, the blood-dissolving protein of the hemolytic streptococcus. This article is published in the *Journal of Infectious Diseases,* where it is seen by Max Gottlieb. Now an immunologist at the McGurk (Rockefeller) Institute in New York City, Gottlieb offers Martin a research position at the Institute. Like de Kruif, Martin accepts and moves to New York. He is by this time married, and it was this marriage that had propelled him into the private practice for which he was so unsuited. His wife, Leora, is believed to represent Lewis's idea of de Kruif's idea of his second wife; de Kruif had divorced his first wife and married her immediately after receiving the ten-thousand-dollar advance from Harcourt.

De Kruif and Lewis produce their most wicked caricature in the person of the director of the McGurk Institute, Dr. A. DeWitt Tubbs. No doubt de Kruif was bitter over his discharge from the Rockefeller Institute for what seemed nothing more than a harmless joke. He took his revenge by mercilessly patterning Tubbs on Dr. Simon Flexner, the director of the Rockefeller Institute.

Flexner was an internationally famous pathologist and bacteriologist. A gifted research scientist, he had isolated the dysentery bacillus, *Shigella flexneri,* and developed a curative serum for cerebrospinal meningitis. During his tenure as director of the Rockefeller Institute, when de Kruif came to know him, Flexner was leading a research team studying poliomyelitis.

But in the de Kruif–Lewis portrait, the brilliant, capable Flexner is transformed into the pompous pooh-bah Tubbs, a man "tremendously whiskered on all visible spots save his nose and temples and the palms of his hands." Tubbs is nothing more than a politician–public relations man, who tries to squeeze profound drama out of even the slightest accomplishments. His own fatuous ambition leads him to become director of the League of Cultural Agencies, an organization with the ridiculous goal of trying to standardize and coordinate all the mental activities in America.

Despite the feverish political activity going on around him, Martin is happy during his first few months in New York. Max Gottlieb admires him and tries to advise him in a fatherly way:

> "But once again always remember that not all the men who work at science are scientists. So few! . . . To be a scientist is like being a Goethe: it is born in you. If you haf, there is only one t'ing—no, there is two t'ings you must do: work twice as hard as you can, and keep people from using you. I will try to protect you from Success. It is all I can do. So . . . I should wish, Martin, that you will be very happy here."

Alone a few minutes later, Martin prays the now-famous prayer of the scientist:

> "God give me unclouded eyes and freedom from haste. God give me a quiet and relentless anger against all pretense and all pretentious work and all work left slack and unfinished. God give me a restlessness whereby I may neither sleep nor accept praise till my observed results equal my calculated results or in pious glee I discover and assault my error. God give me strength not to trust to God!"

The remainder of the book concerns the political struggle within the McGurk Institute and the battle of Martin and Gottlieb to preserve their ideals; the journey to the plague-stricken island of St. Hubert and the death of Martin's wife, Leora; Martin's return to New York and his marriage to the rich and chic Joyce Lanyon; his quitting the Institute and his separation from wife and child; his flight from New York and its society with Terry Wickett, a fellow scientist who shares Martin's ideals. As the story ends, the two are left in the

Vermont wilderness where, unmolested, they will pursue their lonely truths.

In spite of this implausible ending, *Arrowsmith* is considered Lewis's most firmly plotted novel and a masterpiece of American literature. Both *Main Street* and *Babbitt* were more loosely chronicled works with only the most tenuous plot line. In *Arrowsmith,* however, Lewis made some effort to provide dramatic unity to the story. Most of the important characters reappear throughout the book, and in the end there is a quick look back over the earlier scenes. Thus all the loose strings are neatly tied together.

There had been other novels written about doctors, even about those who vacillated between lucrative private practice and professional integrity. *Arrowsmith,* however, is not primarily about a doctor but a research scientist fighting for his scientific integrity. Martin Arrowsmith was a new kind of hero, and scientific idealism a new subject. No subsequent book has portrayed so well the agonies and joys of a medical researcher working in the new world that evolved from the golden age of microbiology.

After *Arrowsmith,* Sinclair Lewis wrote two other famous books, *Elmer Gantry* and *Dodsworth.* Though well received and highly regarded, these are not as widely read as *Arrowsmith.* In 1930 he was awarded the Nobel Prize for literature. But the heavy drinking and the changing times were already taking their toll. Lewis published ten additional novels during the 1930s and 1940s, none of which measured up to the previous ones. After World War II he continued to travel widely, and in September 1949 sailed for Italy. There he took his last drink—one too many—and died in delirium tremens at the age of sixty-five.

De Kruif may well have taken some perverse pleasure from Lewis's tragic demise because of the bad feeling that erupted between the two men after *Arrowsmith* was completed. He expected to receive the acknowledgment "In collaboration with Paul de Kruif" on the title page. Instead, Lewis offered a generous but more qualified blurb on the following page, which de Kruif was ultimately forced to accept. In later editions of the book, Lewis's acknowledgment to de Kruif is replaced by a lengthy introduction by Barbara Grace Spayd or Mark Schorer, detailing precisely the contributions of both authors. Nonetheless, de Kruif refused to collaborate with Lewis again.

And he really didn't need to. During the writing of *Arrowsmith,* de Kruif spent his spare time in libraries collecting material about the

scientists responsible for the germ theory. When he later decided that he did not have Sinclair Lewis's aptitude for writing fiction, he sat down and produced his second and most famous book, *Microbe Hunters,* published in 1926.

Microbe Hunters is a lively, factual account of the men who brought about the golden age of microbiology. By 1971 it had sold more than a million copies and had been translated into eighteen languages. Famous scientists have remarked that they were inspired to enter medical research after reading it. Even a few critics approved of it.

"One of the noblest chapters in the history of mankind," wrote H. L. Mencken.

"A book for those who love high adventure, who delight in clear, brave writing and stirring narrative," said William Allen White.

But other critics were not so generous. De Kruif was faulted for his oversimplification and his verbose, slangy, sometimes ungrammatical prose. He also had the annoying habit of making up dialogue for his famous scientists. One example is an exchange between Giovanni Battista Grassi and Robert Koch.

> "This of that!" shouted Battista Grassi. "Either malaria is carried by one special particular bloodsucking mosquito, out of the twenty or forty kinds of mosquitoes in Italy—or it isn't carried by mosquitoes at all!"
> "Hrrrm-p," said Koch.

Despite these failings, de Kruif was never dull. After *Microbe Hunters,* he wrote eleven more books about science. Among these was *Hunger Fighters,* another work enthusiastically received by the general public and translated into many languages.

Yet the last word about the golden age belongs to Sinclair Lewis. Being nonfiction, *Microbe Hunters* did not ponder the future. *Arrowsmith* did.

Before he is sent to fight the plague epidemic in St. Hubert, Martin Arrowsmith makes a remarkable discovery. In the pus from a carbuncle he identifies a substance capable of killing the bacteria in an infected wound without harming the host tissue. Night and day he works to isolate and purify this material until he is pushed to the borderline of psychosis by the strain. For Martin believes that he has found the long-sought drug which can cure any bacterial infection in

man. Such a drug was, in fact, being assiduously looked for by many scientists.

In fact, what Martin Arrowsmith has isolated is a bacteria-infecting virus called a phage. Because he hesitates to publish until all details have been clarified, he is beaten to priority by a French researcher, Félix d'Herelle of the Pasteur Institute in Paris. And in the end, phage turns out to be worthless as a therapeutic agent.

But in 1928, four years after *Arrowsmith* was published, Alexander Fleming, a British bacteriologist, accidentally discovered a real substance capable of killing bacteria without harming the host; he named his new substance penicillin. The story of how this long-hoped-for new drug finally came into use turned out to be more surprising and ironic than even Martin Arrowsmith could have imagined.

CHAPTER SEVEN

The Chemotherapy of Infection

No medical condition is more unpredictable than bacterial infection. In some cases the tiniest, most insignificant-appearing scratch will begin to suppurate; in others, the deepest, most serious wound will heal without a trace of pus. And when infection does occur, the outcome without antibiotics is equally uncertain. A copiously draining wound may heal completely while a small infection in a superficial cut can prove lethal. Nothing better illustrates the unpredictability of infection than the illness of President Calvin Coolidge's youngest son.

On July 1, 1924, sixteen-year-old Calvin Coolidge, Jr., played a tennis match with his brother John on the White House court. During the game a small friction blister occurred on a toe of young Calvin's right foot. The blister ruptured and infection developed within a few hours. The wound became red and swollen as the boy became feverish. Dr. Edward Brown, the family doctor, was anxiously summoned, and Brown immediately called in a consultant, Commander Joel T. Boone. The prescribed treatment: elevation of the foot, with hot packs of mercury bichloride applied to the wound. Though the local inflammation gradually subsided, the symptoms of generalized sepsis (blood poisoning) quickly appeared.

As the young patient desperately fought for his life, the doctors were virtually useless. Continuous retention enemas and intravenous infusions of salt solution, the standard therapy at the time, were administered to no avail. Four blood cultures and one urine culture revealed a virulent bacterium, *Staphylococcus albus,* an organism that is usually a harmless resident on normal human skin. A blood donor was inoculated with killed bacteria from the cultures, and the boy then received infusions of the donor's blood in the hope that some passive immunity to the infection might be transferred. Intramuscular injections of commercial staphylococcal antitoxin in horse serum were also administered. The patient was even given injections of the new antiseptic mercurochrome, a substance mistakenly believed to possess miraculous powers to kill bacteria in vivo. Nothing helped.

On the sixth day, young Calvin complained of severe pain in the left leg. The shinbone was found to be red and swollen. The infection had been carried by the blood from the right foot to the left leg, where it infiltrated the bone and bone marrow.

The patient was taken from the White House to Walter Reed Hospital. Two eminent Philadelphia specialists, the surgeon John B. Deaver and the bacteriologist John Kolmer, were frantically summoned. Deaver gave the boy a ten-minute anesthetic, then chiseled an opening through the shinbone to allow pus to drain from the marrow cavity. But instead of pus, Deaver found only a mass of lethal staphylococci. The next day witnessed the onset of abdominal distention and vomiting—the terminal signs of sepsis. In the last moments of his life, young Calvin deliriously implored his powerful father to heal him.

Coolidge was totally shattered by the sudden, unexpected death of his favorite son. "When he went, the power and glory of the Presidency went with him," he wrote in his autobiography. "I do not know why such a price was exacted for occupying the White House."

This tragic and totally unpredictable nature of bacterial infection was first observed long before the twentieth century. In the Hippocratic corpus, an ancient Greek physician recorded analogous cases:

> The Cobbler, while piercing a sole, stabbed his thigh with the awl, above the knee, to the depth of about a finger.
>   No blood came out and the wound closed fast, but the whole thigh swelled up, and the swelling gained the groin and the flank. This man died on the third day.

But the one who was wounded by an arrow in the groin, and whom we saw ourselves, was saved most unexpectedly: because neither was the point extracted (it was lying too deep) nor was there any hemorrhage worth mentioning, nor inflammation, nor lameness. When we departed he still had the point, and that was after six years. It was thought that it lay between the tendons, and that no vein or artery had been severed.

In the instance of a relatively minor wound, the Greek doctor witnessed another unfavorable outcome:

About the time when the Pleiades set, the son of Metrophantos—wounded in the head with a shard [ostrakon] by another child—had fever. It was the twelfth day. [The fever occurred] because while washing himself, he hurt the edge of the wound, and caught cold. Soon the lips of the wound swelled up, and all around it the skin became thin. He was promptly trepanned. No pus came out, nor was there any relief. Pus seemed to form near the left ear [the wound was on that side]. But then this abscess did not form, and the left shoulder filled up fast with pus. He died about the twenty-fourth day.

Bacterial infections spreading from skin to bone in children were seen so frequently that the Greeks gave them a special name—
psiloma, "bareness"—which described the resultant bare patch of bony tissue. Here are some grim reminders of life without antibiotics:

The child of Phile, who had the bone laid bare in his forehead, had fever on the ninth day; the bone became livid; he died.
The same happened to the child of Phanias and to the child of Euergetes. The bone becomes livid, there is fever, the skin comes off the bone, and no pus appears.

Elsewhere in the Hippocratic corpus there is an especially vivid description of the agonizing death from a bone infection:

Trepanation brought out of the bone itself a thin ichor, serous, yellowish, stinking, deadly. In such cases vomiting may also occur, and spasms towards the end, and sometimes loud cries, and sometimes paralysis, on the left if the wound is on the right, on the right if it is on the left.

The child of Theodoros exposed himself to the sun on the ninth day. Fever came on the tenth day from a bareness of the bone which was, as one might say, nothing at all. During the fever the part became livid, the skin came off; many loud cries; on the twenty-second day the belly swelled up, especially toward the hypochondria; on the twenty-third he died.

In fifteenth-century Europe the common bacteria to be found in suppurating wounds such as these were joined by a new infectious micro-organism, *Treponema pallidum*—a slender, spiral rod or spirochete that propels itself by bending its body. Syphilis, the result of a *Treponema pallidum* infection, was the first disease caused by a micro-organism that was cured with a specific drug, Salvarsan. The discovery of this drug by Paul Ehrlich began the search that soon produced the antibiotics.

The Great Pox and the Magic Bullet

> . . . the small pox has gone out of late;
>   Perhaps it may be follow'd by the great.
>
> 'Tis said the great came from America
>   Perhaps it may set out on its return—
> The population there so spreads, they say
>   'Tis grown high time to thin it in its turn,
> With war, or plague, or famine, any way,
>   So that civilization they may learn;
> And which in ravage the more loathsome evil is—
>   Their real lues, or our pseudo-syphilis?

Syphilis, the great pox referred to by Byron in this nineteenth-century verse, first appeared in Europe when it struck Naples in 1494. During a fierce battle over the city between the French and Spanish the new disease surfaced suddenly in the form of an acute, infectious skin malady akin to smallpox. The Spanish troops, some of whom had sailed with Columbus, later admitted having acquired the puzzling new illness in the Indies. The ladies of Naples, who contracted it from the Spanish, passed the condition to the French when the city changed hands. Driven off a year later, the French soldiers returned home, and within three years syphilis epidemics swept through France, Germany, Switzerland, Holland, Scotland, Hungary, and Russia. The famous maritime explorers relayed it to India, China, and Japan. Jews and Moslems, driven from Spain, took it with them to North Africa. Thus within a short period, the entire civilized world had become infected.

Where did syphilis originate? No one is sure. The oldest theory holds that, as Byron says, it came from America, where it had been endemic among the natives.

Another theory maintains that a mild variety of syphilis could have long been confused by Europeans with leprosy. In fact, during the first documented outbreaks of syphilis, the disease was often mistaken for leprosy. Not only were appearances similar, but both were also known to be spread by contact.

Still a third theory postulates that syphilis resulted from the introduction of yaws into Spain and Portugal. Yaws is an African disease, bacteriologically identical to syphilis. But unlike the modern form of syphilis, yaws is transmitted mainly by nonsexual contact. It is quite common among children playing together naked. For this reason, yaws is found only in hot climates, where it appears as a horrible skin eruption. The spirochete of yaws, so the theory goes, will cause ordinary syphilis when introduced into a cold climate where people are fully clothed.

One of the earliest clear descriptions of syphilis was written by a German, Ulrich von Hutten, in 1519. According to Hutten, the characteristic acute skin eruption and fever seen in the first cases did not occur after the disease had been prevalent in Germany for about seven years. He also recognized that transmission was by venereal contact.

Hutten's interest in syphilis was more than academic. While in his early twenties, he himself had contracted a peculiarly repulsive case, with "boils that stood out like acorns, from whence issued such filthy stinking matter, that, whosoever came within scent believed himself infected." His physicians treated him with "foreign drugs" and prohibited him from eating peas because of "worms therein which had wings." When he didn't get better, the inflamed pustules on his skin were covered with burning mercury salve, and he was shoved into a large stove filled with glowing coals, where for a month he was kept on a starvation diet. The interior was sealed off from the outside, his only protection against incineration being the large towel that covered him. Hutten managed to survive this treatment, though other less fit syphilitics did not. He then returned for ten more mercury cures—a form of therapy that most patients avoided. Finally he was medicated with guaiac juice, a worthless remedy in vogue at the time, and improved.

"If we ought to give God thanks both for Good and Evil, how much are we bound for his gift of 'Guajacum,'" Hutten wrote ecstatically. "Yea, how much doth the Joy and Gladness for this his Bounty to us, surpass the Pains and Sorrow of our past sickness."

Hutten's "cure" was actually nothing more than a remission. After the skin eruption subsides spontaneously, the disease passes into a latent phase. In the Tuskegee Study, 431 Negro men with latent syphilis were purposely left untreated between 1932 and 1972, when an angry congressional investigating committee ordered that the study be halted. Only 34 per cent of all deaths in the Tuskegee group were due to late effects of syphilis. No doubt Hutten was one of the fortunate 66 per cent never troubled further by their disease.

In 1530, eleven years after Hutten's description appeared, the name syphilis was coined by Girolamo Fracastoro, a physician, poet, physicist, geologist, and astronomer. While living in Verona, Fracastoro published a medical poem, *Syphilis sive Morbus Gallicus,* about an impertinent shepherd named Syphilus who offended Apollo and was suitably chastised:

> He first wore Buboes dreadful to the sight,
> First felt strange Pains and sleepless past the Night;
> From him the Malady receiv'd its name. . . .

In his lengthy poem Fracastoro describes only the generalized skin eruption of secondary syphilis, omitting any mention of the primary genital lesion, the chancre, which customarily erupts and heals weeks before the secondary manifestations appear:

> Yet oft the Moon four monthly rounds shall steer
> Before convincing symptoms shall appear;
> So long the Malady shall lurk within,
> And grow confirm'd before the danger's seen

> The thinner parts will yet not stick so fast,
> But to the Surface of the Skin are cast
> Which in foul blotches o'er the Body spread,
> Prophane the Bosome, and deform the Head:
> Here Puscles in the form of Achorns swell'd
> In form alone, for these with Stench are fill'd

In a second treatise, *De Contagione et Contagiosis Morbis,* written fifteen years later in the pedestrian, droning prose common to medical textbooks, Fracastoro finally recognized the primary lesion: "At last, in the majority of cases, small ulcers began to appear on the sexual organs." And like Hutten, he noted that the disease had changed in character.

Since the days of Fracastoro and Hutten, syphilis has blighted the lives of the common and the great. Charles VIII and Francis I of France were afflicted. The murderous behavior of Ivan the Terrible is attributed to syphilis of the central nervous system. Pope Alexander VII and his nephew Peter Borgia contracted the disease. Among other famous victims have been the artists Benvenuto Cellini and Toulouse-Lautrec; the writers Heinrich Heine, Jules de Goncourt, Alphonse Daudet, and Guy de Maupassant; and the composers Franz Schubert and Robert Schumann. Catherine the Great of Russia, reputed to have been syphilitic, became so frightened of the malady that she took to having her numerous lovers screened through a committee of six women for six months. Cardinal Wolsey was accused of infecting Henry VIII by breathing on him.

For centuries the cause of syphilis was unknown. This ignorance led some physicians to suspect that all venereal diseases, including gonorrhea and chancroid, were merely manifestations of syphilis. John Hunter, the greatest English experimental surgeon of the eighteenth century, tried to verify this notion in a particularly tragic manner. He is said to have infected himself with the pus-filled urethral discharge of a gonorrhea patient, believing that he could effect a quick cure. Unfortunately, the pus contained *Treponema pallidum,* complicating poor Hunter's last years with syphilitic lesions.

In 1905, as the golden age of microbiology was drawing to a close, *Treponema pallidum* was at last identified by two Germans, F. R. Schaudinn and P. E. Hoffmann. Shortly thereafter, Hideyo Noguchi, a Japanese bacteriologist, isolated the same organism from the brains of patients who suffered from general paralysis of the insane. Noguchi had thus provided the link, suspected for half a century, between the early and late stages of syphilis. In 1906–7, the Wassermann test was developed, allowing the disease to be diagnosed even during its latent phases. The stage was now set for Paul Ehrlich's discovery of a cure for syphilis—the first great therapeutic triumph over an infectious disease in man.

"We must search for magic bullets," Ehrlich had remarked during his research. "We must strike the parasites, and the parasites only, if possible, and to do this, we must learn to aim with chemical substances."

"Dr. Fantasy," the young Ehrlich was nicknamed by colleagues who doubted the feasibility of such a goal. But ever since his student days, when he first became interested in organic dyes, Ehrlich was convinced that he was right.

Paul Ehrlich was born March 14, 1854, in the little Silesian village of Strehlen, then in Germany but now part of Poland. His well-to-do Jewish parents sent their son to a preparatory school in Breslau, and from 1872 through 1878 to medical schools in Strasbourg, Freiburg, and Breslau. He presented his doctoral dissertation at the University of Leipzig. Though an indifferent student, Ehrlich had already begun to do his own original research, influenced by the anatomist Waldeyer at Strasbourg. In Breslau he worked with the physiologist Heidenhain and with Koch's supporter, the pathologist Julius Cohnheim. It was Cohnheim's assistant, Ehrlich's older cousin Karl Weigert, who first introduced Ehrlich to the aniline dyes.

Aniline dyes had only recently come into use, though the process of dying was an ancient one. The Egyptians were coloring mummy cloths safflower yellow and indigo blue as early as 3000 B.C. Ancient Britons prized woad, a blue dye extracted from a wild Palestinian plant imported shortly before Julius Caesar's time. Most famous was the dye tyrian purple, long a cachet of royalty, that was obtained from certain shellfish.

Dying remained a small cottage industry until William Henry Perkin, an English chemist, synthesized tyrian purple, the first aniline dye. Ironically, Perkin had been trying to make synthetic quinine, a substance then in great demand. He had been spending evenings and vacations working in a crude home laboratory when in 1856, during the course of an experiment, he oxidized impure aniline with potassium dichromate and obtained a black product, from which he was able to extract synthetic tyrian purple. Perkin went on to synthesize other important organic compounds, and was knighted in 1906.

By this time, however, Perkin's chief economic beneficiaries were not the English but the Germans. Chemists educated in the many fine universities throughout the Prussian Empire immediately took up Perkin's discovery. Within a few years they had produced a veritable rainbow of synthetic dyes and synthetic natural dyes, spawning an enormous industry in Germany. Among these compounds were alizarin red, congo red, the fluorescent bluish-pink rhodamines, and phenolphthalein, the active ingredient in Ex-Lax. The culmination was the Nobel Prize–winning synthesis of indigo by Adolf von Baeyer. Natural indigo, one of the most popular of all colors, was highly variable in quality, even from the same producer. In 1868 Baeyer set to work, and by 1897 German dye factories were turning out the first commercial synthetic indigo. One of the other compounds produced during this era of dye research was used by Ehrlich to make Salvarsan, the first drug effective against syphilis.

Ehrlich initially employed the aniline dyes to stain the cells within blood—work that laid the foundation of modern hematology. He also dyed other tissues for microscopic examination and in 1878 wrote his doctoral dissertation at the University of Leipzig on this research. Dyes soon became the focus of his life, a constant preoccupation. Even in the evening, as his wife played for him on the piano, the tone-deaf Ehrlich continued to think of new medical ways to employ dyes.

Ambitious for an academic post, Ehrlich accepted in 1878 a position as privatdocent at the Second Medical Clinic of the Charité Hospital in Berlin. Here he continued his research until the sudden death of his preceptor, Professor von Frerichs, who was replaced by a far less congenial man. During the difficult period that ensued, Ehrlich discovered he was the victim of pulmonary tuberculosis by staining some of his own sputum. He resigned his position and spent most of the years 1888 and 1889 recuperating in Egypt.

In 1890 Ehrlich returned to Berlin as assistant to Robert Koch. He was just in time to assist Koch in administering tuberculin and witness the furor that followed. Koch, impressed by Ehrlich's brilliance, offered him a position in his new Institute for Infectious Diseases. For a time he was diverted from dye research to help Behring produce immune sera, and though he was later shamelessly flimflammed by the greedy Behring, his reputation from this research led to his 1896 appointment as director of the new Institute for the Investigation and Control of Sera in Berlin.

Ehrlich's new institute was nothing more than an old converted bakery; yet he needed little equipment: bottles of chemicals, shelves, test tubes, water, a Bunsen burner, blotting paper. Never bothered by unprepossessing surroundings, Ehrlich once remarked to a friend, "I can work just as well in a barn!"

In 1899 he received better than that. A large Institute for Experimental Therapy had been created in Frankfurt-on-Main through the efforts of the lord mayor, Dr. Franz Adickes. Ehrlich was appointed its first director, and there, during the last sixteen years of his life, he was to make his greatest discoveries. Among them was his Nobel Prize–winning work on immunity, which included identification of blood-group antigens and blood-group isoantibodies in goats. Working independently, Karl Landsteiner found the same substances in the blood of man, enabling blood transfusions to be made safely. The outcome of these and other studies led Ehrlich to postulate his famous "side-chain" theory of immunity. Chemical side chains produced by the body during infection, he wrote, united like a lock and key with bacterial toxins to neutralize them. Vigorously disputed during Ehrlich's lifetime, this concept is now being incorporated into some of the most recent theories of antibody formation.

Observers who came to watch Ehrlich at work marveled at the success of this unlikely-looking scientist, an almost Chaplinesque figure with detachable cuffs slipping over wrists, who was perpetually showering cigar ash. The laboratory was an indescribable mess, cluttered with test tubes, bottles, journals, bundles of paper—he hated to throw anything away. Every corner was permeated by the smell of cigar smoke and Ehrlich's shrill voice calling for mineral water or a fresh box of stogies.

Long-time associates were those capable of accepting the mercurial temperament of their boss. "Ehrlich is a man whom one can love as a child is loved," said one friend. The great scientist was famous for his irrational rages, his boundless energy, his naïve enthusiasm, and his conviction that all who were not friends were enemies. To subordinates he would hand out instructions on small cards covered with his messy, childish scrawl and underlined with colored pencils. He kept a duplicate of each card so he could be certain that each order was carried out to the umlaut. Grown men were often hostile and resentful toward this highhandedness, but many were

THE CHEMOTHERAPY OF INFECTION

equally fearful of the explosion that protest was sure to provoke. One of Ehrlich's most shameful outbursts, followed by the resignation of part of his senior staff, occurred during the search for Salvarsan.

Ehrlich was prompted to begin this search by the discovery that rats and mice could be infected with trypanosomes, the microbes recently discovered to cause sleeping sickness. In a truly great demonstration of intuitional bravura, Ehrlich plucked a particular bottle of dye from the shelf and instructed an assistant to administer it to an infected mouse. A chemical modification of the dye, trypan red, cured the animal. "Chemotherapy," was the name Ehrlich gave this form of treatment, described as the finding of "substances which have had their origin in the chemist's retort" and are capable of curing infections.

The immediate hope that trypan red might be of value in sleeping sickness was dashed by the first field trials. Ehrlich sent samples of the new drug to doctors working in the tropics and soon learned that the action was too unpredictable for use in treatment. In the meantime, however, two Englishmen had found another substance—atoxyl—that was also effective against the trypanosomes and seemed to help human patients. But this compound had a drawback: a nasty propensity to cause blindness by damaging the optic nerve.

In 1906 Ehrlich began to concentrate his attention on atoxyl, and immediately his unerring chemical intuition again became manifest. Contemporary chemists had worked out a formula for the atoxyl molecule that Ehrlich believed was incorrect. This formula designated a single nitrogen-containing side chain. But because of his knowledge of the chemical reactivity of atoxyl, Ehrlich correctly guessed that the compound had two side chains, only one of which contained the nitrogen atom.

Ehrlich's insight suggested a direct, practical benefit. The old formula indicated that the atoxyl molecule would be difficult or impossible to modify chemically. Ehrlich's formula, however, implied that modifications were possible and might produce a much more useful drug than atoxyl.

Unfortunately, Ehrlich's associates, the senior chemists at his institute, did not agree with him. Three, the doctors Braun, Schmitz, and Bertheim, challenged his apparently facile assumption. In one of his most truculent moods, Ehrlich told them in no uncertain terms that in his laboratory they would do as they were told. "You," he stormed at these well-trained scientists, "cannot judge whether this is right or wrong."

Braun and Schmitz quit on the spot. But Bertheim resolved to wait and see. Indeed, Ehrlich was shown to be completely correct, and the institute soon began synthesizing stable atoxyl derivatives. Bertheim's fame rose with Ehrlich's until the young associate's sudden, tragic demise. In 1914 he joined the army. On his first day in uniform, his spurs tangled in the carpet on a flight of stairs and he tripped. Poor Bertheim was killed by the fall.

Ehrlich was much luckier. As he watched, his assistants produced compound after compound from the original atoxyl molecule. He himself sat in his office for hours on end, dreaming up new possible modifications. His thinking, he claimed, was facilitated by the music of an organ grinder in the street outside his window. The organ grinder, it is said, grew wealthy on the coins that Ehrlich continually dropped into his cup.

No money, however, was made from the early modifications of atoxyl. Some of the derivatives were still capable of curing trypanosome-infected mice, but others produced a fatal jaundice. A few generated a queer alteration in the behavior of the mice—a frantic, jumping, whirling dance that they would perform until they died. Only two of the new compounds appeared of any value. Arsenophenylglycine, the 418th variant synthesized, seemed to be effective against treponemes. And compound number 606, dioxy-diamino-arseno-benzene hydrochloride also engendered some optimism until an assistant tried it and found it to be ineffective.

While this work was going on, a young Japanese bacteriologist, Sahachiro Hata, discovered a way to infect rabbits with *Treponema pallidum*. No one before had been able to produce syphilis in an animal, and even today *Treponema pallidum* cannot be grown on a culture medium. Kitasato, Ehrlich's old associate in Koch's laboratory, had brought Hata's exceptional achievement to Ehrlich's attention.

Hata was brought from Tokyo to the institute in Frankfurt, where Ehrlich gave him the two promising compounds—numbers 418 and 606—from the large array already tested. The young bacteriologist tested these with characteristic patience. After many careful experiments on infected rabbits, he reported to Ehrlich that 606 was effective against *Treponema pallidum*.

Ehrlich was puzzled, since Hata's results contradicted those previously obtained. He ordered that the tests be repeated. Again 606 proved to be of value. On August 31, 1909, Ehrlich watched as Hata injected the compound into a large rabbit with two large syphilitic ulcers on its scrotum. Microscopic examination of fluid from the lesions revealed numerous wriggling treponemes. One day later not a treponeme was to be found, and within a month the ulcers were completely healed.

The most anxious moment had arrived—the first human tests. Other arsenic-containing compounds were known to produce blindness. Nonetheless, two young assistants in the institute volunteered as experimental subjects. They survived unharmed.

Yet Ehrlich still hesitated to treat syphilis with Salvarsan, as he came to call 606. Instead, the first clinical trials were made on relapsing fever, a spirochetal infection recently shown to be curable with atoxyl. Salvarsan samples were sent to Dr. Julius Iverson, a St. Petersburg physician, for use during a relapsing fever epidemic in the city. Of the fifty-five patients treated by Iverson in 1909, fifty-one made a complete recovery after one injection.

Syphilis, Ehrlich soon found, responded equally dramatically to Salvarsan therapy. At first, deafness appeared to be a worrisome side effect of the medication, but careful analysis of the results showed that hearing loss occurred only when Salvarsan was misused. On April 19, 1910, Ehrlich and Hata reported their findings at the Congress for International Medicine at Wiesbaden, Germany.

The demand for Salvarsan quickly became so great that Ehrlich ordered his entire laboratory to do nothing but manufacture the yellow crystalline powder. He himself supervised the dispensing of the thousands of doses. On a cupboard door in his little office he maintained a daily tally, which soon extended down to the carpeted floor. No physician was permitted to use the medicine unless Ehrlich was apprised of the results. And administration was difficult. The powder was dissolved in water at the bedside and then injected into a vein. If the vein should be missed and the Salvarsan injected into the tissue, severe damage to the living cells often necessitated amputation of the patient's arm. The situation was made more amenable when Ehrlich's laboratory came up with compound number 914, Neosalvarsan. It was less active against the treponemes but far safer to administer.

By this time, however, the first tragedies of chemotherapy were coming to public attention—amputated limbs, permanent deafness. The tremendous initial enthusiasm in the press was transformed into harsh criticism of both Ehrlich and his wonder drug. Most virulent was *Die Wahrheit* ("The Truth"), a Frankfurt paper. Its crotchety publisher, Karl Wassmann, claimed that local doctors were becoming rich off Salvarsan, and he accused them of compelling prostitutes to serve as guinea pigs for the therapeutic trials.

In May 1914 the city slapped Wassmann with a libel suit. Ehrlich, in declining health and deeply wounded by the mounting criticism, was called to testify. While he gave his testimony, he was periodically interrupted by shouts from Wassmann and the whores in the courtroom as he reluctantly admitted that the early use of Salvarsan had indeed been disastrous in some cases.

In the end, Wassmann was found guilty and forced to spend a year in jail. Though his own reputation was left intact, Ehrlich had been thrown into a deep depression by the public indignation he was forced to suffer. He never recovered and on August 20, 1915, suffered a fatal stroke. Shortly before his death he was praised by an admirer for his discovery.

"You say a great work of the mind, a wonderful scientific achievement?" Ehrlich replied. "My dear colleague, for seven years of misfortune I had one moment of good luck."

"Sir Almost Right"

Paul Ehrlich's unremitting melancholia in his final months was not only the result of his trial. He had hoped to synthesize a substance which, in one big dose, could destroy all disease microbes within the body. Until a few days before his death, he was still tinkering with Salvarsan, still trying to find the real wonder drug in the short time he knew he had left.

Not everyone in the medical community, however, was so sanguine about the possibility of ever finding such a drug. Chief among the doubters was a British immunologist, Sir Almroth Wright. And it was Wright's distorted viewpoint that shaped the story of penicillin by creating the twelve-year hiatus between its discovery and its eventual isolation. "Sir Almost Right," a number of unkind critics called him.

Wright was a physician of Irish descent who had become professor of pathology at the Army Medical School at Netley on Southampton Water in 1892. Within a short period he had produced a typhoid vaccine from killed typhoid bacilli. The Wright vaccine attracted immediate attention, since many died of typhoid in England every year. The disease was a special scourge of British soldiers in the hot, unsanitary distant corners of the empire.

After some encouraging early clinical trials, Wright tried to convince military authorities to vaccinate all soldiers sent off to Africa during the Boer War. But Wright had broken with the Pasteur tradition by using killed micro-organisms in his typhoid vaccine; as a result, the dubious medical establishment permitted only 16,000 volunteers to be inoculated out of 320,000 soldiers. And further obstructionism made followup of even the 16,000 voluntary subjects quite difficult. It is said that one medical orderly recorded every typhoid victim as having been vaccinated. When asked why, he replied, "The fact that they've got it proves as they've been vaccinated."

Yet the statistics, such as they were, persuaded Wright that his vaccine was effective. Others, however, remained doubtful. The most persistent of these skeptics was Karl Pearson, a distinguished statistician. In the pages of the *British Medical Journal,* Pearson, in a well-argued case, tried to refute Wright's interpretation of his own results. The chagrined Wright fought an angry battle with Pearson and others, producing considerable public stir and private bitterness.

After furiously resigning from the Army Medical Service, Wright secured an appointment as professor of pathology at St. Mary's Hospital, Paddington, in London, where he remained until 1945. Here, as head of the hospital's Inoculation Department, he continued the struggle to have his typhoid vaccine accepted. His personal friendship with Lord Haldane, the secretary of war, finally brought vindication in a somewhat circuitous manner.

"Dear Wright," Haldane is said to have written, "we must have your Typhoid Prophylactic for the Army but I have failed to convince the head man of the Army Medical Service of this. I have, therefore, got to build you up as a Public Figure, and the first step is to make you a knight. You won't like it, but it has to be. . . ."

During his tenure at St. Mary's, Wright's scientific reputation grew on account of his resolution of the controversy over immunity. There were at the time two rival theories of immunity, which Wright managed to combine. Modern ideas of immunity have stemmed directly from this combination. In his enthusiasm, however, Wright became dogmatic and soon had gone too far on a false scent he called the op-sonin theory.

The first of the rival immunity theories, propounded to explain the efficacy of vaccination, maintained that factors in the blood fought off germs. Vaccination, it was believed, produced these factors, though at the turn of the century there was no means for verifying their existence. Much later they were isolated and identified as an-tibodies.

The second of the rival theories evolved from the work of a Rus-sian biologist, Elie Metchnikoff, a brooding, pessimistic, politically radical man who might have stepped out of the pages of a nine-teenth-century Russian novel. During fits of depression, Metchnikoff had twice attempted suicide, once by morphine overdose followed by soaking wet exposure to cold on the Rhône Bridge; on another occa-sion he was even more resourceful, injecting himself with the spiro-chete of relapsing fever, from which—to his dismay—he recovered. These elegant failures were only matched by the elegant success of the simple experiment he conceived to test his theory of immunity.

This famous study was performed in 1882, when an inheritance acquired from his wife's parents allowed Metchnikoff to spend time on the shores of the Mediterranean examining zoological specimens. While using his microscope to observe mobile cells in the transparent larva of a starfish, he conceived the remarkable notion that "similar cells might serve in the defense of the organism against intruders." To test his idea, he pushed rose thorns under the skin of starfish lar-vae. Sure enough, several hours later, the thorns were surrounded by mobile cells. He confirmed his theory by infecting the larvae with bacteria. As he watched, the cells surrounded and engulfed the in-vading germs. *Phagocytosis* was the term that Metchnikoff coined for this process.

After similar studies on the waterflea *Daphnia,* Metchnikoff was convinced that the white blood cells of both the flea and man pro-vided immunity by surrounding and engulfing invading microbes, just as the mobile cells did in the starfish. Vaccination expedited this process, he believed, by gradually strengthening the protective white cells as they attacked the weakened germs, much in the way a prizefighter is strengthened for the big match by sparring partners.

To reconcile Metchnikoff's idea with the blood-factor theory, Sir Almroth Wright postulated that factors in the circulating blood facili-tated phagocytosis. This collaboration between antibodies and phagocytes is now an accepted part of our modern concept of immunity. But Wright then went too far. The blood factors worked, he claimed, by making the germs more appetizing for the phagocytes. A great lover of Greek and Latin medical terms, Wright coined the name *opsonins* for his factors, from the Greek *opsono,* which means "I prepare food for."

The opsonin theory engendered a great deal of controversy and some ridicule. George Bernard Shaw, a good friend of Wright's, included both opsonin and the man who conceived it in a play, *The Doctor's Dilemma.* In the first act Sir Colenso Ridgeon, a gently satiric caricature of Wright, explains his dubious theory to Sir Patrick, a skeptical doctor of the old school:

> RIDGEON: Opsonin is what you butter the disease germs with to make your white corpuscles eat them. . . . What it comes to in practice is this. The phagocytes won't eat the microbes unless the microbes are nicely buttered for them. Well, the patient manufactures the butter for himself all right; but my discovery is that the manufacture of that butter, which I call opsonin, goes on in the system by ups and downs—Nature being always rhythmical you know—and what the inoculation does is to stimulate the ups or downs as the case may be. . . . Inoculate when the patient is in the negative phase and you kill; inoculate when the patient is in the positive phase and you cure.

Even in *Arrowsmith,* the validity of Wright's idea was questioned: "[Gottlieb] had worked for years on the synthesis of antibodies; he was at present in a blind alley, and at Mohalis there was no one who was interested, no one to stir him, but he was having an agreeable time massacring the opsonin theory, and that cheered him."

Wright, however, could not be dissuaded from his belief in opsonin. His laboratory worked out an "opsonic index," which was measured by special techniques. The index was used to gauge treatment by "auto-vaccination"—using the microbe causing the infection to make an antitoxin or vaccine that was administered to the patient.

Perhaps Wright managed to miss the immunologic boat with the opsonin theory because his real abilities lay in the realm of literature rather than science. A great lover of poetry, he was said to be able to recite from memory some 250,000 lines of the Bible, Dante, Goethe, and the great English poets. Figures from the prominent literary, dramatic, and artistic circles were regular visitors to the Inoculation Department. And Wright himself was an able writer, who shamelessly popularized his work in newspaper articles despite the protests of fellow scientists that hoi polloi should not be made privy to laboratory secrets.

There was, however, very little protest in the Inoculation Department itself, which Wright ruled with iron discipline. Though he claimed to preside over a "republic," fief might have been a better description. He was The Professor, lord and master of his domain. Yet he still managed to attract some very brilliant young scientists. At least four became Fellows of the Royal Society and another became a Fellow of the Royal Society of Canada. Sir William Leishman, one of the most famous, is known for his studies of the parasitic infection kala azar.

Two of Wright's other associates in the Inoculation Department, Leonard Colebrook and Ronald Hare, did much to disprove the opsonin theory by showing that whatever the opsonic index measured was not what it was intended to measure. Wright nonetheless continued to cling to the idea. When writing the section on immunity in the 1922 edition of the *Encyclopaedia Britannica,* he included the opsonin theory in full. In *The Doctor's Dilemma* Shaw had a pompous, successful medico, Sir Ralph Bloomfield Bonington, summarize Wright's controversial beliefs:

> Drugs can only repress symptoms: they cannot eradicate disease. The true remedy for all diseases is Nature's remedy. Nature and Science are at one, Sir Patrick, believe me; though you were taught differently. Nature has provided in the white corpuscles as you call them—in the phagocytes as we call them—a natural means of devouring and destroying all disease germs. There is at bottom only one genuinely scientific treatment of all diseases and that is to stimulate the phagocytes. Stimulate the phagocytes. Drugs are a delusion. Find the germ of the disease; prepare from it a suitable anti-toxin; inject it three times a day quarter of an hour before meals; and what is the result? The phagocytes are stimulated; they devour the disease; and the patient recovers—unless, of course, he's too far gone. That, I take it, is the essence of Ridgeon's discovery.

Sir Almroth Wright distilled the essence of his "discovery" even further in his often-quoted adage "Mobilize the immunological garrison." This dubious piece of wisdom pervaded one of the most prominent centers of British medical research, the Inoculation Department of St. Mary's Hospital, at the moment in 1928 that a staff bacteriologist, Alexander Fleming, noted some strange behavior in bacteria growing on a mold-contaminated dish.

Fleming's Discoveries

SIR ALEXANDER FLEMING
Discoverer of Penicillin
was born here at Lochfield
on 6th August, 1881

These words are inscribed on a simple red granite monument at the gate of a farm in Ayrshire, in southwest Scotland. And the man they commemorate had an equally simple childhood and youth. He attended a local grammar school before leaving for London to seek his fortune in a shipping office. A small legacy from an uncle permitted him to leave this dreary job and enroll in the London Polytechnic. Here his high marks resulted in a medical scholarship at London University. From the university, he moved as a medical student to St. Mary's Hospital, the institution in which he was to spend his entire professional career. Fleming chose St. Mary's not on account of its scientific reputation but because he was interested in joining the hospital's rifle shooting team.

Though famous throughout Europe in Fleming's day, St. Mary's would depress any modern scientist. The hospital had only been founded during the nineteenth century and consequently possessed a small endowment. The physical condition of the buildings was deplorable, jammed as they were between Paddington Railway Station and the wharves of the Grand Union Canal—one of the seediest sections of London. The medical school classrooms were dreadfully cold and filthy. The only laboratory outside the Inoculation Department was a tiny room in the basement where the medical clerks tested urine. But very few staff members had much time for research, since most were forced to make a living treating private patients for at least half the week.

The Inoculation Department offered somewhat better facilities, though not much better. It consisted of four floors facing Praed Street, the main thoroughfare to Paddington Station. So fearfully overcrowded were the rooms that even the director, Sir Almroth Wright, was forced to share his office. The appearance of the place at the time of Fleming's discovery of penicillin was later described by Ronald Hare:

> Privacy was completely unknown. . . . The room in which all the glassware was prepared and the media made was not much larger [than fifteen feet square]. The darkroom had been converted from a very small [lavatory] and the hot room was a gas-operated death trap about the same size. Although the Department had appeared much more prosperous and better staffed than the Medical School, it was almost poverty-stricken by modern standards. We had to buy our own microscopes. There was no fume cupboard or sterile room. The nearest approach to a refrigerator was a wooden box about the size of a tea chest into which someone inserted a block of ice if he happened to remember. But one thing the place did possess, and that in abundance, was its smell: an all pervading odour of hot oil reminiscent of an engine room, which was produced by the heated oilbaths in which we sterilised our syringes.

The shortage of space was matched by a shortage of money. Wright paid the salaries of his young researchers out of his fees from wealthy and fashionable patients. These salaries were so pitifully inadequate that everyone was forced to do some private practice of his own. Wright tried to make the outside work seem like a virtue, remarking that it allowed a man to "keep his feet on the ground." But actually it served to strengthen Wright's iron grip on his subordinates, since both pay levels and promotions were entirely dependent on his own whims.

Salaries gradually began to rise as the demand increased for vaccines made by the department. Especially good customers were the private boarding schools, where the upper class and upper middle class children were sent. To prevent the epidemics of infactious diseases that often cost the schools many paying customers, swabs were taken from the boys' throats at the start of term and vaccines prepared from the cultured bacteria. Vaccination of the entire school was real bread-and-butter work, though often long and arduous. Especially tricky was the making of the vaccines themselves.

No one was better at this craft than Fleming. Everyone who knew him attested to the miracles that he could work with only the most elementary equipment. In fact, his amazing manual dexterity had almost led him into surgery before he settled on bacteriology, and he was elected a fellow of the Royal College of Surgeons. Fleming also proved to be an extremely conscientious employee, as one associate recalled: "He was always most meticulous about giving the department the time it paid him for. I remember he would never open the incubator and start handling his own private vaccine work until the clock had struck six."

Wright himself was well aware of these attributes and appears to have been inordinately fond of Fleming. Usually accustomed to taking most of the credit for the institute's publications, he allowed his associate on one paper at least a fair share: "My colleague Dr. Alexander Fleming has given in the treatise which is prefaced by these remarks of mine an admirable summing up of the results obtained by the Inoculation Department at St. Mary's Hospital. . . ."

Fleming's legendary dexterity prompted Wright to make him the department venereologist. In 1910 Ehrlich had come to London to visit his friend Wright, bringing along samples of Salvarsan. Since a slip during the injection of the drug could mean loss of an arm, Wright saw that Fleming was the man to administer the patients' weekly doses. Fleming thus became the first British doctor to use Salvarsan and one of the leading venereologists in London before the war. This enormously lucrative specialty enabled Fleming to accumulate a comfortable nest egg, along with a country home in Suffolk.

At the outbreak of the First World War in 1914 Fleming accompanied Wright's group to a special research laboratory in the casino at Boulogne. It was here, while studying the infectious complications of battle wounds—sepsis, gangrene, tetanus—that Fleming produced one of his finest pieces of research. Unfortunately, the outcome strongly reinforced Wright's dictum "Drugs are a delusion," and no doubt made Fleming all the more willing to later discount the formidable therapeutic possibilities of penicillin.

Since Lister's work a half century before, no one doubted the value of sterilizing surgical instruments to prevent wound infections. Likewise, the covering of an uninfected wound with antibacterial dressings was also accepted as beneficial. The treatment of an infected wound, however, with antiseptics such as boric acid, hydrogen peroxide, and that old standby, carbolic acid, was beginning to be questioned.

Fleming's war studies demonstrated conclusively that the body's own defenses were the only forces that could be depended on to eradicate the infection from a wound. Infected wounds were battlegrounds in which phagocytes massed in greater numbers than in uninfected wounds to fight off the invading bacteria. Antiseptics, Fleming showed, killed these phagocytes—the body's primary defenders—more quickly and effectively than they killed microbes, thus tilting the advantage toward the germs. He strengthened this finding with other studies indicating that antiseptics actually increased the likelihood of gangrene and the rapidity of its development. In other words, dumping antiseptic in an infected wound only made matters worse.

Fleming clinched his argument by the ingenious use of common laboratory glassware. After making a crude glass model of ragged wound tissues in the bottom of a test tube, he applied bacteria. No amount of antiseptic treatment could eradicate these microbes; Fleming could repeatedly infect sterile human blood serum by pouring it over his "disinfected" glass wound.

Wright and Fleming may have been convinced of the worthlessness of chemotherapy by these elegant experiments, but others were not. Wright fought bitter public battles over antiseptics with the Army Medical Service, his old nemesis, and Sir William Watson Cheyne, the president of the Royal College of Surgeons. A *cause célèbre* was mercurochrome, the mercury compound tried on President Coolidge's dying son. This antiseptic was given to Lord Balfour, the man responsible to Parliament for the Medical Research Council, on a visit to America when his lordship developed a sore throat. After gargling with the stuff, Balfour was so impressed that he built a research project around the new wonder drug. Long after Leonard Colebrook and Ronald Hare had shown that mercurochrome was "singularly ineffective even in the test tube, and still more so in the tissues," it continued to enjoy considerable popularity. In his 1940 autobiography Dr. Hugh Hampton Young, the Johns Hopkins urologist, gave it an enthusiastic endorsement.

Another prevalent remedy during the 1920s was Sanocrysin, the gold therapy for tuberculosis. Wright personally discredited this substance by proving that twenty times the normal human dose had no effect on tubercle bacilli in the test tube. Salvarsan, the only antiseptic that worked in the body, seemed to be *sui generis*. Doctors became convinced that an agent active against other infections would never be found.

Fleming further fueled the general spirit of therapeutic nihilism with his discovery of lysozyme in 1922. Identification of this important component of many animal fluids—mucus, tears, egg albumen—was a major achievement. Yet the whole lysozyme story unfolded as such a caricature of the later penicillin discovery that when the real wonder drug came along, Fleming was totally unmoved. Lysozyme had solidified his almost mystical belief that microbes could never be attacked once inside the body.

The best description of the lysozyme discovery is found in the Maurois biography of Fleming. Dr. V. D. Allison, a new laboratory assistant, relates what happened one day while watching Fleming wash Petri dishes:

> As he took up one of the dishes in his hand he looked at it for a long time, showed it to me and said, "This is interesting." I had a good look at it. It was covered with large yellow colonies which appeared to me to be obvious contaminants. But the remarkable fact was that there was a wide area in which there were no organisms; and another further one in which the organisms had become translucent and glassy. Beyond that again were organisms which were in a transitional stage of degradation, between the very glassy ones and those which were fully developed with their normal pigment.

Fleming explained that he had added a little of his own nasal mucus to this dish when he happened to have a cold. The mucus was in the middle zone with no growth. And he guessed that some component of the mucus must have killed the nearby microbes.

"Now that is really interesting," Fleming said again. "We must go into it more thoroughly."

But here the story becomes the inverse of what happened with penicillin. For it was the yellow organisms, not a contaminating mold, that had landed on the plate. And as luck would have it, these

bacteria, "likely to have been in the atmosphere of the laboratory
. . . [or] blown in through the window from the dust and air of
Praed Street," were the one species most easily destroyed by lysozyme. They were previously unknown to science, totally harmless to
man, and named *Micrococcus lysodeikticus* by Fleming, from Greek
words meaning an organism which demonstrates the power of dissolving.

Though disappointed that lysozyme seemed to have no value
against disease-causing microbes, Fleming continued to pursue his
discovery. He proved that lysozyme was found in many plants and
animals, and was apparently the first line of defense against germs.
For this reason, he surmised, it was abundant in exposed areas such
as the mucous membranes of the eyes and nose.

Fleming's report of his discovery points up one of his greatest
failings—his poor ability to communicate. In its introductory para-
graphs, the lysozyme article, entitled "On a remarkable Bacteriolytic
element found in tissues and secretions," inexplicably omits Fleming's two most important findings. It says nothing about how or why
the lysozyme was first noticed, and, even worse, it gives no clue as to
lysozyme's ability to destroy *Micrococcus lysodeikticus*.

Leonard Colebrook, Fleming's loyal former associate, was as puzzled by these strange omissions as everyone else. When writing Fleming's official biography for the Royal Society, he was forced to clarify
considerably the lysozyme paper: "Dr. V. D. Allison, who collaborated with Fleming in much of his lysozyme work, tells me that
Fleming thought these micrococci did not actually come from his
nose, but were chance contaminants blown onto the plate from the
air. . . . It is not quite clear what led Fleming to suspect that there
was something in the nasal mucus which would exert a powerful lytic
action on this microbe. Probably there were some areas on his plate
cultures where the growth of the micrococcus was inhibited or prevented by particles of mucus. At any rate he did suspect it and his
suspicions were confirmed."

Fleming's singular inability to communicate not only was manifest
in his writing but was readily apparent to everyone who met him.
After a first encounter, Professor Ernst Chain, the chemist responsible for the extraction of penicillin, remarked of Fleming, "He had
an almost pathological inability to communicate."

Friends who very much loved him mentioned the same thing. In
an official *Memoir,* Colebrook wrote, "Fleming was a man of few

words—and ideas did not greatly interest him. Women on meeting him for the first time were often nonplussed by the unemotional, 'almost basilisk' stare, which some of them mistook for rudeness, while others were fascinated."

So inadequate was Fleming at getting his ideas across that even at small talk he was a failure. As Ronald Hare recalled:

> Fleming's idea of gossip was different from that of most other people. It usually involved his planting himself in front of the fireplace, with his hands in his pockets, a cigarette dangling from his lips, and looking more or less into space. On rare occasions he would give utterance, usually in the fewest possible words. The information doled out so meagrely might concern anything; that so-and-so had died; that what's-his-name had made a fool of himself again; or how are your Snia Viscosas [stock market shares] doing?

By 1928 Fleming had been appointed professor of bacteriology and deputy director of St. Mary's Inoculation Department. Sir Almroth Wright, over sixty years old, still dominated the place, though he had factionalized his staff by antagonizing one member, Dr. J. B. Freeman. This gifted immunologist, whom Wright once called his "son in science," was angry because the director had put his own name on Freeman's first important paper despite the fact that the work was solely Freeman's. The result was that the staff members on Freeman's side were quick to pooh-pooh the many apparently pointless natural observations that Wright's protégé Fleming was continually making. And the medical community outside the hospital, hostile toward the pompous, argumentative Wright, was equally scornful of new discoveries from his department. In this discouraging intellectual climate, penicillin made its scientific debut.

No one knows the exact date on which Fleming made his first observation of the action of penicillin. Fleming himself was unable to recall, and no written record survives. It seems to have been on a Monday late in August or early in September 1928. Furthermore, the exact details of what happened on that day have been made fuzzy by later hagiography. Only Fleming's official scientific publication of his discovery seems to provide an accurate, unemotional description of what happened. "On the antibacterial action of cultures of a penicillium with special reference to their use in the isolation of B.

influenzae" was published in the *British Journal of Experimental Pathology,* which designated the article as having been "Received for publication May 10th, 1929."

"While working with staphylococcus variants," Fleming tells us in the first paragraph, "a number of culture plates were set aside on the laboratory bench and examined from time to time. In the examinations these plates were necessarily exposed to the air and they became contaminated with various micro-organisms. It was noticed that around a large colony of a contaminating mold the staphylococcus colonies became transparent and were obviously undergoing lysis."

Competent scientists have criticized this first paragraph as being little better than the introduction to the lysozyme paper. Fleming makes no comment on what types of staphylococci were employed, what medium they were grown on, or whether they were incubated. Nor does he reveal the age of the bacteria, the size of the mold colony, the percentage of staphylococci that were lysed, or how far from the mold the effect extended. And nothing is said about the origin of the mold.

Fleming later claimed that his penicillium mold had been blown through the window of his laboratory, which fronted on Praed Street. But others have testified that Fleming, a competent bacteriologist, kept his window closed in order to avoid contaminants. The sill was generally cluttered with plates or test tubes, and so short a man as Fleming would have experienced considerable difficulty opening this particular window.

But directly below Fleming's laboratory, two floors down, an Irish scientist, C. J. La Touche, was studying molds from the houses of asthmatic patients. It was Wright's idea that these molds precipitated asthmatic attacks, and injections of the offending substances could be used to desensitize the patients, thus curing them. Fleming himself appears to have contributed one sample from a pair of moldy shoes in his country home. La Touche had the same penicillium mold in his collection that was found by Fleming on his famous plate, and there is little doubt that it was blown up the staircase from La Touche's laboratory.

In his paper Fleming proceeds to describe how he immediately went on to subculture this mold—no doubt his single most important contribution to the production of penicillin. A former assistant, Merlyn Price, happened to visit the laboratory on the fateful day, and subsequently recorded what he observed: "[Fleming] was busy taking a little piece of the mould with his scalpel and putting it in a tube of broth. Then he picked off a scrap measuring about one square millimetre which floated on the surface of the broth."

In his paper Fleming describes how he went on to grow this little scrap in various nutrient solutions at different temperatures. He found that the rate of growth was markedly affected by both the temperature and the composition of the media. He also discovered that as the mold grew, the medium would become alkaline. These observations were to prove quite important later on by providing clues as to how the mold should be grown and the penicillin extracted.

Fleming's next job was the identification of his mold and the testing of other species for antibacterial activity. In his paper he says that he examined eight additional molds, five of which were penicillium varieties. "Of these," Fleming wrote, "it was found that only one strain of penicillium produced any inhibitory substance, and that one had exactly the same cultural characters as the original one from the contaminated plate." It appears that Fleming obtained these specimens from La Touche.

La Touche played an additional role in the discovery by incorrectly identifying the mold in Fleming's original culture as a *Penicillium rubrum*. When years later the American mycologist Dr. Charles Thom established that the organism was actually a *Penicillium notatum,* La Touche apologized to Fleming and accepted blame for the mistake in the original paper.

Realizing that he had observed a singular phenomenon peculiar to a certain species of mold, Fleming tells in his paper how he went on to test the antibacterial substance that his *Penicillium notatum* produced:

> The simplest method of examining for inhibitory power is to cut a furrow in an agar plate (or a plate of other suitable culture material), and fill this in with a mixture of equal parts of agar and the broth in which the mold has grown. When this has solidified, cultures of various microbes can be streaked at right angles from the furrow to the edge of the plate. The inhibitory substance diffuses very rapidly in the agar, so that in the few hours before the microbes show visible growth it has spread out for a centimetre or more in sufficient concentration to inhibit growth of a sensitive microbe. On further incubation it will be seen that the proximal portion of the culture for per-

haps one centimetre becomes transparent and on examination of this portion of the culture it is found that practically all the microbes are dissolved.

This method, invented by a Swiss scientist named Garré in 1887, was used by Fleming to show that the substance made by his penicillium mold would prevent the growth of staphylococci, streptococci, the gonorrhea-producing gonococci, the meningitis-producing meningococci, the diphtheria bacillus, the pneumococcus of pneumonia, and a few other bacteria that normally do not cause human disease. But he also found that his "mold broth filtrate" was totally ineffective against the bacilli of typhoid and cholera and many normal inhabitants of the bowel. *B. pyocyaneus* and *B. proteus,* organisms commonly causing wound infection, were also untouched. Because *B. influenzae* was similarly unaffected, Fleming suggested that the filtrate might be used to isolate this organism—the only practical application he ever made of his discovery.

Why did the filtrate kill some organisms but not others? One reason appeared to be bacterial cell-wall structure. A Danish scientist, Hans Christian Gram, had previously shown that some bacteria could be colored by a type of stain not accepted by others. It was the cell walls of these organisms that determined whether or not the dye would be retained. Those that did hold dye, the Gram-positive bacteria, were the ones Fleming found vulnerable to penicillium filtrate. Gram-negative bacteria were usually resistant. This differential susceptibility later provided the first clue that penicillin worked by inhibiting synthesis of the cell wall.

In later studies Fleming found that there were some varieties of Gram-positive organisms impervious to his filtrate. He thus became the first to recognize and isolate penicillin-resistant bacterial strains. Today we know that this form of resistance is due not to cell-wall structure but to a penicillin-destroying enzyme produced by the microbe.

Fleming made another important observation in his first paper: the variation in activity of his mold-broth filtrate. When the mold was grown on a new plate, five days were required before any antibacterial action appeared. But the eighth-day filtrate—twenty-five times as strong as the fifth-day filtrate—would still kill staphylococci, Fleming found, when diluted one part to five hundred in water. And under the right conditions a filtrate could be produced that was effective against staphylococci at 1:600 dilutions.

Most surprisingly, this highly powerful antibacterial agent was nontoxic to animals and men—the first such substance that had ever been discovered. The unemotional Fleming makes note of this supremely important characteristic in what almost might be called an aside:

> The toxicity to animals of powerfully antibacterial mould broth filtrates appears to be very low. Twenty cubic centimetres injected intravenously into a rabbit were not more toxic than the same quantity of broth. Half a cubic centimetre injected intraperitoneally into a mouse weighing about twenty grams induced no toxic symptoms. Constant irrigation of large infected surfaces in man was not accompanied by any toxic symptoms, while irrigation of the human conjunctiva every hour for a day had no irritant effect.
>
> In vitro penicillin which completely inhibits the growth of staphylococci in a dilution of 1:600 does not interfere with leucocytic function to a greater extent than does ordinary broth.

The human conjunctiva irrigated every hour belonged to Stuart Craddock, Fleming's young assistant. Craddock had a bacterial infection, which he permitted Fleming to treat with filtrate. One cubic centimeter of the liquid wiped out almost all the infecting organisms. Within a short time Craddock's condition had cleared up completely.

The "large infected surfaces" were those of a woman who had slipped and fallen in front of a bus at Paddington Station. The horrible open leg wound she sustained necessitated amputation, but still sepsis occurred. Fleming was called in as consultant bacteriologist.

"Something very odd has happened in my lab," he told the woman's physician. "At this very moment I have got a culture of mold which destroys staphylococci."

Fleming was permitted to apply a dressing soaked in mold juice over the amputated stump. The patient, however, did not recover. But another of Fleming's assistants, Dr. K. B. Rogers, was completely cured of an eye infection by the filtrate. Fleming was especially pleased, since Rogers was then able to take part in a shooting match with the hospital team.

Though Fleming was held to be a very lucky man after penicillin—
the single most important therapeutic agent in the history of medicine
—was finally isolated in 1940, no one appreciated just how lucky he
really was until many years later, when Professor Ronald Hare repeated the original experiments described in the 1928 publication.
Hare discovered that Fleming had apparently been trying to grow
staphylococci without incubating them when the penicillium mold
dropped from the air onto that first plate. The destructive effect of
the mold on the bacteria, Hare discovered, could not be produced at
temperatures below 68° F or above 90° F. Had Fleming performed
the same experiment just a few days before or after he did, he would
have seen nothing at all. For there had been a heat wave that had
only broken on August 28, 1928, followed by nine days of cold
weather when the temperature rose above 68° F only twice. Fleming not only had the luck to have his plate contaminated with
the one species of mold out of many thousands which makes penicillin; he also had the good fortune to have that mold appear when the
ambient temperature was just right.

And he may have been even luckier than that. In 1971 Dr. Ernst
Chain, who extracted penicillin, lectured on Fleming's discovery before an international symposium.

"Fleming indeed had a stroke of good luck," Chain said, "but not
in the sense of the commonly presented popular accounts of this
event."

What Fleming noted, according to Chain, was not the effect that is
the basis of penicillin's action against animal infections. Instead,
Fleming witnessed a special penicillin effect, seen in only a few bacterial species at just the right age and state of development.

Yet despite his incredible luck, Fleming was unable to believe that
he had somehow stumbled onto the long-sought drug capable of
curing bacterial infection. His own war work and Wright's dictum
"Drugs are a delusion" were too strong an influence. His simple, factual paper—which later won for him the Nobel Prize in Medicine—
aroused no interest at the time, either in fellow scientists or in
members of the pharmaceutical industry. The experiments were regarded as artificial and unlikely to produce results applicable to
human infections.

Nonetheless, Fleming was later very embarrassed by his oversight.
In his Nobel lecture he attempted to exonerate himself in a restrained
manner:

"My only merit is that I did not neglect the observation, and that I pursued it as a bacteriologist. The first practical use was to differentiate between different bacteria. We tried to concentrate penicillin but found, as others did later, that it was easily destroyed, and so, to all intents and purposes, we failed. Had I been an active clinician I would doubtless have used it more extensively."

Privately, Fleming was a bit more candid—and bitter. To a Cambridge colleague he said, "I would have produced penicillin in 1929 if I had had the luck to have had a tame refugee chemist at my right hand. I had to stop where I did."

Penicillin in Limbo

The absence of a skilled chemist at St. Mary's was not Fleming's fault. It was Sir Almroth Wright's philosophy that had led to this situation. "There is not enough of the humanist in chemists to make them suitable colleagues," Wright liked to say. He also frowned upon the results of animal experiments as being not relevant to human beings. This was apparently the reason that Fleming never attempted to inject his filtrate into an infected animal—the next logical step.

But Fleming's own reticent character and inability to communicate kept him from seeking outside advice for his chemical problems. As one associate pointed out, "You have to remember that even if Fleming approached anyone else for help it would have been in a completely offhand way, mumbling almost inaudibly, with the eternal cigarette butt stuck to his lower lip. 'I say, X, I've got something rather interesting in my lab that you might care to look at.' And if there was no response he'd say no more."

Lacking outside help, Fleming set two young men in the Inoculation Department, Stuart Craddock and Frederick Ridley, to work separating the mold filtrate's active principle. Ridley, who had taken a biochemistry course at Birmingham University, had worked with Fleming previously on lysozyme. Craddock had been treated for a conjunctival infection with the mold filtrate. But neither Craddock nor Ridley possessed any real chemical experience.

And the problem they faced was indeed formidable. They had a meat broth containing an agent or agents Fleming named penicillin.

There was evidence that it was quite unstable. If stored for a week or mildly heated, the antibacterial activity was completely lost. Somehow this material would have to be extracted from the broth, concentrated, and characterized.

Today, sophisticated chemical procedures make such an extraction simple. But in 1929 separatory methods were considerably more primitive. The basic technique involved adding another liquid called a solvent to the filtrate and then removing the original liquid by distillation or some other method. With luck, the active principle would pass into the solvent while impurities would remain behind. If the active principle still contained some impurity, the process was repeated with a second solvent added to the first. After each separation Garré's "ditch test" of biological activity was employed to see in which liquid the active principle resided. Finally, when pure active principle had been obtained, the last solvent would be driven off. The residue should be pure, dry penicillin—at least in theory.

In practice, however, nothing was so simple as this. Many different solvents had to be employed, and the temperature sensitivity of penicillin precluded the use of high temperature distillation to drive off the last solvent. The task finally proved too tricky for Ridley and Craddock.

"Ridley had sound and pretty advanced ideas about chemistry," Craddock later wrote, "but when it came to methods of extraction we were driven back onto books. . . . We knew very little when we began. We knew just a little bit more when we had finished. . . ."

Despite their primitive knowledge and the difficult conditions under which they worked, Ridley and Craddock came surprisingly close to success. Unfortunately, the details of their method were not published until 1968. Had Ernst Chain learned what they had found, he might not have begun his own efforts with a complete misconception of the nature of penicillin.

The two young men commenced their work in the largest laboratory in the Inoculation Department but soon found the facilities there inadequate. Because the filtrate was sensitive to heat, they were forced to drive off their solvents—acetone, ether, alcohol—by evaporation in a vacuum. They soon discovered that there was not adequate water pressure in the laboratory to power their crude vacuum apparatus. But Ridley was able to locate a tap outside Wright's office that appeared to be connected to the water main. This tap stood over a corridor sink that had once held dirty bedpans, hot water bottles, and urine jars when the building contained hospital wards. In this narrow, drafty, cramped corridor most of the work was done. Since there was no gas tap, a long tube was used to bring gas from a nearby laboratory to the sink.

The penicillin was made by incubating the mold in "the digest broth of bullock's heart." Mixtures with optimal antibacterial strength were obtained after five days' incubation at room temperature. At 37° C, the normal body temperature at which bacteria grow best, the two investigators discovered that very little penicillin was produced.

The active broth was passed through a Seitz filter, a vacuum device containing asbestos pads to trap the mold and solid meat particles. The filtered mold juice was then placed in a vacuum flask and heated gently to remove the large amount of water from the broth. This process was a slow, tedious one due to the bubbling of the broth. If the frothy bubbles were drawn up by the vacuum with the excess water, much of the penicillin was lost. Frothing remained a thorny problem when the large-scale manufacture of penicillin began years later.

Ridley and Craddock discovered at this point an important characteristic of penicillin. The mold juice with the greatest antibacterial activity was highly alkaline, but this juice lost its activity very quickly during distillation. If, however, the liquid was acidified with hydrochloric acid before distillation, the antibacterial activity was retained. This important finding had to be rediscovered by others years later before penicillin could be successfully extracted.

Though it sounds straightforward enough, the extraction procedure was tedious and time-consuming. One distillation could occupy Ridley and Craddock for an entire day. The reservoir above the Seitz filter was small and needed constant refilling. The flask and water pump had to be watched continually to avoid overheating and bubbling. The acidity of the liquid had to be measured hourly—a lengthy operation involving chemical color changes and reference charts. And when the flask was opened, the inrush of oxygen would erode the activity of the filtrate; to avoid this complication, air had to be replaced with hydrogen when the flask was closed again. This process required a Kipps apparatus—another crude, balky piece of equipment.

The many difficulties notwithstanding, Ridley and Craddock accomplished this part of the extraction handily. On March 20, 1929, an especially good day, they were able to take two hundred cubic centimeters of mold juice that could kill bacteria at dilutions of 1:100 and reduce it to five cubic centimeters that were still lethal when diluted 1:3,000. The dried residue of this distillate was a brown, sticky substance that looked like melted toffee.

The two young investigators tried to purify their extract further with a number of solvents—acetone, ether, alcohol, chloroform. Only acetone or alcohol could dissolve the dried residue, and alcohol was found to work best. An additional benefit: alcohol precipitated the unwanted proteins left from the meat broth.

On April 10, 1929, Ridley produced a solution of penicillin in pure alcohol. After another vacuum distillation, he again found "a small syrupy residue, not more than half a cubic centimeter in volume." Redissolving this in five cubic centimeters of water, Ridley discovered to his amazement that his original extract was active at the enormous dilution of 1:30,000.

But more had been achieved than just concentration. Penicillin had been shown not to be a protein or enzyme, since it had not been precipitated from solution with the other proteins. And its solubility in alcohol, an organic solvent, implied that it too must be a small organic molecule. The extracts, however, were still unstable, even when stored in an icebox.

Hoping to reduce the instability by further purification, Ridley treated an alcohol solution of concentrated penicillin with acetone. Immediately, a yellow-brown precipitate appeared, while the penicillin remained in the acetone. This yellow-brown material, an inert substance called chrysogenin, had imparted to the mold juice and the syrupy extract their peculiar color. At the same time, a full yield of high potency penicillin had been obtained.

"We lost little in the process," Ridley wrote in his notes.

Obviously, Fleming should now have tested his newly concentrated extract by injecting it into normal and bacterially infected mice. But he was literally overpowered by the idea that "drugs are a delusion" and convinced that one must "mobilize the immunologic garrison" to fight infection.

As a consequence, he did nothing. The work of Ridley and Craddock was halted. In his original penicillin paper, their findings are described in only a few lines under the heading "Solubility":

"My colleague, Mr. Ridley," Fleming wrote, "has found that if penicillin is evaporated at a low temperature to a sticky mass, the active principle can be completely extracted by absolute alcohol. It is insoluble in ether or chloroform."

The published report of the work of Ridley and Craddock reveals that though he received itemized accounts of the work, Fleming never played an active role in it. As Craddock later recounted to Hare: "He was 'in' on all we did, but I don't think you can say he directed us in our attempts to concentrate and extract. He tried to help us, but he was as ignorant as we were, and we probably read up the various methods of extracting substances more than he did, and we certainly tried them without his help."

Fleming was later criticized for saying so little about the work of his two young associates in his original publication. Why did he not remark about penicillin's solubility in acetone? Why did he not note the need to use a vacuum or maintain a certain temperature during distillation? Why did he not specify the importance of acidifying the extract? Even his later papers did not rectify these omissions, making the final successful extraction much more difficult for others.

In the spring of 1929, half a year after Fleming's initial glimpse of his famous contaminated plate, the first attempt to extract penicillin ended. The newlywed Craddock, with Fleming's assistance, secured a better position at the Wellcome Research Laboratories in London. Ridley, plagued by recurrent boils, left on a cruise to regain his health. He later became a prominent ophthalmologist.

Fleming made no immediate effort to get anyone to continue the work. No doubt Professor Hare was correct in his assessment of Fleming's lack of motivation: "By the spring of 1929 he was losing interest in penicillin as a chemotherapeutic substance for the treatment of deep-seated infections. It was primarily for the treatment of this type of infection that the work had started at all. Why therefore continue with it if the value of penicillin began to be doubtful?"

Craddock shared Fleming's pessimism: "We could not know at the time we had only one more hurdle to cross. We had been so often discouraged. We thought we had got the Thing. We put it into the refrigerator only to find, after a week, that it had begun to vanish. Had an experienced chemist come on the scene I think we could have got across that last hurdle. Then we could have published our results. But the expert did not materialise."

More Failures

In 1931 a new attempt was made to purify penicillin by Dr. Harold Raistrick, a distinguished mycologist in the London School of Hygiene and Tropical Medicine, who had a lifelong interest in the compounds elaborated by molds. Raistrick was director of the department of biochemistry when he read Fleming's paper, and he assigned the study of penicillin to three associates. Dr. P. W. Clutterbuck, Raistrick's own assistant, was an experienced biochemist. Dr. Reginald Lovell, a bacteriologist, was borrowed from the department upstairs, as was a young mycologist, J. H. V. Charles. The penicillium mold was supplied most willingly by Fleming, but that was all. He told Raistrick nothing about the studies of Craddock and Ridley. In fact, Fleming and Raistrick were not even acquaintances at the time. Raistrick was totally ignorant of the previous attempt to extract penicillin until Professor Hare described it to him thirty-seven years later.

The first accomplishment of Raistrick's group was the straightening out of the mold's true identity. After confirming Fleming's results, they procured another sample of Fleming's penicillium strain from the Lister Institute. Dr. Charles Thom furnished them with a *Penicillium notatum* sample that had been found growing in Norway on a moldy mint plant, and they sent Thom a bit of Fleming's mold. Thom confirmed that it was a *Penicillium notatum,* not a *Penicillium rubrum* as Fleming had reported. But it was indeed a singular species. Raistrick's group found that both a *Penicillium chrysogenum* and the *Penicillium notatum* from Norway produced nothing that inhibited bacterial growth. This ability was possessed only by Fleming's strain.

Raistrick's next discovery was by far his most vital to the eventual successful extraction of penicillin: He demonstrated that Fleming's mold would thrive on an artificial medium. The clumsy bullock's heart broth with its meat chunks and variable content was both difficult to prepare and cumbersome to use when assessing penicillin activity. But standard Czapek-Dox medium, a solution of mineral salts fortified with glucose, proved quite a delicacy for the mold.

Though it grew more slowly than on broth, it elaborated considerably more penicillin.

Clutterbuck filled more than a hundred beakers with the new medium and mold. In a few days he had eight gallons of brownish solution. An experienced chemist, he speedily ascertained the necessity for acidifying the mixture. But in the artificial medium, the addition of sulfuric acid caused a precipitation of brownish flakes—the chrysogenin, as Lovell rapidly demonstrated.

At this point Raistrick, like Fleming, was blissfully unaware of the immense therapeutic implications of penicillin. As a result, much time was expended studying the worthless, inert chrysogenin. Raistrick's group discovered that the medium had to be quickly acidified to precipitate chrysogenin from solution. It was soluble in ether, though it could not be crystallized, and they determined the chemical composition as well as some rudimentary facts about the chemical structure.

More time was spent analyzing a protein extracted from the medium. This alkali-soluble molecule had not been detected by Ridley and Craddock, since in their broth it had been obscured by the bullock-heart protein. Raistrick's group carefully analyzed and characterized their mold-elaborated protein, returning to the study of penicillin itself only after a considerable delay.

In the meantime, though, they had devised—quite by accident—an excellent method for preserving the antibacterial activity of penicillin juice during storage. Because the juice could easily be ruined by bacteria from the air, they kept the excess in a refrigerator. They soon found that adding a pinch of acid to the alkaline juice permitted full strength to be maintained in the cold for at least three months. A little alkali added to a sample again made it suitable for experiments.

It was the attempt to extract the penicillin that discouraged Raistrick's group. Knowing nothing of the work of Ridley and Craddock, Clutterbuck used juice with a different acid content. Contrary to Fleming's report in his original paper, the penicillin in this solution was soluble in ether. This seemed extremely fortunate, since ether evaporates readily at room temperature without the need for a vacuum. Clutterbuck vaporized the ether using sterile air, but with the liquid disappeared the penicillin—and the research project as well.

"Such a thing was never known to a chemist before," Raistrick commented. "It was unbelievable. We could do nothing in the face of it, so we dropped it and went on with our other investigations and experiments."

A few years later, when he discovered what he had narrowly missed, Raistrick was rather annoyed. He vacillated between bitterness on account of his oversight and rationalization—extracting penicillin "was not his job." Once, when asked by journalist David Masters why he had not continued his experiments, he "was averse to discussing the matter."

The truth was that Raistrick, like Fleming before him, was confronted with a sudden loss of the group of men responsible for much of the work. Just as Clutterbuck and Lovell were writing a report of the penicillin study for the 1932 *Biochemical Journal,* Dr. J. H. V. Charles, the project's mycologist, was run over and killed by a bus. A few weeks later, Lovell left for a better position at the Royal Veterinary College.

Fleming later attributed Raistrick's failure to "lack of bacteriological co-operation, so the problems of the effective concentration of penicillin remained unsolved," and his own difficulties to "want of adequate chemical help." But this is a lame explanation, since Raistrick could have procured another bacteriologist just as easily as Fleming could have obtained adequate chemical assistance. In fact, neither Fleming nor Raistrick succeeded simply because both were blind to the possible existence of an antibiotic such as we know it today.

Equally ignorant of the potential value of penicillin was Dr. Roger R. Reid, a bacteriologist at the State College of Pennsylvania. Reid read Fleming's paper shortly after it was published, and in 1930 he obtained a sample of Fleming's mold from Dr. Charles Thom. Twenty-three other strains of mold that Reid tested made no antibacterial agent, a fact he ascertained using his own modification of the ditch test.

Reid found the activity of penicillin against bacteria to be highly variable. Some organisms were affected by the filtrate, others weren't, and he could see no reason why. Though Fleming had correctly observed that his filtrate acted by destroying germs, Reid thought that penicillin only stopped the bacteria from growing. Today we know that some antibiotics—tetracycline, for example—work in this way, but penicillin does not.

Finally Reid made an attempt to isolate penicillin. First he tried to speed its production by passing oxygen through the medium, but the finicky mold produced no penicillin at all when treated in this way. In order to isolate the penicillin he employed collodion bags, doubt-less believing that he was dealing with a very large molecule rather than a very small one. As a result, all he was able to trap with his bags was chrysogenin. Then he employed acetone and ether as sol-vents. After five years of work, he had accomplished less than either of his two predecessors.

One further unsuccessful attempt to isolate penicillin was made by Lewis Holt, a young chemist who came to the Inoculation Depart-ment at St. Mary's in 1934. In his best rifleman's argot, Fleming urged Holt to have another shot at a successful extraction. Though he suggested that Holt study the article by Clutterbuck, Lovell, and Raistrick, Fleming apparently said nothing about what Craddock and Ridley had done. Holt tried amyl acetate as his solvent, a substance that will not mix with water and thus could be separated from the filtrate with a simple device called a separatory funnel. Despite this circumvention of the tedious vacuum distillation, Holt was thwarted by penicillin's instability. When he threw up his hands after a few weeks at the task, Fleming did not urge him to persist.

Early Penicillin Therapy

In 1931, three years before Holt's failure and the same year in which Raistrick's group was studying *Penicillium notatum,* Dr. C. G. Paine employed penicillin therapeutically. Paine, a young English physician working as a hospital bacteriologist in Sheffield, had studied with Fleming at St. Mary's. After reading Fleming's penicillin paper, he sent a letter to his former mentor requesting a sample of the mold. Fleming, as always, gladly complied.

Like the other penicillin investigators, Paine repeated Fleming's experiments and successfully produced the antibacterial filtrate. This he tested on a staphylococcus isolated from a carbuncle, just as Dr. Martin Arrowsmith had tried his antibacterial substance in the Sin-clair Lewis novel. After producing a sufficient quantity of filtrate, Paine set out to use his new drug on patients.

His first three cases, staphylococcal skin infections, were referred by a dermatologist. Paine applied bandages soaked in mold juice to the lesions, just as Fleming had. But after seven days, "the results were uniformly disappointing." Topical antibiotic therapy, such as Paine employed, is widely used today; penicillin, however, is not a very good topical agent for skin infections. Other antibiotics—bacitracin, gentamycin, novobiocin—are far superior. So Paine's poor results are not surprising.

With his next cases, four Sheffield infants, Paine did far better. All the babies had eye infections—two caused by staphylococci, two caused by gonococci received from gonorrhea-infected mothers. After treatment with filtrate at four-hour intervals for three days, both gonococci infections and one of the staphylococcal infections had been cured. The gonococcus, at the time one of the most sensitive organisms to penicillin, will cause blindness in babies if untreated. Other antibiotics must presently be used against this microbe because of the emergence of penicillin-resistant strains. But for many years after Paine's first trials, penicillin was considered the agent of choice in gonococcal infections.

Paine was doubtless puzzled by the persistence of the one staphylococcal infection, but today such an outcome is an old story. Many staphylococcal strains are resistant to penicillin and must, therefore, be treated with other antibiotics.

Paine's next case was his most dramatic: The foreman of a local mine had had his eye penetrated by a piece of stone. So swollen were the man's eyelids that the fragment was impossible to remove. Bacterial cultures of the area revealed large numbers of pneumococci, an organism that Fleming had found to be extremely sensitive to penicillin.

Paine treated the patient with continuous filtrate irrigations for two days. The pneumococci were completely eradicated. As Paine later recounted, "The foreign body was removed and Mr. Nutt [the ophthalmic surgeon] told me subsequently that the man had recovered 6/6th vision in his right eye."

Soon, however, Paine began to experience considerable difficulty producing more penicillin. Some batches of filtrate would prove highly active, while others had scarcely any value at all. Finally he gave up.

"The variability of the strain of Penicillium and my transfer to a different line of work led me to neglect further investigation of the possibilities of penicillin," Paine later commented ruefully, "an omission which, as you may well imagine, I have often regretted since."

The Acceptance of Chemotherapy

Paine's 1931 experiments were never published in a scientific journal and were reported in the press only years after penicillin came into general use. At least four scientific articles dealing with penicillin did appear, however, between 1928 and 1935. Two were written by Fleming, one by Raistrick, and one by Reid in America. All these papers emphasized that penicillin killed bacteria; yet minimal interest was stimulated. No one, including Fleming, Raistrick, and Reid, could believe that any substance capable of killing bacteria in a Petri dish would be of real value in treating an animal infection. The resulting state of medical therapy was best summed up in Dr. Wyndham Davies' book *The Pharmaceutical Industry:* "A pneumonia patient, given a reasonable environment and nursing care, probably stood almost as good a chance of recovery in the days of Galen as he did in 1935."

But the medical profession was indeed striving for improvement. Vaccines were prepared against the strains of bacteria that most frequently caused pneumonia. In the United States, special diagnostic centers had been set up to identify these organisms from pneumonia patients so that the proper vaccine could be administered. To manufacture vaccine, Lederle Pharmaceuticals had constructed the world's largest rabbit-breeding station. The great breakthrough finally came, however, not from the vaccine technology pioneered by Pasteur and Behring. It came, instead—as Ehrlich had predicted—from the retorts of chemists.

And not surprisingly, the chemists involved were Germans, staff members of the enormous I. G. Farben Industrie, which later was to manufacture the dreaded Zyklon B gas used by Hitler to destroy six million human beings. In 1932 the Farben chemists were working to synthesize new colorfast dyes that would act by penetrating more deeply into the fabric than other dyes, thereby being more impervious to light. Among these new so-called azo-dyes was a red chemical, Prontosil.

Dr. Gerhard Domagk, director of research at the German Bayer Company, a Farben subsidiary, tested Prontosil as part of a mass screening program set up to detect chemicals that might be of value in treating infections. Domagk had already found that the best place to test for such substances was the body of an experimental animal. Scientists in his own laboratory had observed that some compounds with no antibacterial activity in the test tube were effective in animal infections.

Though not very effective. In his quest, Domagk had run through most of the compounds of gold, tin, antimony, and arsenic. All were too toxic to be used in man. Sir Almroth Wright, who visited Domagk's laboratory at Elberfeld in the Ruhr near Düsseldorf, came away horrified by the reliance on hit-and-miss, as Ronald Hare described: "Blind groping in the dark in this way was so utterly foreign to someone of Wright's temperament that he looked on it as a form of sacrilege. To him the only method was to think the thing out in the privacy of one's study and then do the experiment to prove the theory."

But Wright's prophecy, "The doctor of the future will be a vaccinator," was finally laid to rest by Domagk when he came to test Prontosil, the red azo-dye. Injected into the abdominal cavity of a mouse infected with deadly hemolytic streptococci, Prontosil saved the animal's life. Similarly infected mice receiving no treatment were dead within four days. The results were equally dramatic in 1,500 treated patients—especially the first, Domagk's own daughter. Little Hildegarde Domagk had pricked her finger with a knitting needle and was dying of septicemia when her father tried his new experimental drug on her as a last desperate measure. In a few days Hildegarde had recovered completely. On February 15, 1935, three years after the initial studies of Prontosil, Domagk's first report of his discovery was published in the *Deutsche Medizinische Wochenschrift*.

The three-year hiatus between discovery and announcement apparently occurred because Bayer wanted ironclad patents on Prontosil and any possible antibacterial chemical derivatives before the drug was released—certainly a sound business practice, but questionable on humanitarian grounds. In fact, their caution was wasted. Nine months after Domagk's announcement, two French scientists discovered why Prontosil was active against bacteria in an animal but not in a test tube.

Dr. Jacques and Madame Trefouel, husband and wife, found that in the body, Prontosil was split into two molecules. Of these, the active one was sulfanilamide. Confirmation came in 1936, when Dr. Albert Fuller detected sulfanilamide in the urine of patients treated with Prontosil. This compound had been discovered in 1908 by Paul Gelmo, a Viennese chemist working on his doctoral thesis, and was thus not patentable. In fact, two Americans studying azo derivatives of sulfanilamide in 1919 had found them to possess some antibacterial activity in the test tube, but this activity was so feeble that they had not pursued their experiments further.

The Trefouels' discovery prevented Farben and Bayer from making a financial killing with Prontosil, but the medical impact was enormous nonetheless. Many of the early studies of the drug were carried out in Wright's own laboratory by Leonard Colebrook. Fleming, too, was quickly converted to the doctrine of chemotherapy, and he published numerous articles on the sulfa drugs between 1937 and 1940.

One of the first patients to be treated in England was Ronald Hare, then one of Colebrook's young assistants. Hare had cut his finger on a glass sliver covered with streptococci. An infection developed, and he was admitted to St. Mary's Hospital on the verge of death from septicemia. Colebrook dosed Hare with Prontosil injections and Prontosil tablets. The patient immediately became bright pink, and later said, "[I] felt so much worse that I began to wonder whether I was dying because of the drug or the microbes." The case appeared so grave that after paying a visit to the bedside, Fleming said to Hare's wife, "Hae ye said your prayers?" But Hare made a complete recovery and regained full use of his infected hand.

As Hare was recuperating, Colebrook made his first extensive human tests of Prontosil. The patients were all women who had developed puerperal fever despite the strict sterile precautions enforced since the time of Semmelweis. Like Emile Roux in the case of diphtheria antitoxin, Colebrook was faced with the dilemma of whether to leave one group of patients untreated as a control. And like Roux, Colebrook made the humane choice: He treated everyone.

"I was no more than a spectator," Hare recalled, "but I soon sensed that a change had come. Patients whom we would have given up before, now recovered easily and without the long drawn-out desperate illness that would have previously been their lot."

"Something we had never seen before in ten years' experience of the disease," Colebrook added.

Unfortunately, sulfanilamide was active against some bacteria but not against others. Unlike penicillin, it seemed to act by interfering with a certain metabolic process, rather than by inhibiting cell-wall synthesis. Chemists made myriad alterations in the molecule to little avail. Today the sulfa drugs are used topically in eye infections and systemically in urinary tract infections; other infections do not respond nearly so well.

These limitations prompted medical researchers to look for still more effective antibacterial compounds, for sulfanilamide had served to break down the prevailing prejudice against systemic antibacterial therapy. And one investigator, Howard Walter Florey, finally managed to come up with the powerful agent that everyone else was seeking so frantically.

Antagonisms

"Of all the things I've done, the most vital is co-ordinating the talents of those who work for us and pointing them at a certain goal."

Nothing better characterizes the role of Howard Florey in the penicillin discovery than this statement; yet it was made not by Florey but by Walt Disney in 1954. Though on the surface the two men may seem to have been very dissimilar—one a showman, the other a pathologist—the part both played in their respective achievements is surprisingly analogous.

Florey was born in Adelaide, South Australia, September 24, 1898. Joseph Florey, a small-time shoe manufacturer, had the money to send his young son to good schools—Kyre College and the fashionable St. Peter's collegiate school in Adelaide. But then the elder Florey's luck ran out. His firm went bankrupt, defrauded by a smart accountant, and on a trip to Melbourne to wind up his affairs Joseph collapsed and died. (Coincidentally, Disney's father, too, was a failed small-time entrepreneur.)

Dependent on scholarships, Howard Florey maintained a grueling pace of study. He won a special prize in chemistry, continued to excel during his first two years at Adelaide University Medical

School, and was awarded a Rhodes Scholarship to Magdalen College, Oxford, in 1922. The grinding exertion, however, was already beginning to tell on him, and he suffered from repeated bouts of pneumonia. Perhaps his frighteningly single-minded pursuit of success is best described by a popular song from the Disney cartoon *The Three Little Pigs*, written only a few years after Florey entered Oxford:

> I build my house of stones.
> I build my house of bricks.
> I have no chance to sing and dance,
> For work and play don't mix.

In England, Florey continued to perform brilliantly. After studying physiology for two years at Oxford with the renowned neurophysiologist Sir Charles Sherrington, he moved to Cambridge to train in pathology. He spent a year in the United States as a Rockefeller Foundation fellow in 1925, and then returned to Cambridge. In 1931 he was appointed professor of pathology at Sheffield, where, coincidentally, he met Dr. C. G. Paine. Florey was unimpressed by Paine's penicillin experiments at the time, and later insisted that his own endeavors had not been prompted by Paine's results. Nonetheless, he sent journalists to Paine when penicillin became famous.

In 1935 the rapidly rising, brilliant young man was offered the chair of pathology at the Sir William Dunn School of Pathology in Oxford—one of the most prestigious medical posts in England. This appointment appears to have been mainly the result of the impression that Florey had made on Sir Edward Mellanby, head of the Government Medical Research Council and a key figure in the British scientific establishment.

Florey came back to Oxford with the express purpose of building a new type of pathology department. His desire was to integrate bacteriology, chemical pathology, and biochemistry in one place in order to derive a new understanding of pathology. Today this would be called the multidisciplinary approach.

The all-important biochemist for Florey's new department, Ernst Boris Chain, had previously worked with Sir Frederick Gowland Hopkins, the scientist responsible for establishing the importance of vitamins in the diet. The German-born Chain, who had almost become a professional concert pianist, had been forced to flee Berlin with the rise of Hitler's wrath against the Jews. Chain looked every inch the part of an Englishman's conception of the continental genius. His face, bushy black hair, and moustache made him almost a dead ringer for the young Albert Einstein.

At Oxford under Florey, Chain continued to study the enzymatic action of snake venom—work he had begun at Cambridge with Hopkins. When this was completed, Florey suggested that he switch to the study of lysozyme, the substance discovered by Fleming in 1922. Florey believed that lysozyme might play a role in natural immunity and also might be somehow responsible for stomach ulcers. Before the end of 1937 Chain was able to demonstrate that lysozyme was an enzyme that killed *Micrococcus lysodeikticus* by acting on the organism's cell wall. Chain was assisted in this research by another young biochemist Florey had hired, an American Rhodes scholar named Leslie A. Epstein.

Lysozyme works by lysing or dissolving the micrococcus, and it was this action that led Chain and Florey to an interest in penicillin, which appeared to do the same thing. But in fact, the destruction of bacteria by *Penicillium notatum* was only one example of a well-known phenomenon, microbial antagonism. Hundreds of others had appeared in the literature since Pasteur and his colleague Joubert had noted in 1887 that a culture of anthrax bacilli was lysed by common airborne bacteria.

Of the many antagonistic microbes, Florey and Chain decided to study two besides penicillin. One was *Bacillus pyocyaneus,* from which two Germans, Emmerich and Löw, had extracted a substance, pyocyanase, that appeared to inhibit the growth of a small number of bacteria. The other was a strange organism called an actinomycete— half bacterium and half fungus—that elaborated actinomycetin. The actinomycetes were quickly forgotten during the course of the penicillin work, but they later yielded the antibiotic streptomycin to another group of investigators.

As the studies of microbial antagonism progressed, an additional type of antagonism appeared—a growing feud between Florey and Chain. During the years of the penicillin work, their relations passed from cordial to bitterly argumentative. "The very walls of Florey's office would shudder with our shouting," Chain said. By the time Chain accepted an offer in Rome to set up a biochemical department for the Institute of Health, he and Florey were not even speaking to each other. Communication between them was carried on strictly in writing.

An even worse problem was Florey's desperate need for money. By the end of 1937 the pathology department was overdrawn at the bank by five hundred pounds. Because he was intent on enlarging his staff, Florey had to forbid the purchase of further equipment or material—even a piece of glass tubing, as Chain recalled. But by 1939 money had become so tight that funds for the gifted associates Florey had recruited appeared ready to run out. Dr. Norman Heatley, an expert on microtechniques from Cambridge, was ready to leave on a grant from the Rockefeller Foundation to study in Copenhagen. The salaries of two other collaborators, Dr. Margaret Jennings and Dr. R. D. Wright, were also in jeopardy.

Realizing that substances elaborated by antagonistic microbes might possibly be of therapeutic value, Florey emphasized the practical implications as well as the theoretical in his appeal for funds. When the university was unreceptive, he approached the Medical Research Council but was rejected. Then on November 20, 1939, he made a formal application for support to the Rockefeller Foundation in New York, at the time one of the largest backers of medical research.

In 1976 the English journalist David Wilson obtained a copy of the Rockefeller application and published it for the first time. The document reveals that Florey was indeed interested in making only a broad study of microbial antagonism. Among the organisms that were proposed for study, *Penicillium notatum* came only third and last—almost an afterthought. Florey was not conscious of a race to produce a new antibacterial agent or the pressures of the impending war, as some sources later asserted.

"We happened to go for penicillin because we had a culture growing at the school," Chain said later.

It is at this point that Florey's role in his achievement so begins to resemble Disney's in his, since both men were essentially impresarios attempting to support talented people working toward a basic goal. To produce *Snow White,* which appeared at almost the same time as Florey's therapeutic penicillin, Disney had assembled a large group of associates, which was in threat of being disbanded because of a shortage of cash. Both Florey and Disney used rather similar techniques to secure funds.

In order to convince the Rockefeller Foundation that he was

worthy of their support, Florey had listed in his application the departmental accomplishments: the lysozyme and snake-venom work done by Chain, the construction of a new type of microrespirator to study metabolism, and others. In the period after the Foundation was first approached, Rockefeller representatives visited Oxford to inspect the work going on in Florey's department.

To raise the money he needed to continue the production of *Snow White,* Disney applied to the Bank of America, then one of the biggest movie lenders. In a 1937 incident that he loved to retell, Disney was forced to show a crude, unfinished print of the film to one of the bank's vice presidents, Joseph Rosenberg, in order to secure the fresh backing. So that Rosenberg could get some idea of the film's continuity, pencil roughs of the unfinished sequences were inserted throughout. The session proved to be a nightmare for the compulsive Disney, a man who loved completed products of perfect smoothness and technical brilliance. Rosenberg appeared unmoved, responding to the film and Disney's accompanying patter with grunts and monosyllables. Afterward, on a tour of the studio, the banker made no comment about what he had just seen. But as he was getting into his car, he turned to Disney and said, "Good-bye. That thing is going to make a hatful of money." Disney got his loan.

And three years later, Florey got his money, too. No record survives as to whether the visiting Rockefeller representatives were as cold as Joseph Rosenberg, but Florey, upon receiving news that his request for aid would be met in full, was probably no less delighted than Disney had been by the Bank of America. The Foundation agreed to provide more than nine thousand pounds for salaries and equipment. Formerly dubbed an "academic highway robber" by colleagues, Florey was never again in need of monetary support.

The Rockefeller money enabled the small-scale studies of microbial antagonism to be considerably enlarged. Chain had already started work on *Bacillus pyocyaneus,* but animal experiments showed the antibacterial substances elaborated by this organism to be extremely toxic. It was at this point that the investigation of penicillin had begun.

Florey's predecessor at Oxford, Professor Georges Dreyer, had secured a specimen of Fleming's mold years earlier, incorrectly suspecting that it might contain bacteriophage, a bacteria-killing virus. As soon as he found that no such virus was present, he lost interest. Chain obtained a sample from Dreyer's cultures and spent the early months in 1939 learning how to grow it so it would make penicillin. Norman Heatley, the skilled Cambridge émigré, then took over this task while Chain turned to the chemical problems of purifying and isolating the penicillin.

Initially, Chain was completely fooled by the behavior of penicillin. The singular instability reported by Fleming and Raistrick had convinced him that he was dealing with a large protein molecule—an enzyme.

"My working hypothesis proved completely erroneous as my first experiments were to prove very soon," Chain said.

These first experiments clearly demonstrated that penicillin was not a protein. Since it passed readily through a cellophane filter, it had to be a small, simple molecule. Chain's curiosity was piqued by such behavior, since no other known antibacterial agent was so unstable. This unusual property—which had thwarted Fleming, Raistrick, and Reid—served to push Chain forward.

The usual method of passing the penicillin from one solvent to another in order to purify it worked best, Chain discovered, if the mixture was maintained at a low temperature. With this modification, he was able to proceed one step beyond Raistrick by getting the penicillin back into water. Still, however, it could not be dried or crystallized without inactivation. This problem was finally circumvented by freeze-drying, a process now very familiar to instant-coffee devotees but then in use only as an experimental means of drying blood serum.

Much to Chain's surprise, the little pile of dry brown powder he ended up with would kill bacteria at the unbelievable dilution of one part in a million. It was twenty times more active than the best sulfa drug.

"Without any optimistic expectations," as Chain later remarked, he decided to test his powder in mice. On Tuesday, March 19, 1940, an eighty milligram pinch of dry penicillin was dissolved in two milliliters of water and injected into the abdominal cavities of two mice. Both animals showed no ill effects. Florey was so incredulous at this result that he repeated the experiment himself. Examination of the animals' urine revealed a high penicillin concentration.

"From this we concluded," Chain later wrote, "that penicillin passed through the body of the mouse without loss of activity and that it was therefore probable that it would display its antibacterial

activity in the body fluids. This looked promising from the chemotherapeutic point of view."

On Saturday, May 25, 1940, penicillin was given the crucial test.
The abdominal cavities of eight white mice were infected with lethal
streptococci. Four of the animals were left untreated, two were
treated with a single dose of penicillin, two with multiple doses. The
laboratory notebook reported the outcome: "All four control mice
which had received no penicillin died between thirteen and sixteen
and a half hours after infection, when the treated mice were alive and
well. The treated mice receiving the smaller dose died after two and
six days, the other two surviving without sign of sickness."

Dr. Norman Heatley was present as Florey performed this experiment. The untreated mice were beginning to look seedy, their coats
puffed out, when Heatley left the laboratory at 3:45 the next morning
for a few hours' sleep. He later remembered being halted on his bicycle by a zealous Home Guard, suspicious of anyone on the Oxford
streets at such an hour.

Heatley returned the next morning to find Florey and Chain examining the four dead controls and the four live, treated animals.
Chain, Heatley remembered, was obviously excited, slightly flushed,
but oddly quiet; he replied to most questions merely by shrugging his
shoulders.

"It looks very promising," was all that Florey would say. But
nonetheless he ordered the production of penicillin to be increased,
and on August 24, 1940, the first paper describing the animal experiments was published in the *Lancet*. Though hard-driving and ambitious, Florey was scrupulously fair in his dealings with associates—a
rarity in science. He insisted that the names of everyone responsible
be listed in strict alphabetical order. Thus he is second on the first
paper, after Chain. On the next paper, reporting the efficacy of penicillin in humans, his name appears fourth, after Abraham, Chain,
and Dr. Charles Fletcher, who joined the group to administer the
drug to human patients.

Sadly, Florey's domestic life had reached a low ebb just at this
time. His wife, Ethel, a strong-willed physician like her husband, had
grown increasingly deaf. Their always-strained relationship was now
further compromised by her inability to understand anything that was
not shouted into her ear trumpet. Guests at the home would see her
eyes fill with tears when her husband raised his voice in anger at her;
some were so embarrassed by these exchanges that they vowed never

to visit the Florey home again. Florey himself began spending more and more time in his office, while Ethel was left alone. The two Florey children had been evacuated to America on account of the bombings.

The Sunday after the first *Lancet* paper was published, Alexander Fleming telephoned Florey, asking to visit the Oxford laboratory. "Fleming?" Chain said when he heard the news. "Good God; I thought he was dead."

The next day Fleming appeared, a short, white-haired man with a gay little bow tie. "Hullo," he said, holding out his hand, "I hear you've been doing things with my old penicillin. I'd be interested to look around." This was the longest sentence that he produced during the entire visit.

Fleming was taken through the laboratory and explained the step-by-step procedure of the extraction technique. He was given a sample of the purified concentrate, but Chain suspected that he did not understand the explanations of the concentration method. "He looked a lot," Chain remarked, "but he said very little." Fleming went back to London, never to return.

On January 17, 1941, five months after Fleming's visit, the first human trial of penicillin was made. The volunteer was an unnamed woman dying of breast cancer. Charles Fletcher made the injection —100 milligrams, or five times the dose found harmless for a mouse. Immediately, the patient developed chills and fever, indicating that impurities, perhaps produced by the mold, were still left in the penicillin. A more ominous possibility was that the penicillin itself had caused this reaction.

So further efforts at purification were made. Chain's assistant Abraham passed a penicillin solution through a chromatographic column—a long glass tube filled with alumina powder. The penicillin separated by this method was tested on rabbits and this time found to be free of the impurity that had caused the chills and fever.

Now the problem was only to produce enough penicillin. The resourceful Heatley grew the mold in every vessel he could lay his hands on: bedpans, crockery, glass soft-drink bottles. Many of the cultures were stored on old bookshelves from the Bodleian library. It was with the first large batch of penicillin that the most famous case was treated.

The patient, Albert Alexander, was a burly, forty-three-year-old constable who had scratched the side of his mouth with a rose thorn.

The tiny wound became infected with *Staphylococcus aureus,* and two months later the patient was dying. He lay in the Radcliffe Infirmary, his body covered with draining abscesses, one eye gone. Sulfonamide treatment had not helped.

On February 12, 1941, Dr. Fletcher gave the man 400 milligrams of penicillin in a vein, followed by a constant intravenous drip of the drug. By the fourth day, the effect was striking. The infected wounds were drying up and the fever had disappeared. These improvements continued into the fifth day, when a grim entry was made in the chart: "Penicillin supply exhausted. Total administered: 4.4 grammes in five days." Fletcher had been returning the patient's urine to the laboratory, where the penicillin was extracted from it and reused. But finally there was just not enough.

For ten days, the man seemed to be holding his own. Then he deteriorated quickly. His lungs became infected and he died on March 15, a month after the start of the treatment.

A plaque was later placed in the Radcliffe Infirmary, designating this tragic case as the first to have been treated systemically with penicillin (though in the text on the plaque, "systematically" is mistakenly substituted for "systemically"). In fact, the first systemic penicillin therapy was administered by Dr. Martin Henry Dawson at the Presbyterian Hospital in New York City, four months prior to Fletcher's injection of the woman dying of cancer.

Dawson had obtained a sample of Roger Reid's mold after reading Florey's first *Lancet* paper. Assisted by Gladys Hobby, a microbiologist, and Karl Meyer, a chemist, Dawson had begun to produce penicillin by stacking bottles of mold in the classrooms of Columbia University. To obtain an even higher-yielding mold, Dawson wrote to Chain, enclosing an international money order for five dollars to cover shipping costs. On May 5, 1941, Dawson reported to the Society for Clinical Investigation the promising results he had obtained on the first twelve cases treated.

By 1943 the use of penicillin in American and British troops had dramatically increased survival after wound infections. Though no wounded German soldier ever received this drug, Hitler, in a propaganda move, awarded the Iron Cross to his quack personal physician, Dr. Theodor Morell, for discovering penicillin. When penicillin finally did become available in German hospitals after the war, it was produced by the Berlin firm of Scherring from the urine of American soldiers. The scale of General George Patton's famous gesture—he urinated into the Rhine as his victorious tanks crossed into Germany —had thus been expanded.

The Fight Over Streptomycin

The discovery of penicillin brought about a revolution in medical therapeutics. Formerly fatal infectious diseases—septicemia, pneumonia, meningitis, diphtheria, scarlet fever, rheumatic fever—could be successfully treated. And the venereal diseases—syphilis and gonorrhea—could also be easily eradicated. Previously, a year of unpleasant Neosalvarsan therapy had been required to cure syphilis. In 1945 Fleming, Florey, and Chain received the Nobel Prize for their discovery. Within a few years, modifications of the penicillin molecule made it effective against an even wider range of bacteria.

But one formidable microbe—the tubercle bacillus—was impervious to all forms of penicillin therapy. The first antibiotic effective against tuberculosis came from an unlikely location—the throat of a sick chicken. This antibiotic, streptomycin, was to become the center of one of the more acrimonious quarrels in the science of healing.

The streptomycin work was done in the Rutgers University laboratory of a soil microbiologist, Selman Waksman. Born in Priluki, a poor peasant village near Kiev, in 1888, Waksman had to struggle from the beginning. His father, Jacob, was something of a ne'er-do-well, and the family was supported by his mother, Frieda. Despite the strict czarist restrictions that forbade Jews to attend Russian schools, Waksman was able to obtain a diploma from an Odessa gymnasium before emigrating to the United States in 1910.

The first years in America were spent in a peasant environment similar to the Russian one. Waksman lived with cousins on a five-acre farm in Metuchen, New Jersey. He milked their cows, fed their chickens, weeded their vegetable garden, and picked up English from their children.

Waksman's curiosity about the soil was stimulated by these early experiences. "I used to go out in the field and watch the peasants plow the land," he later recalled. "I loved the smell of the soil, the crops, the chickens, the cows."

With this love of dirt, it was natural that Waksman should enter an agricultural college—Rutgers. After graduating in 1915, he went to the University of California at Berkeley, where in 1918 he was awarded a Ph.D. in biochemistry. He then returned to Rutgers to do research.

In the course of his work, Waksman investigated soil microbes to determine whether any might manufacture chemicals capable of killing bacteria harmful to man. In 1940 he discovered his first antibiotic, actinomycin. Unfortunately, it proved too toxic in animals to be of use in the treatment of infections. Though it was later shown to be of great value in treating some forms of childhood cancer, actinomycin was a great disappointment at the time.

"There was nothing to do but lay it aside," Waksman lamented. "It was a terrible blow."

Waksman continued to study soil cultures in order to find an antibiotic useful in human disease—especially tuberculosis, which was untouched by the newly discovered penicillin. In 1943 a graduate student, Albert Schatz, identified such a compound in a clump of dirt taken from the throat of a sick chicken. The agent—streptomycin— was elaborated by *Streptomyces griseus,* a microbe that Waksman had coincidentally discovered and named during his days as a Rutgers student. Schatz proceeded to study streptomycin's antibacterial activity, while another graduate student, Elizabeth Bugie, was assigned the investigation of the biology and chemistry of *Streptomyces griseus.*

On November 20, 1944, a young woman dying of tuberculosis at the Mayo Clinic in Rochester, Minnesota, became the first patient treated with streptomycin. Extensive lung surgery had been used to no avail. The drug saved her life. Within ten years, deaths from tuberculosis in the United States had decreased fourfold—a decline largely due to streptomycin and the antituberculous agents that followed it. Throughout the world, Waksman was hailed as the discoverer of streptomycin. The two associates, Schatz and Bugie, were largely forgotten.

In later years, Waksman liked to use a story to illustrate the secret of his success. A famous rabbi, he recounted, was asked, "How did you come to accumulate so much knowledge in a single lifetime?"

"I owe a great deal to my teachers," the rabbi replied. "They taught me well. But I owe more to my friends. They encouraged me, they stimulated me. And most of all I owe to my students. They questioned me. They made me realize I didn't know it all."

Waksman had an odd way of showing his gratitude to his students. On February 9, 1945, a joint application was made for letters patent on streptomycin by Waksman and his student Schatz. Then, according to Schatz, Waksman asked him to assign the patent rights to the Rutgers Research and Endowment Fund. Schatz refused at first, but he was in no position to put up much of a fight. To assure himself of future employment, Schatz said, he eventually agreed.

On March 10, 1950, when the royalties from streptomycin had grown to more than $1,000,000 per year, Schatz filed suit against Waksman and the Rutgers Research Foundation. In this action he accused his former mentor of "fraud and duress" and asked for a portion of the streptomycin royalties.

"Baseless and preposterous," replied Russell E. Watson, Waksman's attorney. "The trial of Dr. Schatz's unfounded action will conclusively demonstrate that his charge is false." Moreover, Watson added, Waksman had also assigned all patent royalties to the Rutgers Research Foundation.

On March 25, 1950, at a closed pretrial hearing, Waksman finally admitted that he had indeed made money from streptomycin. Before he had turned the patents over to Rutgers, he had earned $350,000 from the drug and he still held a 10 per cent interest. But he continued to deny that Schatz was codiscoverer, insisting that his former student had been only one of many who helped with experiments. Schatz, he added, just happened to be "in at the finish."

This lame argument was doomed from the start, since Schatz had been the senior author of the paper announcing the discovery of streptomycin. Waksman was listed as third author, after Elizabeth Bugie. No doubt realizing that they were involved in a losing battle, Rutgers and Waksman agreed to a settlement. Schatz was given $125,000 and 3 per cent of future royalties, a share estimated to be worth another $500,000. Fifteen other scientists and twelve laboratory assistants also received awards, including the widow of a dishwasher. In the end, the drug earned more than fifteen million dollars.

The settlement also forced Waksman to admit that Schatz was "entitled to credit legally and scientifically as codiscoverer of streptomycin." Until his death in 1973 Waksman was galled at being forced to make this admission and forever insisted that the settlement was unjust. The Royal Caroline Medico Chirurgical Institute apparently agreed with him. In 1952 it named Waksman sole recipient of the Nobel Prize in Medicine for the discovery of streptomycin.

CHAPTER EIGHT

*The Search
for Invisible Poisons*

One class of infectious diseases untouched by the antibiotic and antibacterial agents remained a mystery during the golden age of microbiology. Though these maladies seemed similar to bacterial illnesses, no causative agent could be identified. After devising an effective mode of therapy for one of them—rabies—Pasteur guessed that they must result from an invisible infectious agent. "Virus" was the term he coined, from the Latin word for poison. Only in the last few years, however, with the aid of the electron microscope, have scientists been able to see the tiny particles that constitute Pasteur's invisible poisons.

But two centuries before its causative agent was identified, an effective means was devised for preventing another of the viral diseases—smallpox. The lessons learned from smallpox—and subsequently from rabies, yellow fever, and polio—have formed the basis for bacteriology's companion science, virology.

Smallpox

No one is certain when or where smallpox first appeared, since the disease was not even distinguished from measles until the tenth century A.D. One school of medical historians holds that the malady was present in Greece and Rome. These scholars assert that the sixth-century B.C. plague of Athens and second-century A.D. plague of Galen were both smallpox. Contradicting this theory, however, is the fact that no known ancient Western sculpture depicts a pock-marked face. There is likewise no mention of such disfigurement—an unmistakable sign of the disease—by any Greek or Roman author.

Two more probable sites of origin for smallpox are widely accepted today. One is China, where the disease may have been introduced by the Huns as early as A.D. 49. It was certainly the disorder described by Ko Hung, a Chinese who lived A.D. 265–313. But its most likely source was India. From the dawn of history, the Hindu goddess Shitala was invoked for protection against smallpox.

The routes of spread, like the origins, are also murky. Smallpox seems to have reached Western Europe by A.D. 581, when Gregory of Tours recorded what was undoubtedly an early epidemic. In A.D. 980 the Japanese coped with one of their first outbreaks by establishing special isolation hospitals. The recommended therapy: wall hangings of red cloth.

In the tenth century A.D., as medieval Arabic civilization was rising toward its zenith, the most authoritative early account of smallpox was written. The author was one of the outstanding physicians of the period, Abu-Bakr Muhammad ibn-Zakariyya al-Razi, known as Rhazes.

Rhazes was born in the Persian city of Rai about A.D. 865. As a young man he appears to have devoted himself mainly to music, physics, and alchemy. But at the age of thirty, during a visit to a Baghdad hospital, he became fascinated by the practice of medicine, and to this he devoted the remainder of his life.

The society that produced Rhazes was considerably more developed than that of the contemporary West. Among its many great achievements were algebra, alcohol, and the Arabic number system. In medicine it remained unsurpassed until the sixteenth century, producing many famous medical authors. Of these men, Rhazes is considered the greatest because of his inventiveness and keen powers of observation.

Though director of a large Baghdad hospital and a court physician as well, Rhazes found time to write an astounding 237 books—a one-man medieval Book-of-the-Month Club. He dealt with all the sciences in his works, but his principal interest was medicine. Much influenced by Hippocrates and Galen, he still demonstrated great independence and originality, including in his texts a wealth of personal experience. In one monograph he describes a lead catheter of his own invention, in another an instrument for the removal of foreign bodies from the esophagus. His treatise *A Dissertation on the Cause of the Coryza Which Occurs in the Spring When the Roses Give Forth Their Scent* is one of the first descriptions of hay fever.

Of Rhazes' thirty-six surviving books, the most famous is his treatise on smallpox and measles. The work's great merit is twofold: the clear, accurate descriptions of both diseases—a first in medical literature—and the emphasis on the features which allow differentiation:

> When, therefore, you see these symptoms, or some of the worst of them (such as pain of the back, and the terrors of sleep, with the continued fever) then you may be assured that the eruption of one or other of these diseases in the patient is nigh at hand; except that there is not in the measles so much pain of the back as in smallpox; nor in the smallpox so much anxiety and nausea as in the measles, unless the smallpox be of a bad sort; and this shows that the measles came from a very bilious blood.

So good were Rhazes' descriptions that they differ only slightly from those in Osler's textbook written a thousand years later. The principal error was Rhazes' assumption that both illnesses were manifestations of the same disease.

For reasons not entirely clear, the smallpox described by Rhazes is not the fearsome, lethal illness so widely prevalent in eighteenth- and nineteenth-century Europe. Indeed, many of Rhazes' contemporaries regarded measles as considerably more dangerous. One explanation might lie in the fact that smallpox exists in three distinct forms.

Variola major is the true, virulent smallpox. Variola minor, also called alastrim, is a relatively benign illness. Variola vaccinae, or cowpox, is mainly a disorder of cattle. Perhaps the disease known to Rhazes was alastrim rather than Variola major.

In 1518 smallpox reached America. The Indian population of Hispaniola was so devastated that a Spanish witness, Bartolomé de Las Casas, reported only a thousand survivors. From Hispaniola, smallpox was carried to Mexico by the relief expedition that joined Cortez in 1520.

The conquering Spaniards could not have asked for a more effective ally. When Montezuma had been killed and the Aztecs were preparing to repulse the Spanish invaders, smallpox struck Tenochtitlán. Within hours after the Spaniards had been driven from the city, the native leader and his followers died of the disease. The remainder of the population proved too sick to expel the tiny band of Spaniards from the land. In this interval of breathing space Cortez was able to rally his forces, recruit allies from among the Aztecs' subject peoples, and return to administer the *coup de grâce* to the capital. "Clearly, if smallpox had not come when it did," writes Dr. William H. McNeill in *Plagues and Peoples,* "the Spanish victory could not have been achieved in Mexico."

Smallpox served as an equally powerful ally for Pizarro, the Spanish conqueror of Peru. After spreading to Guatemala in 1520, the disease continued moving southward, finally penetrating the Inca domain in 1525 or 1526. The sufferings of the Incas were every bit as great as those of the Aztecs. The reigning chieftain succumbed to smallpox while away from his capital on campaign in the north. His designated successor also died. The absence of a legitimate heir precipitated civil war, and during the havoc that ensued, Pizarro and his men were able to reach Cuzco and plunder its treasures. They encountered practically no military resistance along the way.

"The Indians die so easily that the bare look and smell of a Spaniard causes them to give up the ghost," remarked one missionary.

Smallpox appears to have served the Spanish conquerors as such an efficient weapon because in sixteenth-century Europe it was principally a disease of childhood. Confronted by the adult Spaniards' immunity, the highly susceptible Indians were forced to believe that the white newcomers had divine approval for all they did. So no matter how small their numbers or how brutish and squalid their behavior, the Spaniards prevailed. Native authority structures crumbled at the apparent abdication of the old gods.

But by the end of the seventeenth century, Europeans, too, began to suffer dearly from smallpox. Previously a comparatively benign illness of children, it became the most lethal infection of the very young. Throughout the eighteenth century, smallpox destroyed more infants than any other disease. A late-eighteenth-century Swedish physician recorded that every year the malady killed one-tenth of Swedish children in their first twelve months of life. Adults were stricken as well when smallpox was introduced into a susceptible community. A single epidemic in Iceland wiped out 40 per cent of the population. Even London, where many were immune, lost 4 per cent of its inhabitants to smallpox between 1760 and 1770. In the face of this frightful death toll, inoculation, an old preventive measure, was revived.

Inoculation was probably first introduced by Chinese physicians at the beginning of the eleventh century. The practice stemmed from the common observation that some diseases, particularly smallpox, would attack a patient only once in a lifetime. No doubt the Chinese reasoned that transplanted tissue or secretion from a mild case would confer immunity by inducing another mild case. Transplantation was accomplished by removing scales from the drying smallpox pustules and blowing them into the nose of the person to be protected. A new wrinkle was added to the old technique by Giacomo Pylarini of Smyrna, an eighteenth-century Greek physician. Pylarini removed matter from the pustule and rubbed it into a small needle scratch. Another Greek doctor, Emanuel Timoni of Constantinople, communicated Pylarini's method to a London physician, Dr. John Woodward, who had it published in the *Philosophical Transactions* of the Royal Society in 1714. This paper stimulated some interest in Britain and America, but only after the experiments of Lady Mary Wortley Montagu was inoculation widely accepted.

In 1717 Lady Mary was the twenty-eight-year-old wife of Edward Montagu, the new English ambassador in Constantinople, a tedious, miserly career diplomat. Turkey might have proved dull to many English women, but not to Lady Mary. Instead of spending most of her time behind the embassy shutters, she became a regular tourist.

Many of the local customs met with her immediate approval. An active feminist, she heartily endorsed the property rights of married Turkish women; on divorce, the woman was entitled to keep her own money while still receiving support from the ex-husband. She also recorded that after childbirth Turkish women were out of bed the same day and returning calls in a fortnight, turned out in their jewels and finery.

So congenial did Lady Mary find the ambience that she had her portrait painted in Turkish dress. After a visit to a Turkish bath, she was thoroughly delighted and wrote that "if it was the fashion to go naked, the face would hardly be observed."

But scarcely any man could have failed to notice Lady Mary's beautiful face, though when she was undressed her exquisite, amply proportioned body would certainly have presented a distraction. Indeed, many men did more than just ogle, as Lady Mary's intimate diaries and letters revealed. Some of these spicy documents were so shocking that they were later destroyed. According to Alexander Pope, she was an Eve who tasted not one apple, but robbed the whole tree.

Her beauty was matched by her charm and wit, making her a great favorite at the Court of St. James's. One of her most famous observations concerned the mistress of the new German king of England. The monarch's lover, Lady Mary remarked, was "duller than himself and consequently did not find out that he was so."

It was Lady Mary's influence at court that eventually provided her a place in the history of medicine by making her inoculation experiments possible. She had herself contracted smallpox when young, and though her beauty had been dimmed, she managed to hide the worst effects. Therefore, she watched and recorded with great interest the efforts made by some of the citizens of Constantinople to prevent the disease.

In September, after the heat of summer had passed, Lady Mary noticed a group of old women going from house to house. Each of these women carried nutshells filled with pus from a mild smallpox case. The customers extended their arms, a vein was scratched open with a large needle, and pus from a nutshell was smeared on the open vein. The crone would then close and bind the subject's wound with a piece of nutshell. Lady Mary's notes on this preventive ritual, known as "ingrafting," recorded the outcome:

> (The children or young patients) play together all the rest
> of the day, and are in perfect health to the eighth. Then
> the fever begins to seize them, and they keep their beds

two days, very seldom three . . . and in eight days' time they are as well as before their illness. . . . Every year thousands undergo this operation; and the French ambassador says pleasantly, that they take the smallpox here by way of diversion, as they take the waters in other countries. There is no example of any one that has died in it; and you may believe I am very well satisfied of the safety of this experiment, since I intend to try it on my dear little son.

And try it Lady Mary did. In 1718 little Edward Wortley Montagu was the first recorded English subject of smallpox inoculation. The successful procedure served not only as a preventive measure, but as a means of identification as well. The child frequently ran away from his school, Westminster. In one advertisement offering a twenty-pound reward for his recovery, he was described as having "two marks by which he is easily known; viz., in the back of each arm, about two or three inches above the wrist, a small roundish scar, less than a silver penny, like a large mark of the smallpox."

Returning home in 1721, Lady Mary was convinced that every English subject should be inoculated. She was able to persuade Dr. Charles Maitland, the embassy physician in Turkey during part of her stay, to adopt the practice. But soon the medical profession and the Church of England raised a resounding outcry against the "heathen" procedure.

Lady Mary, however, was simply too well connected to be deterred by mere physicians and clerics. One of her admirers and a possible recipient of her favors, the Prince of Wales, was a strong supporter. Surprisingly, Caroline, Princess of Wales, was also a friend. Even that "honest blockhead," the king, had risen in Lady Mary's estimation. With the backing of these powerful patrons and the help of Sir Hans Sloan, secretary of the Royal Society, Lady Mary was able to conduct the experiment that made her famous.

Promised a reprieve for participation, six condemned criminals at Newgate Prison volunteered to be inoculated. All survived unscathed. The procedure was then repeated—one step up the social scale—on six young orphans, who also survived. George I, impressed by these successful results, ordered the inoculation of his two grandchildren. The royal example made this first method of smallpox prevention immediately fashionable. The technique spread throughout

Europe, and Lady Mary became a celebrity almost as exalted as the Beatles.

But not for long. The attack of smallpox that resulted from inoculation was not always a mild one and would usually prove fatal in two or three cases out of a hundred. Moreover, many people rightly suspected that the procedure made smallpox epidemics more probable by multiplying the foci of infection. For these reasons, European physicians had all but abandoned inoculation by 1728.

In America, however, which was more sparsely settled, the method was accepted with much greater alacrity. Cotton Mather, the fire-and-brimstone minister, became the first advocate after reading of Pylarini's experiments in the *Philosophical Transactions*. During a 1721 smallpox epidemic in Boston, Mather suggested to the local physicians that they try the new technique. But only one, Dr. Zabdiel Boylston, evinced any interest.

Boylston began by inoculating his six-year-old son and two Negro slaves. Thirty-five inoculations later, he still had caused no deaths. He was nonetheless accused of propagating smallpox, and on one occasion narrowly escaped a lynch mob. Gradually, however, the procedure was accepted. In 1738 it was successfully employed by Dr. James Kirkpatrick during a very severe smallpox epidemic in Charleston, South Carolina. After losing a son to smallpox, Benjamin Franklin, too, became a prominent convert. And during the Revolutionary War, George Washington ordered the establishment of special inoculation clinics for his troops.

European interest in inoculation was again stimulated when Dr. Kirkpatrick visited London in 1743 with a report of his experience. Kirkpatrick attributed his success to an improved method, which had a mortality rate of only 1 per cent. His report prompted the founding of the Smallpox and Inoculation Hospital with a generous grant from the Duke of Marlborough. Two other Englishmen, Robert and Daniel Sutton, made many improvements in Kirkpatrick's technique and were able to report 2,514 cases without a single fatality. This imposing track record soon attracted a large clientele of affluent Londoners. In his private clinic, Daniel Sutton was reported to have earned 2,000 guineas in 1764 and 6,500 in 1765.

So many inoculators were English-trained in the following years that the method became a virtual British monopoly. English inoculators were summoned by Maria Theresa to Vienna and by Frederick the Great to Potsdam to instruct local physicians in the technique.

Since the patients were drawn mainly from the upper classes, the arrival of these foreign specialists often generated intense excitement. In 1756, when a professional inoculator was summoned to Paris to treat the family of the Duc d'Orléans, second in rank only to the king, a queue of elegant carriages formed at the specialist's door. One observer later commented that the scene was reminiscent of the hubbub in the street before a performance of the Comédie Français.

This sudden upsurge in the popularity of inoculation was not merely the result of a fad. Smallpox epidemics had continued to occur with sickening regularity, striking both the poor and the rich indiscriminately. Voltaire was stricken at the age of twenty-nine but survived. Maria Theresa did not contract the disease until age fifty-two; she also survived. Louis XV of France was not so lucky. Smallpox felled him at age sixty-four after two weeks of intense suffering. Because of the politically turbulent atmosphere, his malodorous corpse was rushed to the grave at night for fear that the pomp of a king's funeral might cause a popular uprising. Louis XVI was so horrified by his predecessor's macabre demise that he ordered the entire royal family inoculated.

By the eve of the French Revolution the method of inoculation had been so refined that a small pinprick and a drop of thin pus introduced by lancet served the purpose. Most well-to-do Europeans had been inoculated. The phenomenal increase in European population of the late eighteenth century has even been attributed by some demographers to the prevalence of inoculation. But the chance of dying from the procedure was never completely eliminated and thus prompted the search for a safer method of smallpox prevention.

The safer method—vaccination—resulted from a part of the same body of folk knowledge that had led to inoculation. For centuries peasants had recognized that an infection with cowpox, a pustular disease of the teats of cattle, conferred immunity against smallpox. Milkmaids and milkmen commonly contracted cowpox pustules on their fingertips and finger joints. The infection would then extend to other parts of the body, accompanied by a few days of mild fever.

The first use of cowpox to prevent smallpox was made by an English farmer and cattle breeder, Benjamin Jesty, in the little Dorset village of Yetminster. Jesty, aware of the folk belief that cowpox prevented smallpox, had watched two of his own servants with cowpox nurse several smallpox victims without becoming ill themselves. During a severe epidemic in 1774 Jesty scratched his wife and two sons with a darning needle, then rubbed in material from the pustules of an infected cow. None of the three subjects contracted smallpox, but Jesty was severely criticized for making an inhuman experiment on his family. Fifteen years later the two sons received a proper inoculation with matter from a smallpox pustule; neither boy had any reaction at all.

In 1791 another deliberate cowpox vaccination was made. Peter Plett, the tutor to a landowner's family, performed the procedure on his employer's children. Three years later an epidemic of smallpox struck the village where the family lived. Plett's vaccinated children are said to have been the only ones in the village to escape infection. But neither Jesty nor Plett altered the practice of medicine with his experiments, since neither published his results. Edward Jenner, the first vaccinator to publish, now is accorded scientific credit for the discovery.

Jenner was born May 17, 1749, the son of the Reverend Stephen Jenner, vicar of Berkeley, in Gloucestershire, England. When he was five, his father died, and he was brought up by his older brother, also a clergyman. During early life, young Edward had his first experience of smallpox prevention—and a bad one it was. Before being inoculated, he was bled to be sure "his blood was fine," purged until he was emaciated, and put on a starvation diet. This series of unpleasant experiences may have played a role in the shaping of Jenner's rather unconventional nature. Like Semmelweis, he had a cyclothymic personality, marked by wide fluctuations in mood. He would pass from varying periods of elation and great mental activity to dark fits of melancholy and introspection.

At the age of thirteen, while apprenticed to a local surgeon, Jenner had already begun to demonstrate the intense curiosity in natural phenomena that was later to make him famous. He was especially interested in the behavior of birds, and on one occasion expended considerable effort proving that the robin, and not the lark, announced the coming of dawn. In addition, he determined the order of appearance of the songs of the raven, the jay, the swift, and other English birds.

The cuckoo, however, was the bird that most fascinated the young Jenner. Naturalists at the time believed that the cuckoo's victim, the hedge sparrow, would push its own young from the nest so that the infant cuckoo could survive. But after a great deal of observation, Jenner discovered that the infant sparrows were forced from the nest by the fledgling cuckoo itself. Utilizing a concavity in its back as a spoon, the little usurper tossed out the rightful inhabitants. The paper describing this discovery, addressed to Dr. John Hunter, won for Jenner a fellowship in the Royal Society.

Hunter, the famous experimental surgeon who purposely infected himself with syphilis, had taken on Jenner as his first house-pupil at St. George's Hospital in London. The two men became lifelong friends, and Hunter encouraged Jenner's interest in natural phenomena, comparative anatomy, and research. "Why think? Why not try the experiment?" Hunter once told his famous pupil. But Jenner was considerably more circumspect about self-experimentation than his teacher had been, though prodded frequently by letters from Hunter demanding this investigation or that specimen.

An interest in biology earned Jenner the job of classifying and arranging the specimens brought back by Joseph Banks from Captain Cook's first Pacific voyage in 1771. But when asked to join Cook's next expedition, Jenner refused, preferring to return to Gloucestershire and establish a medical practice. It was here that the cowpox studies were made.

In 1788 a smallpox epidemic erupted in Gloucestershire, and a great demand for inoculation ensued. While administering the inoculations, Jenner noted that individuals previously infected with cowpox showed no reaction. He had heard the old wives' tale that cowpox conferred immunity to smallpox, and now was confronted with confirmatory evidence. Intrigued, he spent the next several years carefully observing further examples of this phenomenon.

An under-gardener to the Earl of Berkeley, Joseph Merret, was Jenner's first recorded case. In 1795, twenty-five years after a cowpox attack, the man showed no reaction to a smallpox inoculation. Even after Jenner had made several tries, a small swelling on Merret's arm was the sole result. And during one smallpox epidemic, Jenner observed that the gardener remained healthy while caring for his sick family.

The same observation was made in the case of Sarah Portlock, a servant girl, who had contracted cowpox twenty-seven years before. During a smallpox outbreak, the girl nursed one of her own sick children, yet remained healthy. Jenner inoculated both her arms with smallpox, yet produced no visible effect.

The seventeenth patient in this series, James Phipps, turned out to be the crucial one. "The more accurately to observe the progress of the infection I selected a healthy boy," Jenner wrote, "about eight years old, for the purpose of inoculating the cow-pox. The matter was taken from the sore on the hand of a dairymaid, who was infected by her master's cows, and it was inserted on the 14th day of May, 1796, into the arm of the boy by means of two superficial incisions, barely penetrating the cutis, each about an inch long.

"On the seventh day he complained of uneasiness in the axilla and on the ninth he became a little chilly, lost his appetite, and had a slight headache. During the whole of this day he was perceptibly indisposed, and spent the night with some degree of restlessness, but on the day following he was perfectly well."

As he had in his other cases, Jenner challenged the boy's immunity with smallpox. "He was inoculated on the 1st of July following with variolous matter, immediately taken from a pustule. Several slight punctures and incisions were made on both his arms, and the matter was carefully inserted, but no disease followed. The same appearances were observable on the arms as we commonly see when a patient has had variolous matter applied, after having either the cowpox or smallpox. Several months afterwards he was again inoculated with variolous matter, but no sensible effect was produced on the constitution."

Young James Phipps was lucky. Other subjects of the experiment, however, were not, and Jenner has been criticized for his risky human tests. The patients appear never to have been informed that they were being used as guinea pigs, and at least one died.

Mistakenly confusing cowpox with "grease," an infection of horses' heels, Jenner obtained a batch of infected material from the hand of a sick farm worker, who appeared to have contracted his disease from the horses he tended. On March 16, 1798, some of this material was used to vaccinate a five-year-old child from the local parish poorhouse, John Baker. But things went awry, and, as Jenner wrote, "the boy was rendered unfit for inoculation from having felt the effects of a contagious fever in a workhouse soon after this experiment was made."

In fact, the child had died. Jenner, however, conveniently omitted any mention of the death in his original report. He also made no comment on the appearance of the vaccination vesicle and failed to supply any description of the boy's "fever."

Shortly after the demise of John Baker, Jenner submitted a paper to the Royal Society describing his cowpox studies. So revolutionary were his findings that fellow Society members advised him "not to risk his reputation by presenting . . . anything which appeared so much at variance with established knowledge, and withal so incredible." But Jenner knew better, and in June 1798 published his observations in a little pamphlet, *An Inquiry into the Causes and Effect of the Variolae Vaccinae.* The dedication was from Lucretius: *Quid nobis certius ipsis sensibus esse potest, quo vera ac falsa notemus*—"What can we have that is more reliable than our senses to distinguish between truth and falsehood?"

Jenner's little pamphlet made quite a big splash. Within a year Dr. M. Woodville of London's Smallpox Inoculation Hospital had made an extensive trial of the new method and was so impressed that he sent four hundred samples of the life-saving "matter" to practitioners throughout England. A hundred thousand Englishmen had been vaccinated by 1801. But Jenner was not pleased by his colleague's enthusiasm, for he was convinced that Woodville was trying to make off with some of the credit.

In America cowpox vaccination was also enthusiastically accepted. Dr. Benjamin Waterhouse, a professor at the Harvard Medical School, received a copy of Jenner's pamphlet in 1799 and subsequently became the first American to employ the method. He vaccinated seven subjects, among them his own children, and then inoculated each with smallpox. As in all of Jenner's cases, the smallpox produced no effect. Deeply impressed, Waterhouse wrote glowing newspaper letters to publicize the practice and tried to enlist the support of the President. John Adams, though an old friend, turned out to be politely unhelpful; but not so the new President-elect. Thomas Jefferson was as fascinated by vaccination as by all other new ideas and immediately sought to vaccinate his own family. At the time, vaccine was usually transported as a thread impregnated with matter from a cowpox pustule and often was inactivated by heat. Jefferson and Waterhouse had to make several tries before a sample in working order finally arrived. To remedy the problem, the inventive Jefferson suggested that the thread be placed in a bottle inside a larger bottle filled with water—a sort of eighteenth-century thermos.

A more vexing problem than deterioration was the confusion of cowpox with other more harmful diseases. Jenner had compounded this predicament by referring to cowpox as "cow small pox." After reading his pamphlet, some physicians in India believed that Jenner was referring to cattle plague, an extremely deadly condition. Patients that they mistakenly inoculated with cattle plague died in great numbers before the error was rectified.

But probably the greatest obstacle to widespread vaccination was the early failure to recognize that the effect—unlike smallpox inoculation—was not lifelong. As time passed, a growing number of smallpox cases occurred in people who had been vaccinated. Jenner himself claimed that such mishaps were due to "spurious smallpox" or inept vaccinators. Then in 1811 the Honorable Robert Grosvenor almost died of smallpox despite having been personally vaccinated by Jenner some ten years before. To his great dismay, Jenner was forced to defend his technique before the House of Lords. Thereafter he had to endure the pamphlets, lampoons, and caricatures published by the antivaccinators, some of whom even argued that infecting humans with a cattle malady had caused men to bellow like bulls and women to grow hairy.

Jenner spent the remainder of his life writing in defense of vaccination and trying to extend his theory. In later years, when the technique had proved a great boon, he was showered with honors and money. Oxford awarded him an honorary Doctor of Medicine degree. Parliament granted him ten thousand pounds later raised to thirty thousand, in recognition of his discovery and as reimbursement for the time he devoted to the public good at the expense of private practice.

Benjamin Jesty, the farmer who had vaccinated his wife and children twenty years before Jenner had used the method, did not fare nearly so well. Learning of Jenner's parliamentary award, Jesty sent letters to the Jennerian Society to substantiate his claim to the discovery. But after being invited to London, all that Jesty received was a portrait of himself and a pair of gold-mounted needles. Quite rightly he was awarded no scientific credit since he had not bothered to publish his results.

In the two centuries since Jesty's experiment, vaccination has proved so effective that smallpox now appears to be the first infectious disease to have been eliminated from the earth. Since there is no known animal or insect reservoir of the virus, for infection to persist in a population one sick person must transmit the microbe to a susceptible contact, and that contact must in turn transmit it to another in an unbroken chain. The smallpox patient can transmit the disease only from the time his rash appears until the scabs drop off, a period of about a month. Improved vaccines and vaccination methods coupled with the efforts of the World Health Organization seem to have finally broken the fragile transmission chain.

By 1966 smallpox had been eradicated from Europe and most of America except for Brazil. In the rest of the world only three remaining reservoirs of disease existed: the Indian subcontinent, all of Africa south of the Sahara, and the Indonesian archipelago. An intensive vaccination campaign mounted by WHO has now banished smallpox from these regions.

Though not without considerable difficulty. Fighting between government forces and various dissident groups was a perpetual problem. Two Ethiopian health workers were shot and killed; vaccinating teams were forced to withdraw for months at a time. Small village epidemics would appear and have to be contained.

Nonetheless, great progress was made in the four years after 1967. In 1971 only sixteen countries reported smallpox cases. Brazil's last case occurred in April 1971 and Indonesia's in January 1972. The final campaign in the battle was fought against the last reservoir of the disease in Asia, a region that stretched from Bangladesh through northern India and Nepal into Pakistan. Support for the program by local health authorities was halfhearted, since so many former efforts to control the malady had failed. Smallpox was considered inevitable and impossible to eradicate.

But WHO mobilized all available health personnel for a house-to-house search, which revealed many previously undisclosed cases. Containment vaccination around each outbreak eliminated smallpox from the affected areas within weeks. Special surveillance teams asked questions at markets and in schools to uncover additional cases. Rewards were offered to anyone reporting a case of smallpox and to the health worker receiving the report. As the incidence of the malady declined, the size of the reward was increased, always with extensive publicity. Local guards were posted night and day at the homes of smallpox patients to prevent the patient from leaving and to see that all visitors were vaccinated.

The battle now appears to have been won. Afghanistan was smallpox-free by 1972. Pakistan's last case was reported in October 1974. After a 1974 epidemic, the last case of smallpox in India was reported May 24, 1975. Bangladesh, the final stronghold, proved more difficult than the others until a national emergency program was launched by presidential directive.

On October 16, 1975, one of the world's last known cases of smallpox was reported in Bangladesh—a three-year-old girl named Rahima Banu. Twelve thousand health workers supervised by nearly a hundred epidemiologists searched the country house by house, but could find no additional cases. At the present time, WHO is pressing its search for new cases in the remote Simyen Mountains of Ethiopia's Begemdir Province. If none is found, smallpox will be declared to have been eradicated from the earth—the first such achievement in medical history.

Mad Dogs and Frenchmen

Rabies, as old a disease as smallpox, has been known in Europe and Asia since ancient times. Sirius, the Dog Star, was commonly believed to be the cause; during the days of its heliacal rising—"dog days"—dogs were said to be especially liable to attacks of madness. Animals ordinarily docile and friendly would become extremely vicious and aggressive, apparently for no reason, and after a period of maniacal behavior would convulse, become paralyzed, and die. The ancient Egyptians, Greeks, and Romans quite understandably attributed rabies wholly to supernatural causes.

What else, indeed, but an angry god could inflict such a terrible malady? A rabid human, after a short period of restlessness and fever, becomes uncontrollably excited and salivates excessively. Excrutiatingly painful spasms of the throat muscles, triggered by the attempt to drink water, suggested the name "hydrophobia." Tortured by an unquenchable thirst, the victim dies within three to five days from asphyxia, exhaustion, or general paralysis. Few diseases bring about a more gruesome, horrible death.

Rabies in animals was first described by Democritus in the fifth century and later by Aristotle in the third century B.C.; the connection with human rabies was recognized in the first century A.D. by Celsus, who realized that the condition was incurable. Prophylactic cauterization was the treatment he recommended for wounds inflicted by a mad dog.

Other ancient authors, less impressed by the smell of burning human flesh, advocated different remedies. The pharmacologist Dioscorides enthusiastically endorsed the ashes of a seahorse. The naturalist Pliny had even more exotic ideas:

> It is universally agreed, too, that when a person has been bitten by a dog and manifests a dread of water and of all kinds of drink, it will be sufficient to put under his cup a strip of cloth that has been dipped in menstrual fluid; the result being that the hydrophobia will immediately disappear. This arises, no doubt, from that powerful sympathy which has been so much spoken of by the Greeks, and the existence of which is proved by the fact, already mentioned, that dogs become mad upon tasting this fluid.

Rabies has never been a significant public health problem, though it is quite prevalent in wild animals. As early as 1271 it was known to be common among wolves in France. The first recorded epidemic in domestic dogs occurred in Italy in 1708. These outbreaks often provoked panic because of the dread consequences of a human bite. Sometimes persons bitten by rabid dogs were hunted down by a mob and killed like wild beasts. Strangling and suffocation were especially popular means of dispatching a victim.

Such was the attitude toward rabies until 1879, when Victor Pierre Galtier, a professor of veterinary medicine at Lyons, France, began to study the disease. In a series of experiments Galtier succeeded in infecting rabbits with rabies. Previous attempts by many other investigators to accomplish this had failed miserably. Galtier was thus able to prove that the infectious agent was contained in the saliva. In addition, he found that the virus was propagated through the nerves and—most important—that animals could be immunized by intravenous injection. But his further progress was hampered by two obstacles: the long, irregular incubation periods of the disease and his inability to transmit it by means of the liquid matter extracted from the brains of mad dogs.

One year after Galtier's experiments, the attentions of Louis Pasteur were focused upon rabies. A former French Army veterinary surgeon, Pierre Rose Bourrel, impressed with Pasteur's previous successes, gave him two rabid dogs to study. Bourrel had long been interested in *la rage,* and had suggested filing down the teeth of all domestic dogs to prevent them from inflicting deep bites. Unfortunately, this remedy proved far from satisfactory, and shortly after proposing it, Bourrel himself contracted rabies and died.

Even before he received Bourrel's gift, however, rabies was nothing new to Pasteur. As a boy of nine in Arbois he watched the bite wounds of a man named Nicole seared with a red-hot iron by the local blacksmith. A mad wolf had raged through the village, attacking people and animals. Eight persons with bites on their hands and faces died of rabies, but Nicole survived.

On December 11, 1880, Pasteur began his studies of rabies. In the Sainte-Eugénie Hospital a five-year-old child bitten by a mad dog the previous month was dying of the disease. All the characteristic symptoms were present: the restlessness, the fear of liquids, the terrible spasms of the throat. A few hours after the child died, Pasteur removed a small amount of mucus from the palate and a blood sample from the thigh.

This material turned out to be a bacteriologic red herring. Pasteur inoculated it into rabbits, and within three days the animals had all died, but with no symptoms of rabies. In their blood he found a microbe shaped like a figure-eight and surrounded by a mucous capsule. Pasteur believed that this organism was the cause of rabies until he again encountered it in the bodies of children who had died of other diseases. Refusing to be sidetracked, he put the new microbe aside. Four years later Albert Frankel demonstrated that what Pasteur had found was the pneumococcus—the bacillus that causes lobar pneumonia.

And what of the actual rabies virus? Pasteur never was able to see it since the light microscope he employed was not sufficiently powerful. But he was eventually able to isolate it and deduce correctly that he had found an ultramicroscopic germ.

It was from a dog belonging to the unlucky Dr. Bourrel that Pasteur managed to obtain a good sample of rabies-virus-filled saliva. Two of Bourrel's assistants threw a rope around the raging animal's neck, dragged him foaming from his cage, and proceeded to pinion him to a table. With a glass tube between his lips, Pasteur aspirated a small amount of the infected saliva from the dog's mouth.

With this saliva Pasteur succeeded in transmitting rabies to other animals—sometimes. But often the experimental animal remained healthy, and when the disease did finally appear, days or weeks might have elapsed. All in all, ordinary injection proved to be a highly inefficient tool for laboratory work.

The transmission problem was ultimately circumvented in an ingenious manner. Remembering that rabies was primarily a disease of the nervous system, Pasteur substituted ground-up spinal cord for saliva. The result: experimental infections could be induced with greater certainty, but still the incubation period was long. Emile Roux, Pasteur's assistant famous for his studies of diphtheria antitoxin, introduced the final wrinkle. His clever innovation, however, had two unforeseen consequences. It brought loud protests from an army of outraged antivivisectionists, and it created a split between Pasteur and Roux.

Roux's method was to put the ground-up nervous tissue directly into the brain of a healthy animal. Before using the tissue, he placed it in an elegant little flask in which it could be hung to dry. Roux's flask was equipped with two openings that allowed air to flow through freely. He would test the tissue in the vessel day after day in order to determine how long the dried virus retained its infectiousness.

One day Pasteur and his young nephew Adrien Loir, who had recently begun to work in the laboratory, happened through the room in which Roux kept his flasks. Suddenly, Pasteur stopped and picked one up. "Who put this there?" said Pasteur to Loir.

"It could only be Monsieur Roux. It's his shelf space," Loir replied.

Pasteur held the flask up to the light and examined it silently for several minutes before replacing it on the shelf. Returning to his own laboratory, he immediately ordered his glass-blower to make twelve identical vessels—only larger.

Pasteur's idea was to use Roux's flask to weaken the rabies virus by drying the infected tissue over potash. He set his nephew to the task. Loir was clumsy at first as he tried to suspend pieces of rabbit spinal cord within the flask. But after a day he had assembled three successful preparations and placed them in the incubator to dry.

Roux was furious when he discovered that his boss had appropriated his idea.

"Who put those flasks there?" he angrily asked Loir, indicating the new larger vessels.

"Monsieur Pasteur," Loir answered.

"He went into the incubator?"

"Yes."

"He saw the flask on my shelf?"

"Yes."

Roux had never completely forgiven Pasteur for the scene in the laboratory before the final day of the anthrax experiment at Pouilly le Fort when Pasteur, learning that the trial might prove a failure, had said angrily that Roux would have to face the ultimate humiliation before the crowd of spectators. The plagiarism of Roux's design for the flask was the last straw.

Besides Roux's hostility, Pasteur was forced to contend with the ire of the antivivisectionists. Proper English ladies wrote him letters denouncing his crimes. And Pasteur himself was hesitant. Though not fond of dogs, he found the idea of perforating the animal's skull for an experiment most disagreeable.

Finally, however, he overcame his scruples, and the procedure was a great success. After the virus had been inserted directly into the brain, the first dog became rabid in fourteen days and died five days later.

The next step involved the passage of rabies through rabbit brains. The virus was injected serially into the skulls of a hundred rabbits, and the incubation period progressively shrank to a minimum—six days. The microbe had now reached its maximum virulence for rabbits. In Pasteur's terminology, it had become "fixed." At the same time, it had become much less harmful to dogs.

Now Pasteur proceeded to induce immunity to rabies. With Roux's flask he dried a rabbit spinal cord for fourteen days and injected it into a dog. The next day he repeated the process with a slightly more virulent thirteen-day-old cord. This repetition continued until the fourteenth day, when one-day-old cord was used. Thus treated, a healthy dog could be bitten by a rabid one with no ill effect. The immunized animal proved impervious to rabies even when highly virulent spinal cord was inserted directly into its brain.

Elated by these results, Pasteur was nonetheless hesitant and uncertain of his next step. Should all two and a half million dogs in France be vaccinated against rabies? The fourteen-day period required made such a plan impractical. And where would one get enough rabbits to make thirty-five million doses of vaccine?

Another possibility existed. The vaccine could serve as a form of treatment. Since rabies has a very long incubation period—sometimes weeks or months—and since immunity could be induced in two weeks with vaccine, a person bitten by a mad dog could be inoculated prophylactically.

But how safe was the vaccine for humans? Only a test on a human volunteer could tell, though Pasteur was considerably more reluctant to experiment on human beings than Jenner had been. He considered using a condemned criminal as a subject, promising the man a pardon if he survived. Unfortunately, the French judicial system would not countenance such a bargain. The only other alternatives were more forbidding.

"I have not yet dared to treat human beings after bites from rabid dogs," Pasteur wrote a friend, "but the time is not far off. I am much inclined to begin by myself—inoculating myself with rabies, and then arresting the consequences, for I am beginning to feel very sure of my results."

Roux was not so certain, however, and maintained that too little testing had been done to warrant a human experiment. In medical school he had been taught that rabies was incurable. But Pasteur knew otherwise, and on July 4, 1885, a chance to test the new vaccine materialized in a highly dramatic fashion.

A little boy, nine-year-old Joseph Meister, was walking to school at Meissengott, in Alsace, when he was attacked by a mad dog. The animal had thrown him to the ground and bitten him repeatedly while he buried his face in his hands. A bricklayer witnessing the attack had beaten the dog off with an iron bar. It had then run home to its master, a grocer named Theodore Vone. Vone had shot and killed the dog, but not before it had managed to bite him on the arm.

The bricklayer carried little Joseph, covered with blood and saliva, to his parents. Dr. Weber, the local physician, cauterized the boy's fourteen wounds with carbolic acid and advised the mother to take the child to Pasteur in Paris. Though the famous scientist was not a physician, Dr. Ville said, he would know best what to do.

On Monday, July 6, Joseph Meister, his mother, and grocer Vone appeared on the doorstep to Pasteur's laboratory. Vone's case was not serious. His shirtsleeve had not been pierced, indicating that saliva had not entered the bite marks on his skin. Pasteur soothed him and sent him home.

But Joseph Meister was in worse shape. He was in so much discomfort from his wounds that he could hardly walk. After finding a room for mother and son, Pasteur consulted colleagues on the action he should take.

Roux was adamant against the use of the vaccine. He wanted nothing to do with a human trial. Months later, even after Pasteur had proved the efficacy of his preparation in humans, Roux remained dubious. To a woman who offered to pay for rabies treatment, he is said to have remarked, "I can assure you, dear Madame, that all my services are free, including autopsies."

Two other scientists were more sanguine. Dr. Edmé Vulpian, a physiologist on the government commission investigating the vaccine, and Dr. Jacques Grancher, a physician, told Pasteur what he wanted to hear. After examining the boy's deep bites, the two men affirmed that the child would certainly die from rabies if not vaccinated. And so that evening, Pasteur and Grancher administered the first injection.

Little Joseph was terrified before the procedure, but calmed down considerably upon learning that nothing worse than a skin-prick in the side was involved. Over the next eleven days, eleven more injections were given.

"There is some reaction," Pasteur wrote to his son, "which is becoming more intense as we approach the final inoculation, which will take place on Thursday, 16 July. The lad is very well this morning. . . . He had a slight hysterical attack yesterday."

Pasteur was much edgier than his patient. He slept fitfully, was plagued by nightmares and tormented by anxiety over the outcome. On the evening before the last injection, little Joseph insisted, "Dear Monsieur Pasteur, kiss me good night," and then slept soundly. Pasteur had insomnia.

For the next ten days, Grancher kept the child under observation. Then he was sent home perfectly well. A few years later Joseph Meister went to work as doorman at the Pasteur Institute, no doubt having acquired a taste for city living during his first short visit to Paris. The job proved to be a stable one, and Joseph was still on duty at the age of sixty-four. When the Nazis invaded Paris in 1940 and ordered him to open Pasteur's crypt, he committed suicide.

Not all the early cases had such a favorable outcome as that of Joseph Meister. In November 1885 Pasteur was brought a ten-year-old girl, Louise Pelletier, who had been bitten around the head by a mountain lion thirty-seven days previously. He believed the case to be hopeless, but, faced with the child's pleading parents, gave in and administered his vaccine. Eleven days later, after returning to school, Louise was seized by the terrible signs of rabies. Pasteur stood by her bedside in the rue Dauphine and watched her die. In the street outside her home he burst into tears. Not without reason did the physicians of antiquity refuse to touch a hopeless case.

But even in curable cases such as Joseph Meister's, many scientists were not convinced that Pasteur's vaccine was of value. For not everyone bitten by a rabid dog will die, as Pasteur himself well knew. Yet the vaccine treatment turned out to have a mortality rate of ½ per cent. An additional complication was a vaccine-induced inflammation of the brain that often produced permanent paralysis.

Pasteur's critics made the most of this situation. How could Pasteur claim a clear success rate, they asked, when he was not certain whether his patients were really infected with rabies. Since Grancher was administering the injections, he, too, was disparaged.

The most cogent critic was Dr. Michel Peter, a professor of medicine at the University of Paris. Peter emphasized how rare a disease rabies really was by citing the very small number of cases he had seen in thirty-five years of practice—two to be exact. In Dunkirk also, Peter pointed out, only one person had died from rabies in the previous twenty-five years. And since the adoption of the Pasteur treatment one year before, there had been one death in the same city. Peter echoed the sentiments of many others when he suggested that Louise Pelletier had actually died of "laboratory rabies" inflicted by Pasteur.

By this time, however, Pasteur had personally treated a large number of patients. Citing his own statistics, he pointed out that of the 350 persons treated as of March 1, 1886, only one had died. And an official inquiry mounted by the city of Paris had determined the mortality rate from rabid dog bites to be 16 per cent.

These figures, however, did not quell the controversy. There were more deaths at the Pasteur clinic. The father of one child who had died after antirabies treatment sued Pasteur and Grancher. Crank letters poured into the laboratory; insulting newspaper articles appeared, insinuating that Pasteur was keeping his failures secret. "I did not know I had so many enemies," Pasteur remarked to Vulpian.

The situation abroad also appeared unfavorable. In April 1886 a British commission was organized to evaluate Pasteur's claims. Though it did find his treatment efficacious, it did not recommend adoption of vaccination. Since the annual number of rabies deaths in Britain was a mere forty-three, the commission advocated only stricter police regulation of dogs as a means of rabies prevention.

But finally, as more and more experience with the new vaccine accrued, its worth could no longer be doubted. The French statistics revealed that from 1880 to 1885 sixty patients had died of rabies in Paris hospitals. From November 1885 to August 1886, when the vaccine was in use, only three patients had died, and two of these had not been vaccinated.

In July 1887, his rabies treatment at last acclaimed a great success, Pasteur was elected life secretary of the Academy of Sciences—the highest honor bestowed upon him during his career. Public adulation reached a new peak. During a theater benefit that featured Gounod conducting his *Ave Maria,* the composer, "in an impulse of heartfelt enthusiasm, kissed both his hands to the 'savant.'" But misfortune soon struck the aging scientist. In October 1887, as he sat writing a letter in his room, Pasteur had a second paralytic attack. He attempted to speak to his wife but had lost the use of his tongue. A week later he suffered an even more serious stroke. Like Dr. Max Gottlieb in *Arrowsmith,* Pasteur was forced to spend his final days as a pathetic, helpless invalid.

Yellow Jack

Pasteur's shrewd guess that rabies was caused by an ultramicroscopic agent soon led to the understanding of a much more common disease —yellow fever. In light of the germ theory, rabies and smallpox were easily explained, since both were directly transmitted. But yellow fever was an enigma to the early microbe hunters, and for obvious reasons. It was caused by a virus they couldn't see and was transmitted by a vector—the mosquito. Thus yellow fever resembled the malaria puzzle doubly compounded.

And a terrible puzzle it was. For reasons that no one could explain, yellow fever was notoriously a disease of seaports and sailing ships. It would decimate a city and then disappear for years. During an epidemic that swept through Philadelphia in 1793 four thousand people—one out of every ten inhabitants—perished within three months. The malady was nicknamed "yellow jack" because ships infected with it were quarantined and forced to fly a yellow flag.

Though sometimes confused with malaria, yellow fever has a

unique appearance. The headache, backache, chills, and nausea appear suddenly. The combination of a high or rising fever accompanied by a slowing of the pulse rate—just the opposite of what would be expected—is called Faget's sign after Jean Charles Faget, the nineteenth-century French physician who first described it. The intensely restless victim develops a bright red tongue, swollen lips, flushed face, and inflamed eyes. After three or four days a period of deceptive improvement begins. The patient feels better and his fever diminishes. But suddenly the fever returns, the complexion assumes a dusky yellowish pallor, and the sufferer begins to choke up *el vomito negro*—a dreaded sign. This black vomitus is blood from the stomach wall that has been discolored by stomach acid. Death usually occurs on the sixth or seventh day. Should the patient survive, however, he is left with a solid immunity to the disease.

Like smallpox and rabies, yellow fever is of uncertain origin. Most medical historians believe that it was brought from Africa by ship to America and the West Indies in the early sixteenth century. But a few others maintain that the disease originated in Central America and was then transported to Africa. Though this may seem a minor point, two men are known to have murdered each other over it.

One of them, John Williams, had been surgeon to a slaving ship plying the route between Guinea and the West Indies. While in practice in Kingston, Jamaica, Williams wrote what is now regarded as the first account of African yellow fever—a description of an outbreak that seems to have occurred sometime around 1740. Williams' account engendered great hostility in Jamaica—an island inordinately proud of its reputation for being the source of yellow fever. As a result, Williams entered a duel with Dr. Parker Bennet, his principal critic, and both men were killed.

Wherever yellow fever may have originated, by the mid-eighteenth century its vector, the mosquito *Aedes aegypti,* had established itself in many parts of the world. This highly domesticated insect, which uses collections of still water as its breeding place, is actually said to prefer manufactured containers—water casks, cisterns, gourds—to natural bodies of water. Thus it was carried to every port of call in the water casks of ships and could establish itself ashore in any location where the temperature remained above 72° F.

The special fondness of *Aedes aegypti* for water casks meant that mosquitoes transmitting yellow fever from sailor to sailor could remain on board ship for weeks or months at a time. Even on the lengthiest voyages, the disease could continue to attack crew members. This characteristic made it uniquely feared, since most other infectious diseases, if they did break out on board, would quickly burn themselves out. Either everyone got sick and recovered simultaneously, as when influenza occurred; or else only a few crew members lacking immunity fell ill. But most adult Europeans contracting yellow fever died and therefore few sailors had any immunity. As a consequence, a long voyage could be haunted by an endless series of yellow fever deaths. No one could know who would sicken next and die in his turn. No wonder "yellow jack" was so dreaded by seamen.

And it horrified city dwellers as well. There were 135 major yellow fever epidemics in American port cities alone between 1668 and 1893. Scarcely a port in the Western Hemisphere, in fact, escaped the disease. And those people who had survived one epidemic lived in terror of another. During outbreaks in the South, thousands of citizens would flee to the North by train. The town of Jackson, Mississippi, instituted a shotgun roadblock to prevent the entry of people from areas where yellow fever was reported. Blacks crossing the fields were shot. And in cities where the disease appeared, officials would often order the burning of clothes, household goods—even homes of stricken families. Sulfur, believed to ward off the malady, was sometimes burned in the streets and houses. At least the bad smell did no harm, which is more than can be said for many of the other medical measures that were employed.

Dr. Benjamin Rush, a signer of the Declaration of Independence and a leading colonial physician, came under especially harsh criticism for the treatment he administered to yellow-fever victims during the Philadelphia epidemic of 1793. Dr. Wilson G. Smillie, a professor of public health at Harvard, characterized Rush as "a fool of the highest order," adding, "it becomes quite clear that he did more to retard medical progress in the United States than any other one man."

At the time of the epidemic, Rush was extremely busy with a large private practice. Most of his patients were poor, since he never received referrals from other physicians. They had been alienated years before by the hot-headed, tactless, stubborn Rush, who could never resist publicly attacking colleagues whenever the opportunity arose.

In August 1793 Rush began to see the first patients die with "a serious bilious fever." While an apprentice twenty years before, he had seen cases of yellow fever and so was immediately able to recognize the disease. In his copious notes Rush recorded the characteristic symptoms: the nausea, violent chills and fever, languor, slow pulse, bloodshot eyes, vomiting, yellowness, stupor, delirium. He noted vivid spots on the body "that resembled mosquito bites" and "a bleeding at the nose, from the gums and from the bowels, and a vomiting of black matter in some instances close to the scenes of life."

Soon thousands of citizens were fleeing Philadelphia. Officials of the federal government hastily departed along with many prominent physicians. Rush, however, stayed on to witness the hysteria and chaos that ensued. Despite frantic conferences among city officials, municipal activities ground to a halt. The only wheels left turning belonged to carts hauling away the dead. Husbands and wives abandoned sick spouses; parents deserted sick children and vice versa. Sick patients were left to starve or die alone, unattended.

But unattended sufferers were considerably better off than those ministered to by Rush. He purged them with jalap and calomel, dosed them with tincture of cinchona bark, bled and blistered them. One favorite remedy: dousing the feverish with buckets of cold water. He reluctantly set this method aside after killing a few patients with the chilling shock. In its place he substituted cold-water enemas and a cold cloth on the head.

He never gave up bleeding, however. When the fever was highest, he took the most blood—three quarts in some cases. One historian, James Thomas Flexner, wrote that Rush "shed more blood than any general in history."

Controversy erupted when Rush wrote about his techniques in the local papers. Colleagues bitterly criticized his harsh methods. But patients didn't. They flocked to his door by the hundreds. He had little time to sleep or eat. People woke him at night begging him to come at once. In the daytime they flooded into his living room and followed him into the dining room.

By mid-October, Rush estimated that a minimum of six thousand Philadelphians were sick with yellow fever, and "only three physicians were able to do business out of their houses." A hundred people a day were dying—among them Rush's sister and three of his five young apprentices. Rush himself became seriously ill with the disease, but miraculously survived a vigorous application of his own treatments. While in his sickbed he continued to prescribe for his patients. The epidemic did not finally subside until the onset of frost.

A year later Rush published a book describing his experiences, *An Account of the Bilious Remitting Yellow Fever, As It Appeared in the City of Philadelphia in the Year 1793*. Yellow fever, he insisted, was not contagious, as everyone believed, and was not spread by personal contact. According to his theory, the disease was one of the blood system due to such factors as miasma and violent emotion. The Philadelphia epidemic, Rush wrote, had resulted from the smell of a heap of spoiled coffee that had been tossed on Mr. Ball's wharf in the Delaware River. But, he claimed, almost any decaying matter—cabbages, for example—could produce a similar noxious effluvium, though rotting vegetables were definitely more dangerous than rotting meat.

Surprisingly, Rush remained totally oblivious to a fact that some people had noted even then: The yellow fever had been brought in from the West Indies on a sailing ship that had tied up at Mr. Ball's wharf. Rush did record that the weather that summer had been hot and dry, and that much stagnant water lay in streams, springs, rain barrels, and cisterns. "Moschetoes, the usual attendants of a sickly autumn," he wrote, "were uncommonly numerous." Yet he attributed no special significance to the mosquitoes. The fever had disappeared with the frost, Rush explained, because people shut their windows to keep out the chill and so excluded the miasma as well.

Rush went on to live through three other yellow fever epidemics—in 1794, 1796, and 1798. Amid the repeated scenes of horror and chaos, he continued to bleed and purge his fellow citizens. But as he came under increasing criticism from colleagues, his medical practice shriveled away. In 1797 he was saved from penury by his friend President John Adams, who appointed him treasurer of the United States Mint. During his last years Rush wrote another book, *Medical Inquiries and Observations Upon the Diseases of the Mind*. In it he advocated his old standby, bloodletting, as a treatment for insanity. He also recommended that unco-operative patients be strapped in his "tranquilizer"—a cruel, uncomfortable chair with headpiece, no doubt patterned after the apparatus used for stamping coins.

In 1804 Rush's miasma theory of yellow fever was questioned by another American physician, Stubbins ffirth. While an undergraduate medical student at the University of Pennsylvania, ffirth performed a series of horrifying, disgusting experiments to determine whether the disease was contagious. First he injected himself with blood, urine, sweat, black vomit, and other material from yellow fever victims. He then swallowed this material along with all manner of other repulsive substances taken from patients dying of yellow fever. But since he used samples from people in the last stage of the infection, when there is no virus in the blood, he did not become ill. ffirth's natural but completely erroneous conclusion was that the agent producing yellow fever was not to be found in blood, sweat, urine, feces, or black vomit.

Ten years after ffirth's experiments, Dr. David Hosack, a New York physician, noted that during every epidemic a period of eight to fourteen days would usually elapse between the appearance of the first case and the development of subsequent cases; yet he failed to appreciate the significance of his supremely important observation.

In 1850 the mosquito was finally implicated in the transmission of yellow fever (and malaria, as we have noted) by the Mobile, Alabama, physician Josiah Clark Nott. Nott's other distinction: He delivered "Willie" Gorgas in 1854. Nott incurred considerable ridicule for his theories; but Gorgas was destined to show the world that his mother's physician had been right.

Long before, however, yellow fever had become a rare visitor to seaports in the temperate zone. Two nineteenth-century technological innovations served to confine the disease to the tropics. Both worked by separating the mosquito from man.

One, the piped municipal water supply, limited the number of dry land sites in which the insect could reproduce. The *Aedes aegypti,* inordinately fond of manufactured storage containers full of clean, nonsalty water, were gradually left homeless in the Western Hemisphere by the installation of water faucets. But in Latin America they still thrived, especially in one favored breeding place: the holy water fonts in village churches. In West Africa, too, they persisted near human habitations in a favorite spot—the clay juju pots the natives kept by their doors to ward off evil spirits.

The second innovation, the modern steamship, denied the small, silvery mosquito suitable travel accommodations. The open water casks on sailing vessels, a perfect place to reproduce, were replaced by closed water systems on steamships. Thus, even before its cause had been discovered, yellow fever had been circumscribed in habitat. But in the areas it continued to haunt, it was as troublesome as ever. And one, Havana, became the proving ground for the mosquito transmission theory.

Dr. Carlos Finlay, a Cuban physician, made the first attempt to implicate *Aedes aegypti* experimentally as the vector of yellow fever. Finlay was born in Puerto Principe, Cuba, to a French mother and a Scottish father, who was a practicing physician and coffee-grower. Young Carlos received his early schooling from a paternal aunt. Then he was sent to France to continue his education—an unlucky decision, for in Le Havre he suffered an attack of chorea. He went home to recover but was left with a residual stammer for the remainder of his life.

In 1848 the young man returned to France to continue his schooling, but decided to enroll in London because of the unsettled conditions on the Continent. He subsequently spent a year on the Rhine in Mentz before trying France once more. In Rouen illness again struck him. An attack of typhoid fever sent him home—without his liberal arts degree. Because the medical school at the University of Havana would not accept a college dropout, he enrolled at the less demanding Jefferson Medical College in Philadelphia.

His experiences at Jefferson appear to have decisively directed Finlay toward the study of yellow fever. For he quickly fell under the influence of one preceptor, Dr. John Kearsley Mitchell—an early proponent of the germ theory of disease. Mitchell's son, Dr. S. Weir Mitchell, urged the young medical student to consider opening a New York office. But Finlay always seems to have been possessed by a bit of wanderlust. After graduation in 1855 he worked in both Paris and Lima, Peru, before returning to settle in Havana.

In 1881 Finlay reported the results of his experiments on yellow fever. Having been struck by the fact that the disease and *Aedes aegypti* always seemed to be found together, he deduced that the bite of the female mosquito must be responsible. To prove his point, he raised mosquitoes and used them in more than a hundred experiments, allowing the insects to bite yellow fever patients and then healthy subjects. In five cases he claimed to have been able to transmit the infection experimentally.

But since childhood Finlay had been unlucky with diseases, and yellow fever proved to be no exception. Medical colleagues regarded him as nothing but an eccentric. When he persisted, they demanded an incontrovertible proof. This Finlay was never able to produce because he was totally unaware of the one important fact that had also eluded Stubbins ffirth: The virus is present in the blood of a patient for only the first three days of the illness. Finlay made many further attempts, and a few subjects came down with yellow fever, but the results were so erratic that other physicians could not be convinced. The mosquitoes, they maintained, had not transmitted the disease. Only Finlay's wife and his assistant believed him. And so the mosquito theory was once again forgotten.

Then in 1898 the problem was taken up by Dr. Henry R. Carter, a physician in the United States Public Health Service. While working many years as a quarantine officer, Carter had made the observation, similar to Dr. Hosack's, of a fact that had been common knowledge among sailors for more than two centuries. When a man aboard ship contracted yellow fever, his crewmates did not develop it until a few days after he had recovered or died.

Carter's chance to verify his finding statistically came during an epidemic of yellow fever in Mississippi. Again he observed that people living with the first yellow fever victim in an outbreak did not come down with the disease for two or three weeks. Why should this be?

Carter had no explanation. He referred to the puzzling break in time as the "extrinsic incubation" period, implying that the disease was harbored somewhere in the environment. Where? Carter made no guess, though perhaps one might have helped. He submitted his carefully researched paper with its fussy tables and statistical analysis to an American medical journal. Back it came with the reason for rejection: "Too long."

At the conclusion of the Spanish-American War in 1898 Carter was reassigned to Havana as quarantine officer. At the same time, Major William C. Gorgas was ordered to the city to serve as a U. S. Army sanitary officer: Though initially ignorant of both Carter's work and the mosquito theory, Gorgas had an open mind and learned quickly.

Born into the Army, Gorgas was the son of Major Josiah Gorgas, an ordnance officer in command of the Mount Vernon Arsenal near Mobile, Alabama. The elder Gorgas, a sympathizer with the southern cause, had resigned his commission at the outbreak of the Civil War and joined the Confederate Army as chief of ordnance. When young Willie later applied for admission to the United States Military Academy at West Point, he found that having a Rebel for a father was no help. Rejected for officer training, he enrolled in the Bellevue Medical College in New York, and, after his graduation and internship, gained appointment to the Army Medical Corps.

Gorgas spent twenty years in the routine life of an army surgeon, moved like a pawn to forts in Texas, North Dakota, and Florida. He cut a wide swath among the ladies on the various posts, who called him the "Gorgeous Doctor." His only unpleasant experience seems to have been an attack of yellow fever at Fort Brown, Texas. But the immunity he acquired served him well during his tour of duty in Cuba.

When the forty-four-year-old Gorgas arrived in Havana, the city had been reduced to a cesspool by Spanish oppression and the war. Sick natives and the carcasses of dead animals littered the stinking streets. Homeless beggars and orphan children wandered forlornly about while flocks of black vultures circled overhead. Though yellow fever was on the wane, typhoid and dysentery were rampant.

Gorgas quickly proved himself the most efficient sanitary officer in memory. Within two years he had managed to clean up the entire city. Cooing with adulation, the American press printed before-and-after stories and pictures. But then yellow fever struck.

The infection appears to have been brought in by several thousand Spanish immigrants. Gorgas believed it to be a disease of filth, transmitted by fomites—clothing, patient bedding—and he acted accordingly. Keep calm and clean harder, he advised.

Nothing helped. The natives ridiculed Gorgas, for yellow jack did not touch the dirty, impoverished shanties but the parts of the city that were most sanitary. High American officials succumbed. The wife of one threw herself across her husband's body as he died hawking up *el vomito negro;* after attending his funeral, she ran home and killed herself with his pistol. Distraught clerks at Camp Columbia outside Havana burned sulfur, hoping to drive away the disease. At the mess nearby, officers drank a toast: "Here's to the ones who have gone. Here's to the next to go."

General Leonard Wood, the Army's chief sanitary officer, was distressed. He ordered that every dirty native be scrubbed clean. In the meantime, yellow fever continued to wipe out his staff. When more than a third of his men had died, he frantically cabled to Washington for help. On June 25, 1900, Major Walter Reed was ordered to Cuba with instructions to "give special attention to questions relating to the cause and prevention of yellow fever."

The forty-nine-year-old Reed, selected because of his bacteriologic expertise, was the son of an itinerant Methodist minister. He had been an academic prodigy, a master of the Greek and Latin classics, and at age seventeen the youngest graduate of the medical school of the University of Virginia. But as a scientist he was a late bloomer, who did not publish his first paper until the age of forty-one. His early years in practice were spent as an inspector for the Brooklyn Board of Health, then as an army doctor on the western plains and mountains. Like his father, he was a strongly moral man, and he shunned routine military diversions: beer, bottle pool in the officers' mess, and alcoholic nights at draw poker.

After fourteen dry, dreary years on lonely military posts, Reed was ordered to Baltimore to study pathology and bacteriology with Dr. William H. Welch at Johns Hopkins. Here he spent the next three years exposed to the new discoveries in bacteriology. In 1893 he was appointed curator of the Army Medical Museum; and during the Spanish-American War he headed a committee responsible for the important finding that typhoid fever was propagated in military camps by flies carrying infected waste.

Reed arrived in Cuba to study yellow fever with Dr. James Carroll, who had been his assistant at the museum. Two other men had also been assigned to help. One, Dr. Jesse W. Lazear, a southern physician, had studied the mosquito transmission of malaria and was in charge of the Las Animas Hospital Laboratory at Camp Columbia. The other, Dr. Aristedes Agramonte, the son of a Cuban revolutionary, had been Lazear's classmate at New York's College of Physicians and Surgeons; he was in charge of the laboratory at Military Hospital No. 1 in Havana. These four men—Reed, Carroll, Lazear, Agramonte—constituted what came to be called the United States Army Yellow Fever Commission.

Reed and Carroll encountered their first case of yellow fever the day they arrived at the Las Animas Hospital. The Army's chief surgeon in Cuba had it. Over the next month, the four investigators studied eighteen other patients and performed eleven autopsies looking for "*Salmonella icteroides*," a chimerical organism postulated to cause the disease. After a fruitless search, Reed concluded correctly that no such bacillus was involved.

Lazear's mosquito experience suggested the next step. The commission went to call on Carlos Finlay, still licking his bites after his ignominious scientific defeat. He told them, as he told anyone else who would listen, why he believed mosquitoes carried yellow fever; he showed them the records of his discredited, muddled experiments that had so far convinced nobody; he gave them some tiny, black, cigar-shaped eggs of *Aedes aegypti*.

"Those are the eggs of a criminal," he warned Reed grimly.

By this time, Reed, too, was suspicious of an insect vector. For he had repeatedly watched nonimmune nurses handle yellow fever cases and yet remain untouched by the disease. Such a thing was unheard of in bacterial infections—cholera and plague, for example. Moreover, the yellow fever distribution pattern was also quite different from that of an ordinary infectious disease. In Quemados, Reed had seen a man in a house in 102 Real Street become ill; then the infection jumped around the corner to 20 General Lee Street, and from there it hopped across the road. Yet these families had no contact with each other whatsoever.

Reed's suspicions were confirmed when his fellow Virginian Dr. Henry Carter came to see him. Carter showed Reed the results of his Mississippi study documenting the extrinsic incubation period. Usually, there was a short time lag between the first appearance and the second outbreak.

"Are you sure your dates are accurate?" Reed asked.

Carter replied that he was.

"Then it spells an insect host," Reed answered. Ronald Ross, incidentally, had found the same time lapse in the mosquito transmission of malaria. For the mosquito must digest the infected blood before it can transmit the disease.

Now Reed was faced with his most difficult decision. He would have to repeat Finlay's discredited human experiments, since no animal besides man was known to contract yellow fever. But trying to give human beings yellow fever was extremely unsettling to a man of Reed's stern morality. In some epidemics the mortality rate was 85 per cent.

Human experimentation in medicine was nothing new, of course. Jenner had done it. Pasteur had done it. So have many scientists before and since who were far less ethical.

Armauer Hansen, for example, who discovered the bacillus of leprosy in 1873, conducted a uniquely horrible experiment. Convinced of the transmissibility of leprosy but unable to find a susceptible experimental animal, he tried to infect an unwilling subject. Without getting permission, indeed against her strongly expressed plea, he twice pricked into the surface of the eye of a thirty-three-year-old woman, material from the nodules of a leprous patient. In the ensuing uproar, Hansen was interrogated and admitted he had only told the woman that he would give her a prick in the eye without disclosing the purpose of this treatment. Hansen was tried but was acquitted with merely a minor reprimand.

A much greater outcry occurred when an article on unethical human experimentation from the June 16, 1966, issue of *The New England Journal of Medicine* was reported on the front page of the New York *Times*. The author, Dr. Henry K. Beecher of the Harvard Medical School, related a series of recent cases even more horrifying than Hansen's. In one, melanoma, a highly malignant skin cancer, was transplanted from a daughter to her mother "in the hope of gaining a little better understanding of cancer immunity. . . ." The daughter's condition was described as terminal, and she died the day following the transplant. The tumor was excised from the mother on the twenty-fourth day after implant, and she died a little over a year later—of diffuse melanoma conclusively shown to have come from the transplanted tumor. Beecher went on to cite other equally disturbing cases—among them a study in which live cancer cells were injected into twenty-two hospitalized patients. These subjects were "merely told they would be receiving 'some cells.' . . . The word cancer was entirely omitted."

Yellow fever, too, had its share of unethical experimenters. Professor G. Sanarelli, who in 1897 mistakenly identified the chimerical *"Salmonella icteroides"* as the cause, tested his conclusion on five human subjects without their permission or consent. After he had injected ten cubic centimeters of his toxin, one subject experienced incessant vomiting, cessation of kidney function, delirium, and coma; another reacted similarly after the injection of five cubic centimeters. But to one patient, not so susceptible, Sanarelli gave an eye-popping forty-four cubic centimeters of his poison. Many physicians were stunned by such callous cruelty, especially William Osler, who wrote, "[These] experiments . . . have been characterized . . . as ridiculous, but I beg to say that is not the term to use. . . . To deliberately inject a poison of known high degree of virulency into a human being, unless you obtain that man's sanction, is not ridiculous, it is criminal."

Walter Reed was determined not to deal with experimental subjects the way his predecessor Sanarelli had. Even during animal experiments, Reed was known for his humanity. When an antivivisectionist complained to a U. S. Senate committee in 1896 about the horrible things he believed were being done to dumb animals in Reed's laboratory, a former researcher there, Dr. J. C. McConnell, replied, ". . . at no time during my connection with the Army Medical Museum, from about 1870 to the end of the year 1895, have any experiments been performed upon animals in which an anesthetic was not used, unless one of the ordinary inoculation experiments, which were practically painless, nor were animals kept in a mutilated condition."

And Reed was reluctant to experiment on human beings at all. This was well demonstrated at an 1897 medical meeting in Washington, D.C. After Reed had presented his results on a study of splenic leukemia, Dr. A. F. A. King, a member of the audience, rose to suggest the following frightening procedure: "Since leucocytes destroyed micro-organisms, it might be an interesting experiment . . . to inject bacteria into the blood of a leukaemic subject and note whether the large number of leucocytes would so far increase phagocytosis as to protect the system from bacteric infection."

Undoubtedly horrified, Reed replied, "I should be afraid to try Dr. King's suggestion upon human beings. We do not know what the injection of bacteria into the blood of human beings suffering with leukaemia might do. . . ."

In the case of yellow fever, Reed would allow the vital human experiments on only one condition: that the members of the commission would themselves be bitten and thus subject to the risk that necessity compelled them to impose on others. Moreover, the scrupulously honest Reed insisted on "informed consent" in all volunteers. To this end, he drew up and signed a compact with each, explaining precisely the risks and hazards involved. Under the terms of the agreement, each volunteer would receive one hundred dollars in gold for being bitten, plus an additional hundred dollars in gold should he contract the disease. And "in case of his death because of this disease," the compact added, "the Commission will transmit the said sum (two hundred American dollars) to the person whom the undersigned shall designate at his convenience."

An additional concern was for the age of the volunteer, since yellow fever was more likely to end fatally in an older person. Surgeon General George Sternberg had either ordered or advised the forty-nine-year-old Reed not to experiment on himself. Reed, therefore, ruled that no subject over the age of forty should be used.

Lazear was given charge of the mosquitoes and soon had a large stock of both adults and larvae. He placed each female in a labeled test tube stoppered with a wad of gauze. He then allowed the insects to bite yellow fever patients, and with the other commission members proceeded to expose nine volunteers—mostly soldiers, who grew more and more doubtful of their chances of getting yellow fever as the failures accumulated. But getting bitten was easy. The subject merely pulled the stopper and clapped the test tube to his forearm. If the mosquito was hungry, she would alight on the skin and suck her fill.

In early August, while Reed was in Washington finishing a report on his typhoid studies, the one eligible commission member, thirty-four-year-old Jesse Lazear, allowed himself to be bitten. Carroll, forty-six, and Reed were ineligible because of age. Agramonte was immune on account of a previous attack. The insect used was a mosquito that ten days previously had fed on a yellow fever patient during his fifth day of illness. Nothing happened. The commission had yet to learn that the virus disappears from the blood after three days.

The first successful transmission, finally accomplished on August 27, almost ended the study. A mosquito that had fed on a patient in his second day of illness would not eat. Lazear repeatedly tried to feed the apparently debilitated insect that morning. In the afternoon, Lazear mentioned the problem to Carroll. Carroll picked up the tube, held it to his own forearm for a few minutes, and was bitten.

Two days later he felt ill. The next day, August 30, he had chills and fever. When Agramonte and Gorgas came to examine him, they witnessed a familiar sight. Carroll was thrashing restlessly in bed, his fever high, his eyes bloodshot. Soon he was delirious with yellow fever. His eyes turned yellow but *el vomito negro* never appeared. A week later he was much better. After Reed's death in 1902 Carroll was criticized for disobeying orders, having been declared ineligible. For the experiments would no doubt have been immediately terminated had his infection ended fatally.

When Carroll recovered, the inevitable question arose: Had the mosquito bite caused the disease?

"We decided to test it upon the first nonimmune person who should offer himself to be bitten," Agramonte wrote. At that moment, a soldier named William H. Dean happened by, saluted, and watched Lazear cajole a mosquito from one test tube to another.

"You still fooling with mosquitoes, Doctor?" Dean asked.

"Yes," Lazear replied. "Will you take a bite?"

"Sure, I ain't scared of 'em."

Lazear and Agramonte looked at each other.

Five days later Dean had yellow fever, the second experimental case. Fortunately, he recovered. The news was immediately cabled to Reed in Washington. With the other three members of the commission, he decided that the investigators themselves should incur no further risks. One hero among them was enough. But it was already too late.

Five days previously, Lazear had been bitten by an infected mosquito. He claimed it was a stray one that had landed on his hand, though Reed later suspected him of having made up this story after experimenting on himself without his collegues' knowledge. Poor Lazear's case was the worst Gorgas had ever seen. It terminated in wild delirium and *el vomito negro*. Two men had to hold Lazear in bed as he died the morning of September 25, 1900—the first of six investigators to perish of yellow fever. "Accident in the line of duty" was the description in the final report.

In early October Reed returned to Havana. With Agramonte and Carroll he agreed that three cases, the first questionable and the third "accidental," were not sufficient to convince anyone. To avoid Finlay's fate, they needed a larger, better controlled series.

So a new experimental site, Camp Lazear, was built in an isolated area a few miles from Camp Columbia. Here the commission conducted two experiments in November and December. In one, seven American volunteers were exposed to the soiled clothing, towels, and bedding of yellow fever victims for twenty consecutive nights, yet remained well. This experiment confirmed that yellow fever was not transmitted by fomites. In the second experiment thirteen volunteers, mostly paid Spanish immigrants, were bitten by mosquitoes carrying yellow fever.

The immigrants themselves were eager for the money, but the Havana newspapers raised a terrible outcry. "Horrible . . . if true," screamed *La Discusión,* blasting the "criminals" said to be taking advantage of unsuspecting Latinos. In two red-hot articles, the paper accused the commission of all manner of inhumanity and barbarity. But all the noise had no effect at all, as Reed wrote to Sternberg:

". . . the Spanish Counsel [sic], a most courteous and intelligent gentleman, assures us that we shall have his support, as long as we do not use minors and the individual gives us written consent. . . ."

Of the thirteen volunteers, eleven came down with yellow fever.

The means of transmission was now certain, but a more puzzling question still remained. What was the organism responsible? All efforts to identify a germ microscopically, cultivate it on an artificial medium, and transmit it to an experimental animal failed.

The clue to the viral nature of yellow fever came from the French studies of rabies, for Pasteur had postulated an ultramicroscopic agent as the cause. Supporting Pasteur's notion was the research of Friedrich Löffler and Paul Frosch in 1898. These two Germans had discovered that hoof-and-mouth disease in cattle is transmitted by a filtrate of infected blood serum that has been passed through a porcelain filter able to catch the smallest visible living cells and bacteria. As a result of this work, Reed and Carroll surmised that yellow fever, too, was caused by an ultramicroscopic agent. Nearly half a century later the electron microscope revealed the yellow fever virus to be a spherical particle, from one to two millionths of an inch in diameter.

The work of Pasteur also suggested that a vaccine for yellow fever might be prepared. In August 1901 Reed asked Carroll to attempt this, but the results were disastrous. With Dr. Juan Guiteras, a Havana health officer, Carroll began the inoculation experiments. Patterning their method after direct smallpox inoculation, they obtained material from a series of mosquitoes that had transmitted mild cases of yellow fever during one series of tests. Of the eight volunteers they inoculated with this material, three died.

But Carroll did manage to confirm that yellow fever was caused by an ultramicroscopic organism. Blood from a Spaniard infected with one of Guiteras's mosquitoes was carefully filtered. The filtrate was then injected in three American volunteers. The result: One developed only mild headache and fever, but the two others came down with yellow fever. All survived.

A Man, a Plan, a Canal, Panama

No one had been watching these experiments with greater interest than Gorgas. "If it is the mosquito," he proclaimed, "I am going to get rid of the mosquito."

"It can't be done," Reed replied, and with good reason. Havana was teeming with millions of the ubiquitous insects. Moreover, no one was certain that other insects or animals did not also carry the disease.

Undaunted by Reed's distaste for the project, Gorgas, with his usual enthusiasm, commenced his campaign against yellow fever early in 1901. He employed two main tactics. All yellow fever cases were confined to a tightly screened room; subsequently the room was fumigated to kill any lingering mosquitoes. And a concerted effort was made to annihilate the entire adult mosquito population. Gorgas, who believed these measures to be sufficient, would have failed had he not instituted one more tactic—almost as an afterthought. This was a house-to-house attack on the insect's breeding places.

Aedes aegypti were to be found multiplying within most of the barrels, jugs, vases, and gourds in town. So Gorgas persuaded the city council to rule that all water containers in the city had to be either empty, fully covered, or partly filled with kerosene, since a thin layer of kerosene on the water surface was lethal to the mosquito larvae. Any person with mosquitoes reproducing on his premises was fined ten dollars, a stiff penalty in those days.

The natives regarded the whole operation as one great joke. They laughed at the "Yanqui" mosquito-hunters and hid their water containers from them. The inspectors countered by listing every water vessel on an index card. During repeat inspections, the señora had to show that all vessels were mosquito-free. Kerosene was immediately poured into those that were not.

The volatile Latin temperament might not have long tolerated this probing nuisance but for Gorgas. Because he spoke Spanish, he was able politely to smooth rumpled native feathers while continuing the monthly inspections of every house, hotel, barroom, and hut. A genuine diplomat, he rarely fined anyone; yet, with his mild manner and zeal for detail, he managed to wipe out yellow fever in Havana—a truly remarkable feat.

For almost a century and a half—from 1762 to 1901—the city had not gone a day without a new case of yellow fever. In March of that year Gorgas commenced his campaign, and by October the disease had disappeared. For the next nine months not a single case was reported. One more outbreak occurred in 1905 but was speedily quelled by reapplication of Gorgas's techniques. Thereafter, yellow fever was only an unpleasant memory to the grateful citizens. "No hay mosquitos aqui, señor"—"There are no mosquitoes here, señor"

—they would happily report to the municipal inspectors. Soon other Latin American cities followed suit. In 1908 Dr. Oswaldo Cruz used identical methods to eradicate yellow fever in Rio de Janeiro.

In the meantime, however, Gorgas recognized an especially dramatic place to eliminate yellow fever and malaria as well—Panama. During the year Gorgas had spent cleaning up Havana, Theodore Roosevelt had become President. And the young, vigorous Roosevelt was determined to build an interoceanic canal across the Panama Isthmus.

The idea of a Panama Canal was not a new one, having been conceived shortly after Balboa crossed the Isthmus of Panama in 1513. But no such project was physically feasible until the perfection of the steam engine. In 1881 the French began to dig, in an ill-fated effort organized by the seventy-six-year-old Ferdinand de Lesseps. The unlucky Balboa had been beheaded after a row with a superior; Lesseps's men, however, were defeated by two deadlier assassins—malaria and yellow fever—and the result was one of the greatest scandals in the history of capitalism. French investors lost 1.435 billion francs, or about $287 million. Lesseps, who had been a French national hero after successfully completing the Suez Canal, died a broken man soon after the revelation of the graft, corruption, and payoffs that had occurred during the Panama fiasco.

Yet Lesseps might have triumphed at Panama as he had at Suez had there been no malaria and no yellow fever. These two diseases had rendered the region a pesthole since the days of the Spanish settlements. During the building of the Panama railroad in 1850 fever was said to have felled a laborer for every railroad tie laid along the forty-seven miles of track between Colón on the Atlantic and Panama City on the Pacific. In some versions of this story the dead men were Irish, in others, Chinese. Certainly this number is too high—there were some seventy-four thousand ties along the Panama line—but it may not be far from the correct one. No one will ever know, since the company kept no systematic records.

Surely, however, it is small when compared to the number of Lesseps's workers who perished during the abortive French attempt to build a canal. At first the company tried to keep this number a secret, but soon too many parents had been informed of the deaths of their sons. Professional engineers in Paris began advising their young colleagues not to go to Panama, saying that it would be suicidal. And one in a series of chief engineers, Jules Isidore Dingler, paid an especially terrible price for his devotion to the doomed French cause.

In 1883 Dingler brought his family with him to the Isthmus—Mme. Dingler, a son, a daughter, and the daughter's fiancé. They moved into a large, comfortable house on the site. Arriving in the fever-free dry season, Dingler had imported magnificent horses from France. There were family excursions into the hills, accompanied by servants and huge picnic hampers. In one old photograph the daughter appears as a pretty, dark-haired girl about eighteen, sitting side-saddle in a full skirt and little Panama hat.

But in January, as the wet season commenced, the daughter contracted yellow fever and died within a few days. "My poor husband is in a despair which is painful to see," wrote Mme. Dingler to Lesseps's son Charles. "Our dear daughter was our pride and joy."

The young woman's death had a deep effect on everyone—canal officials, workers, the local citizens. Dingler and the fiancé rode at the head of a large procession to the cemetery following the funeral in the crowded cathedral.

A month later Dingler's twenty-one-year-old son died of yellow fever, followed shortly by the daughter's fiancé. By summer forty-eight officers of the canal company were dead of the same disease. According to one American naval officer, laborers were dying at a rate of about two hundred a month. It was a despondent Dingler who wrote to Charles de Lesseps, "I cannot thank you enough for your kind and affectionate letter. Mme. Dingler who [knows] that she is for me the only source of affection in this world, controls herself with courage, but she is deeply shaken. . . . We attach ourselves to life in making the canal our only occupation; I say 'we' because Mme. Dingler accompanies me in all my excursions and follows with interest the progress of the work."

Mme. Dingler died of yellow fever on New Year's Eve 1884. The morning after her death her husband was so distraught that he could barely speak, yet he somehow managed to appear at his desk at the customary hour. After the funeral he led all the family's horses, including his own, into a mountain ravine and shot them. By late August, close to physical and mental collapse, he resigned his position and sailed for France, never to return to the spot in which all his family lay buried.

After a bloodless revolution fostered by the presence of American gunboats, Panama seceded from Colombia and immediately agreed to allow the United States to build a canal. The French equipment on the site, the Panama Railroad, and the exhaustive plans and surveys for the failed French effort were purchased by the U.S. government for forty million dollars. "I took the isthmus," Roosevelt liked to brag in later years when describing his role in the coup. And when informed of the dissatisfaction of some academics over his heavy-handed intervention, Roosevelt responded, "Tell them that I am going to make the dirt fly."

On March 4, 1904, four months after the Stars and Stripes had been raised over the old French administration building, Roosevelt named Dr. William Gorgas sanitary officer of the Canal Zone. That such an officer should have been appointed at all was due primarily to the intervention of Dr. William Welch, the Johns Hopkins pathologist. During a personal call at the White House, Welch urged the President to eradicate the sources of disease on the Isthmus before the work began.

Unfortunately, many construction officials were dubious of Gorgas's Havana methods. And the most prominent doubter was John F. Wallace, the chief engineer. Convinced that degeneracy and inefficiency had been responsible for the French downfall, Wallace allotted very little money for Gorgas's cleanup efforts. He did not believe the mosquito theory and maintained that clearing the refuse, dead cats, and other detritus from the streets would be sufficient.

Yet Wallace still lived in mortal terror of disease. With his wife he moved into the old French official residence of the chief engineer, Dingler's former home, and there heard of the frightening deaths in his predecessor's family from servants who were holdovers from the French regime. Soon his assistant, William Karner, was taken ill with malaria, followed by the valet and cook. During a short trip to Washington in September 1904 the apprehensive Wallace took the precaution of purchasing two expensive metal caskets for himself and his wife.

On November 21, 1904, the first case of yellow fever for the year was brought into the Santo Tomás Hospital in Panama City. More cases appeared in December. In January the disease broke out on the cruiser *Boston,* anchored in Panama Bay. "YELLOW JACK IN PANAMA," screamed the newspaper headlines.

In vain Gorgas tried to get rid of the mosquitoes. They were breeding in almost every office in small glass receptacles containing brushes used for copying letters. Efforts at eradication were met with little or no co-operation. Wallace ignored repeated pleas to screen office windows and doors. And his chief architect, M. O. Johnson, declared himself too busy with serious matters to worry about window screens. The architect joked about the fuss being made, having "little faith in modern ideas pertaining to yellow fever transmission," as one witness recounted.

In early 1905, while Wallace was away in Washington, yellow fever struck the administration building. Among the first to die was Johnson. Gorgas personally attended the case but could do nothing; even today, no treatment exists for yellow fever. The twenty-nine-year-old architect, who had given up his job with the Illinois Central Railroad to come to Panama, was buried in Wallace's expensive metal casket.

As the number of deaths quickly mounted, a feeling of alarm, almost amounting to panic, spread among Americans on the Isthmus. Many resigned their positions to return to the United States. Those who stayed were convinced that they were doomed, just as had been the French before them. As the fever wards filled to overflowing, local undertakers piled stacks of coffins in plain view at the railroad depot. One funeral procession after another passed through the streets. And James Stanley Gilbert, an American resident of the Isthmus, composed some appropriate verse:

> You are going to have the fever,
>   Yellow eyes!
> In about ten days from now
> Iron bands will clamp your brow;
> Your tongue resemble curdled cream,
> A rusty streak the center seam;
> Your mouth will taste of untold things,
> With claws and horns and fins and wings;
> Your head will weigh a ton or more,
> And forty gales within it roar!

Finally, all unscreened windows in the administration building were ordered closed. The building was fumigated again and again. Discovering mosquitoes to be breeding in the holy water font of a nearby cathedral, Gorgas ordered that the water be changed daily. But his manpower and supplies had been so limited that he could accomplish little.

At the height of the panic in mid-June Chief Engineer Wallace resigned. With his wife he hastily packed and sailed for New York. He spent the rest of his life trying to live down the damage to his reputation done by this flagrant dereliction of duty. But at least he had managed to depart the Isthmus in a stateroom rather than a coffin. To replace him, Roosevelt appointed John Stevens, a former construction engineer on the Great Northern Railroad.

Recommended to Roosevelt by James J. Hill, the Great Northern's crusty founder, Stevens was one of the toughest, most resourceful men ever to lay a rail. He had built railroad lines through swamps and pine forests while managing to survive Mexican fevers, Indian attacks, Michigan mosquitoes, and Canadian blizzards. On one occasion he had been treed by wolves. Restless and temperamental, he had no patience with slackers.

"There are three diseases in Panama," he told his workers. "They are yellow fever, malaria, and cold feet; and the greatest of these is cold feet." While he was surveying the shambles that had been left by Wallace, one of his aides pointed out to him that at least no collisions had occurred on the Panama Railroad in more than a year.

"A collision has its good points as well as its bad ones," Stevens replied. "It indicates there is something moving on the railroad."

At first the new chief engineer was unimpressed by Gorgas and his great sanitary success in Havana. "We are not here to demonstrate any theories in medicine," he told his sanitation officer, informing him that he had four months to eradicate yellow fever in Panama. But, unlike Wallace, he backed Gorgas to the hilt and gave him all the supplies he needed, regardless of the cost.

Wallace had limited Gorgas's budget to fifty thousand dollars a year; Stevens would approve requisitions for ninety thousand dollars' worth of wire screening alone. As a consequence of this new affluence, Gorgas was able to fumigate the cities of Panama and Colón house by house. Enormous sanitary brigades traipsed through the streets, loaded with ladders, paste pots, buckets, cans of mosquito-killing kerosene and pyrethrum powder. All cisterns and cesspools were oiled weekly. Towns on the Isthmus were provided with running water, thus dispensing with the mosquito-breeding water containers.

Stevens and Gorgas got on well together from the start. When efforts were made in Washington to have Gorgas removed, Stevens resisted and was backed by Dr. Welch. Yet initially, the chief engineer made no open declaration of confidence in Gorgas's notions. "Like probably many others I had gained some little idea of the mosquito theory," he recalled, ". . . but like most laymen, I had little faith in its effectiveness, nor even dreamed of its tremendous importance."

He was soon pleasantly surprised. Once Gorgas had been adequately equipped, yellow fever dropped off with the same dramatic rapidity as at Havana. Within a year and a half the disease had disappeared from the Isthmus.

On November 9, 1906, Roosevelt sailed for Panama on the new battleship *Louisiana* to inspect the construction. He was deeply impressed by the progress that he witnessed. And he had special praise for the advances in sanitation made by Gorgas. The situation was especially surprising, the President said, in light of Panama's past.

But, in fact, Panama had become a paradise of health only for the white workers. The black workers continued to die at an alarming rate. For every dead white there were ten dead blacks. The causes were varied—railroad accidents, alcoholism, dysentery, suicide, syphilis, tuberculosis. Viral pneumonia, however, was the chief killer. Since the disease was unknown in Barbados, where most of the black laborers came from, they were exceedingly susceptible.

They were also plagued by malaria. The brush-burning, swamp draining activities had eliminated the anopheles mosquitoes in the towns and along the construction line. But the insects were still very much in evidence in the jungle, only a short distance away. And since this was where most black workers lived, in rude, unscreened huts, the incidence of malaria among them was high.

Roosevelt said nothing publicly, but in private correspondence he was quite candid. "The least satisfactory feature of the entire work to my mind was the arrangement for feeding the negroes," he wrote on returning to Washington. "These cooking sheds with their muddy floors and with the unclean pot which each man had in which he cooked everything, are certainly not what they should be. . . . Moreover, the very large sick rates among the negroes, compared with the whites, seems to me to show that a resolute effort should be made to teach the negro some of the principles of personal hygiene. . . ."

Despite this single sore spot, Roosevelt was quite pleased overall with his trip and his chief engineer's accomplishments. In a message to Congress on December 17, 1906, he expressed his great faith in Stevens. And so he was extremely annoyed when on February 12, 1907, a six-page letter from Stevens arrived at the White House expressing great discontent with the situation at Panama.

Stevens was by this time an exhausted and embittered man. He complained of "enemies in the rear" and of being "continually subject to attack by a lot of people . . . that I would not wipe my boots on in the United States." Though he did not formally resign, one paragraph in the letter sealed his fate. "The work itself . . . on the whole, I do not like. . . . There has never been a day since my connection with this enterprise that I could not have gone back to the United States and occupied positions that, to me, were far more satisfactory. Some of them, I would prefer to hold, if you will pardon my candor, than the Presidency of the United States."

"Stevens must get out at once," Roosevelt wrote to an aide, and cabled to Panama that the "resignation" was accepted. As a replacement, the President chose George W. Goethals, a cool, capable, correct and dignified army officer; it was he who was to complete the canal in 1914.

Gorgas, one of the few American officials to remain with the project from the beginning, continued to fight yellow fever in South America. During World War I he was appointed surgeon general of the Army. When asked by a doctor friend the first thing he would do if he received a telephone call that the war had ended, Gorgas replied, "I would ring off, call New York City, and order a passage for South America. I would go to Guayaquil, Ecuador, the only place in which yellow fever is prevalent, exterminate the pestilence, and then —and then return to Panama, the garden spot of the world, and end my days writing an elegy on yellow fever."

"A man, a plan, a canal, Panama," goes the famous palindrome. Though the man and the plan are usually taken to be Roosevelt and his dream of an interoceanic passage, they might equally well be Gorgas and his method for eradicating yellow fever.

Yellow Fever: Germ and Vaccine

The cause, however, still remained uncertain. Dr. James Carroll had shown that the organism would pass through a porcelain filter capable of trapping the smallest bacteria. But he could neither see nor grow it. By the mid-1920s a lively dispute over the exact nature of the yellow fever germ had arisen, chiefly on account of the work of Dr. Hideyo Noguchi.

Noguchi had achieved world fame as a bacteriologist while part of Dr. Simon Flexner's original staff at the Rockefeller Institute for Medical Research. Though he had dabbled in rabies, polio, Rocky Mountain spotted fever, trachoma, hog cholera, and even snake venom studies, Noguchi was best known for his studies of syphilis. He reported that he had grown the spirochete of syphilis in a test tube; no one up to the present time has been able to repeat his results. He also reported cultivating the rabies virus, the polio virus, and the trachoma organism, but these results were never confirmed, either. Nonetheless, he was greatly revered at the Rockefeller Institute despite his rather dubious experimental ability and humble origins.

Seisaku Noguchi was his name at birth. Born in Japan to a poor servant family, he quickly caught the eye of his teachers, who couldn't decide whether he was a genius or just plain crazy. His consuming passion, he always maintained, was "to accomplish the impossible." Impressed by his zeal, one professor suggested the name Hideyo, the Japanese for "great man of the world." As a medical student in Tokyo he intended to train further in Germany. But on his way through the United States he took a small detour to meet Flexner, then at the University of Pennsylvania.

In his prime, Noguchi was known as quite a character. He had a cheerful manner, a small stature, an enormous ego, and a deformed left hand, which was almost fingerless from burns as an infant. A confirmed workaholic and prolific writer, he was never able to master the intricacies of English grammar. He was idolized by friends and associates, but often spoke of himself as "funny Noguchi."

In 1918 Noguchi arrived in Guayaquil, Ecuador, to study the raging yellow fever there. With him he brought an enormous quantity of laboratory equipment and sixty guinea pigs. On his legs he wore puttees to protect himself from mosquito bites. Ecuador had statutes forbidding the entry of both Japanese and guinea pigs, but in Guayaquil these were graciously waived by city fathers anxious to rid the town of its reputation as a pesthole.

Noguchi worked quickly. Though his excessive secrecy embarrassed both American and Ecuadorian physicians, within nine days he found what he suspected to be the cause of yellow fever. A month after his arrival, he reported to the newspapers that he had transmitted yellow fever to guinea pigs.

Noguchi's yellow fever organism was, of all things, a spirochete, and nine years were to pass before this totally erroneous finding could be refuted. For he had confused another condition, Weil's disease, with yellow fever—an easy mistake to make, since during an epidemic the two can appear remarkably similar. And Weil's disease is caused by a spirochete, *Leptospira icterohaemorrhagiae*.

Medical historians today tend to be critical of Noguchi for his error. He had himself worked previously with *L. icterohaemorrhagiae* and was known as a specialist in the spirochete field. Why did he not try to make certain that the organisms he found in Guayaquil were not really different from the spirochete of Weil's disease? Why did he use guinea pigs, animals known to be susceptible to the leptospira of Weil's disease and known also to be impervious to yellow fever? No doubt he really believed that he was Hideyo, the great man of the world, and that he could not fail.

At first Noguchi managed to convince almost everyone that a spirochete was the cause of yellow fever. He even claimed that the organisms could pass through a porcelain filter and could be transmitted by a mosquito. But gradually, papers appeared that failed to confirm his findings. The tide of observation and opinion increasingly swung away from him. At a Kingston, Jamaica, conference in 1924 he was soundly drubbed. Among his chief critics was old Aristedes Agramonte, the last surviving member of the Yellow Fever Commission. It was a dark day for Noguchi.

For three years Noguchi brooded over the crushing defeat he had suffered. Finally, on November 17, 1927, he sailed to Africa to vindicate himself despite mild diabetes, an enlarged heart, and generally failing health. He hoped to prove that African yellow fever was also caused by a spirochete.

At Accra, the capital of the Gold Coast, he was met by a delegation of doctors and various officials. "Gentlemen, I shall do my best," he told them. "The results—I cannot say—they are not with me."

Everyone treated Noguchi with the greatest respect. Dr. William A. Young, director of the British Medical Research Institute in Accra, volunteered his laboratory. Noguchi was given the spacious, specially screened bungalow of another doctor; he was waited on by a staff of native servants, including a former cook for the Prince of Wales. Nothing was too good for this man whom Flexner ranked with Robert Koch.

In the laboratory Noguchi was again his usual secretive self. He announced that he would work nights, to be less disturbed. He permitted no scientists in the room, only untrained helpers. Soon he had isolated himself from the other Americans and began referring to colleagues as spies.

At Christmas Noguchi became ill and was taken to a hospital. No precise diagnosis was made, though he considered himself to have a mild case of yellow fever. His life had been saved, he said, by injection of a vaccine he had made in New York against the Guayaquil organisms. In the hospital he gave the nurses trouble and behaved like a petulant child. "I am Noguchi," he would say to explain his misconduct. On the fifth day of his illness, he ordered a monkey injected with his blood. The animal died of what Noguchi claimed to be yellow fever, though the other scientists thought this doubtful.

During the late winter and spring, Noguchi was again working at a frantic pace while continuously sending cablegrams to New York. One message cost $250, and the cable bill was sometimes $1,800 a month. Some of the cables contained important pronouncements; others he filled with rambling, pathetic fantasies: "I am sitting on my bed looking at the wall. . . . My work is so revolutionary that it is going to upset all our old ideas of yellow fever. . . ."

Much of the news of his work that appeared in the United States came from the long letters that he sent to his wife and friends. He wrote of his discovery of the African yellow fever germ, more deadly even than the South American one. His own illness, he claimed, had led to this breakthrough. These revelations often filled the pages of the New York *World*.

Noguchi had made plans to sail for home during the third week in May. Shortly before his departure, he stopped to visit a nearby medical research laboratory at Lagos. He looked very tired and felt ill. A blood smear was made to identify malarial parasites. None were found. He asked to be sent back to Accra. On the overnight boat trip he had a chill and appeared quite sick on the morning of his arrival, May 12. The sea was rough and rain was falling as the crew lowered him by chair into a surfboat. He made a dangerous landing.

He was put to bed in the home of a friend, but soon was taken to a hospital. There he was found to have the typical high temperature and low pulse rate of yellow fever—Faget's sign. On May 13 he vomited dark blood. By the sixteenth he felt better and his temperature had dropped, but the doctors suspected that this was only the well-known false remission. They were right.

For the next three days Noguchi's condition continued to vary: "much improved," "rational but no better," "quite well." He talked freely and asked about his laboratory. Then on the ninth day he suffered a seizure and bit his tongue. "I don't understand," he murmured. That night his condition deteriorated. The following morning he was confused and had convulsions. Death came at noon, Sunday, May 20, 1928. A fatal case of yellow fever customarily lasts a week; Noguchi had taken ten days to die.

Hideyo Noguchi was the fourth yellow fever investigator to succumb to the disease. Jesse Lazear had been the first. In 1921 Howard Cross, a Rockefeller bacteriologist studying yellow fever in Mexico, was the second.

The third victim was Dr. Adrian Stokes, a forty-year-old professor of pathology in Guy's Medical School, London. While studying yellow fever in West Africa, Stokes had made the discovery that monkeys could be infected with the disease. He was a kindly, tweedy sort of Englishman, charming with the ladies, an athletic type who played tennis. He became ill on September 15, 1927, and died on the night of September 19. The autopsy was performed by a colleague and friend, who wept at the assignment.

Dr. William A. Young, the director of the British Medical Research Institute in Accra, was the fifth victim. Young died on May 30, 1928, ten days after Noguchi. He had taken blood from Noguchi at the beginning of the latter's illness and inoculated it into a monkey, which died. Colleagues believed that Young might have accidentally infected himself with this blood sample.

A fifty-year-old Rockefeller bacteriologist, Dr. Paul A. Lewis, was the sixth victim. Lewis shared the conviction of Flexner and Noguchi that yellow fever was caused by a spirochete. He was at work in a laboratory in Bahia, Brazil, trying to grow the organisms in a test tube when he became ill. At first he had cabled Flexner in New York saying he was sick with influenza. The second cable said he had yellow fever. On June 26, 1929, a third cable reported that he was dead.

Other infectious diseases had proved dangerous to investigators. Typhus had killed two scientists studying it—Howard T. Ricketts and Stanislas von Prowazek. But none was worse than yellow fever. Only after years of work was a vaccine finally discovered.

Following up on the work of Stokes and others, Dr. Max Theiler and his associates at the Rockefeller Institute developed two strains of attenuated live yellow fever virus. One, known as the French strain and grown in mouse brains, is widely used today as a vaccine, especially in Africa. But since this vaccine sometimes causes serious reactions, Theiler grew another strain in chick embryos to produce another vaccine known as 17D. From 1940 to 1947 the Rockefeller Foundation made more than twenty-eight million doses of the 17D vaccine, many of which protected American soldiers from yellow fever during World War II. In 1951 Theiler was awarded the Nobel Prize in Medicine.

Poliomyelitis

Unlike yellow fever and most of the other epidemic diseases, all associated with centuries past, poliomyelitis is primarily a disease of this century. True, it has existed a long time and may have afflicted an Egyptian pharaoh, but for hundreds of years it attracted little attention. Ironically, epidemic polio was brought about by the very advances in sanitation that had all but wiped out cholera, typhoid, and other infections, though no one realized this at first.

The victims were primarily children in the industrialized countries with high living standards—the United States, Great Britain, and Sweden. The permanent paralysis polio left in its wake engendered great emotional terror, and those people wealthy enough would evacuate their children to an isolated spot during the dreaded polio season. Victor Fleming, director of *The Wizard of Oz* and *Gone With the Wind,* spent the summers with his two daughters on an island he had bought in British Columbia in order to keep them safe.

Little could be done for those children unlucky enough to come down with infantile paralysis, as polio came to be called. The afflicted limbs were massaged, the paralyzed legs stiffened with steel braces. But the most fearsome form of aid was the Drinker respirator, also called the iron lung. This device was employed to keep children alive after their muscles of respiration were permanently paralyzed.

In the nineteenth century paralytic polio was quite rare. Doctors and scientists paid little attention to it, preoccupied as they were with the epidemics of diphtheria, typhoid, and tuberculosis. But when filth came to be seen as associated with disease-producing organisms, cleanliness achieved new popularity. Daily bathing, long considered unhealthy, was energetically endorsed. Laws were passed protecting citizens from "dirty" food. Babies in particular were fiercely sheltered. Everything intended for contact with baby was scrupulously scrubbed free of germs. Milk was boiled, pabulum was steamed. The polio virus, which produces only a mild intestinal infection in an infant, was also kept away. Older children without the immunity acquired from a mild, early infection became susceptible to infantile paralysis. And just when many Americans were beginning to feel smugly superior to the poor, filthy unfortunates in less enlightened countries who knew nothing of hygiene, the first great polio epidemic struck the United States.

The year was 1916 and the result was panic. In some parts of the country, New York in particular, people behaved as though confronted by the Black Death. Thousands attempted to flee the Big Apple; many were turned away by armed townsfolk elsewhere, fearful of contagion. Before the outbreak was over, some twenty-seven thousand cases and six thousand deaths had occurred. Poliomyelitis had been suddenly transformed from a medical curiosity into a real threat.

No more innocuous name could have been devised for such a frightening malady. *Polio* is a Greek word meaning gray, and *myelitis* means inflammation of the spinal cord. Thus the full name refers to the inflammation of the gray matter which occurs in the spinal cord.

Almost forty years were to pass between the 1916 epidemic, which burned the name polio into the public consciousness, and the discovery of an effective immunization technique. To provide the funds that paid for much of the research, public hysteria was skillfully manipulated by a single organization, the National Foundation for Infantile Paralysis. The result was the largest privately funded program ever mounted to abolish a single infectious disease. But so desperate was the public for an end to the great scourge that inordinate pressure was applied to the scientists involved. The carefully controlled scientific method was repeatedly tossed to the wind. And many disasters occurred before a safe vaccine was finally produced.

The National Foundation for Infantile Paralysis may be said to have grown out of the illness of one man—Franklin Delano Roosevelt. In 1920 Roosevelt was a rising young politician, the handsome albeit distant relation of a popular former President, and the Democratic candidate for Vice President in the election that year. In spite of the Democratic defeat, he stood out as a sure winner in future elections. Then tragedy struck.

Roosevelt and his family had gone for a vacation that summer to Campobello Island. There, after an exhilarating day of swimming and boating, he awoke with a fever and was soon found to have a bad case of polio. His legs were permanently paralyzed, and his inspiring efforts at recovery again brought the disease into the public awareness. Polio by this time had been all but forgotten, since the next great outbreak did not occur until the late 1920s.

A very wealthy man, Roosevelt could have retired to his home at Hyde Park to live the refined life of a Dutchess County gentleman. His protective, solicitous mother, indeed, pressed him to do so. But instead he fought fiercely to overcome his handicap. When he rose on his paralyzed legs to nominate Al Smith, "The Happy Warrior," at the 1924 Democratic Convention, a thrill of awe and admiration swept through the convention delegates and the country as well. Roosevelt, in his battle against polio, appeared to embody the noblest elements in the American spirit, and he was to provide the most powerful emotional appeal in the history of fund-raising.

The cause to benefit from his efforts began in the form of a seedy, run-down resort hotel in the little town of Warm Springs, Georgia. Roosevelt went frequently to swim in the warm, buoyant mineral waters, hoping for some improvement in his condition. Finally he bought the hotel with the idea of making it a health resort. A Wall

Street lawyer and partner, Basil O'Connor, reluctantly agreed to run it after Roosevelt was elected governor of New York in 1928.

But the little hotel stubbornly refused to remain solvent. The many crippled people who patronized it, polio victims for the most part, were poor; and the people who did have money had no desire to pass their vacations staring at invalids. In 1929 another blow to the hotel came in the form of the stock market crash. Most former sources of private philanthropy quickly dried up. By 1932, when Roosevelt was elected President, the situation looked desperate.

It was O'Connor who saved the day. He had become fond of the Warm Springs Hotel and conceived the idea of soliciting public contributions to support it. With Roosevelt he approached public-relations and advertising firms, convinced that the ploys used to sell dentifrices, deodorants, and detergents could sell a worthy cause, too.

And he was quite right. The first fund-raising campaigns were a series of "President's Birthday Balls" promoted by means of a clever slogan, "To dance so that others may walk." In spite of the Depression, these affairs that took place throughout the country brought in over a million dollars in 1934. In the two following years, however, Roosevelt had made enough enemies to become a temporary liability. Closely associated with the Democratic Party as well, the balls did not bring in much.

Casting about for a fresh approach, Roosevelt, O'Connor, and a new public relations firm hit upon the concept of the National Foundation for Infantile Paralysis. This organization, Roosevelt announced, would "ensure that every responsible research agency in this country is adequately financed to carry out investigations into the cause of infantile paralysis." Appeals for money would be made directly to the public, since 1938, the opening year, was still a bad one for the depression-battered large private philanthropies.

One problem still remained: another catchy slogan. Madison Avenue agencies were once again consulted, but the winning idea came from Hollywood this time. Eddie Cantor, the popular banjo-eyed radio and film comedian, suggested "The March of Dimes." This was a sly allusion to "The March of Time," a pompous, neoconservative movie newsreel with commentary delivered in a voice that sounded as though God above were narrating. Cantor also suggested that radio stations donate time for broadcast appeals. People were requested to mail their dimes to President Roosevelt in the White House—a simple address to remember.

On January 30, 1938, the President's birthday, the first series of appeals reached its climax, and for the next forty-eight hours the March of Dimes seemed to be a phenomenal flop: Exactly $17.50 had been received. But on February 2 the situation abruptly reversed itself, and in the following days the White House corridors were literally awash in mailbags. So choked was the White House mail room that official letters, such as communications from foreign heads of state, were lost in the great heaps of sacks. Dimes had been mailed baked in cakes, gift-wrapped in boxes, and wrapped in yards of tape. In all, more than 2.6 million dimes had been received, along with other currency; altogether, almost two million dollars was collected. The problem was no longer how to get the money but how to spend it. Indeed, caution was imperative, for money from the first Birthday Balls had already financed one disaster.

In 1935 O'Connor and the Birthday Ball Commission had appointed Paul de Kruif, the popular author of *Microbe Hunters,* to find someone who could make a polio vaccine. De Kruif chose Maurice Brodie, a young scientist at the New York University School of Medicine. If O'Connor had second thoughts about the project, he did not admit them, having previously been stung by de Kruif's criticism that too much money was being poured into Warm Springs. No one, the famous writer pointed out, had ever been cured of polio there. But de Kruif was soon to learn just how poor his advice had been, since almost nothing was known about the polio virus, or any other virus.

Brodie began by injecting polio virus into the spinal cords of monkeys. The ground-up cords were then immersed in formalin, a solution that was supposed to kill the virus within the tissue. Brodie proceeded to make the claim that this preparation could confer immunity to polio. To prove it he injected the preparation into monkeys, and even into himself. When the inoculated monkeys were challenged with live polio virus, he asserted, they did not develop polio because they were immune. And since he was still alive after his injection, his preparation was assumed to be safe. The Birthday Ball Commission and the public hailed Brodie as a new Pasteur; certainly the similarities between the methods he used and the methods Pasteur used to prepare rabies vaccine were striking.

But the hoopla came to a sudden halt when one child died and three more developed paralytic polio after receiving Brodie's vaccine. Other scientists who tried to repeat Brodie's experiments found that monkeys "immunized" with the vaccine quickly succumbed to polio when injected with live polio virus. This debacle was in part responsible for the disappointing outcome of the 1936 Birthday Balls. And polio research was further hindered by a second disaster unrelated to the Birthday Ball Commission.

Dr. John Kolmer, the eminent bacteriologist at Temple University in Philadelphia who had been called to treat President Coolidge's dying son, also claimed to have made a polio vaccine. Kolmer was well known for a special syphilis blood test he had invented. His polio vaccine, Kolmer claimed, was made from live viruses altered so that they would produce immunity but no disease symptoms. The thousands of children injected with this vaccine developed no immunity at all; yet six of them died and three were paralyzed.

O'Connor and the commission learned a painful lesson from these two spectacular failures. A great deal of basic research was necessary before another attempt was made to produce a vaccine. And perhaps no vaccine would ever be discovered.

To review the research, a Virus Research Committee was organized. Dr. Thomas M. Rivers, a distinguished virologist, was appointed its chairman. Rivers, director of the Rockefeller Hospital since 1929, had written several books on virology. His achievements, however, stood in strong contrast to his appearance, for he had been born in rural Georgia, and he looked and sounded more like a redneck cracker than a scientist. A brusque, profane man, he had a pronounced knack for making enemies. Controversy and crisis swirled around him continuously until his death in 1962, since he was virtually the czar of polio research financed by the National Foundation for Infantile Paralysis.

And the amounts of money he had to dispense were enormous. From 1938 until 1945 no other research foundation was nearly so successful in generating cash. A large segment of the public believed that the National Foundation for Infantile Paralysis was a federal agency and that President Roosevelt's birthday was a national holiday. To perpetuate its success, the foundation spewed out torrents of encouraging publicity hinting at miracles just around the corner. More disasters were to occur when this publicity campaign suddenly backfired.

Virology was still a relatively primitive science when the foundation began pouring money into it. In the 1930s there were few full-time virologists. Most were bacteriologists who dabbled in virus research. The occasional hard facts that had been learned about virus behavior were almost lost among the ill-founded theories. And these theories were zealously defended by scientists who had built careers on them.

In fact, no one was even sure what a virus was. In some circles they were referred to as organisms; elsewhere this term was disparaged. "Organism" means "living thing," and viruses had never been shown to be alive. While some scientists considered them miniature bacteria, others maintained that they were a poisonous liquid—a point of view dating from the days of Jenner.

The existence of microbes smaller than the smallest bacteria had first been suggested in the 1890s by two scientists working independently—Martinus Beijerinck in Holland and Dmitri Ivanovski in Russia. While studying tobacco mosaic disease, a disorder of tobacco plants, both men had extracted a fluid from the leaves which was capable of inducing the disease in healthy plants. They forced the fluid through a porcelain filter able to trap the smallest known bacteria, yet it retained its infectiousness. Whatever had caused tobacco mosaic disease passed right through the filter, and thus was named a filterable virus. Pasteur had correctly guessed that rabies was caused by such a substance, and Dr. James Carroll had proved this for yellow fever by filtering the blood of a yellow fever victim and demonstrating that it was still infectious.

The filtering experiments triggered considerable controversy over whether a virus was solid or liquid. A partial resolution occurred in 1931 when William Elford, an English scientist, succeeded in making a filter with pores small enough to trap viruses. This work, indicating that viruses were particulate, was reinforced by the research of Wendell Stanley, an American biochemist. From a ton of tobacco leaves infected with tobacco mosaic disease Stanley laboriously isolated a tablespoonful of white crystalline powder. Though apparently no more alive than a spoonful of sugar, the powder could produce the disease when rubbed on a tobacco leaf and was considerably more infectious than the liquid extracts.

Stanley's results highlighted in bold relief the puzzling nature of viruses. They behaved like a living, infectious organism, yet they would crystallize like salt. They would only grow in living cells and not on the media used for bacteria. No drugs were effective against them. And by the late 1930s only three viral diseases—smallpox, rabies, and yellow fever—could be prevented with a vaccine.

That polio was also caused by a filterable virus had been determined in 1908 by Karl Landsteiner, also known for his discovery of human blood groups. Moreover, since polio appeared to be a disease of the nervous system, the assumption was made that the polio virus traveled to the central nervous system from the peripheral nerves in the same manner as rabies virus. This assumption fostered a bizarre effort to control the malady.

Convinced that the polio virus entered the body through the nose and traveled along the olfactory nerves to the brain, Edwin Schultz, a Stanford University microbiologist, postulated that polio could be prevented by spraying a substance into the nose that would block the entry of the virus. He selected zinc sulfate because of its ability to coagulate some proteins in the mucous membranes of the nasal passages. This material was dutifully sprayed into the noses of a few thousand people, mostly children, during a 1937 polio epidemic in Toronto. A few recipients permanently lost their sense of smell, but the epidemic was not curtailed.

Now there seemed to be no way to prevent polio. Spraying didn't work. The Brodie and Kolmer vaccines had proved a disaster. And there was no safe method of growing sufficient quantities of virus to make an effective vaccine. Since the time of Pasteur and Koch, scientists had been able to cultivate bacteria abundantly on artificial media. But polio virus could be readily grown only in the spinal cords of monkeys.

The disadvantage here was the one shared with the rabies vaccine. For there was no way to separate all the bits of spinal cord from the solution. When these bits were injected, a fatal inflammation of the brain called encephalitis sometimes resulted. Of course, to a person bitten by a mad animal, the risk of encephalitis was more acceptable than the alternative—inevitable, agonizing death from rabies. But the decision to employ the rabies vaccine was exceptionally difficult in so-called "bite and run" cases, where the biting animal may not have been rabid. And injecting millions of healthy children with polio vaccine-containing bits of spinal cord was totally unacceptable; yet the virus could be produced in no other medium.

The depressing certainty of this situation was reaffirmed by a set of careful experiments performed at the Rockefeller Institute in 1935 by Albert Sabin, a young researcher, and Peter Olitsky, a widely respected American virologist. Working with cultures of live cells taken from a stillborn embryo, Sabin and Olitsky attempted to grow polio virus in vitro. The experiments confirmed what was widely believed. The virus flourished in nerve cells but would not propagate in liver, kidney, skin, or any other cell variety. This finding appeared to quash any hopes for producing a safe polio vaccine.

Nonetheless, the National Foundation for Infantile Paralysis continued to raise funds for the support of polio research. Much of this support went for basic investigations in virology, because Thomas Rivers had convinced Basil O'Connor that this was the best approach. Some support also went for studies of the epidemiology and pathology of polio. The epidemiologists attempted to discover how the disease was spread, while the pathologists tried to determine its effect on tissue.

The epidemiologists and pathologists eventually helped to upset some of the most firmly entrenched errors in the understanding of polio. But the old ideas took a long time to die. In the 1930s, for example, it was discovered that large amounts of virus could be found in the stools of individuals with nonparalytic polio. This finding strongly suggested that the virus must proliferate in the cells of the intestine. Still, the dogma that declared polio solely a nervous-system disease persisted. The olfactory nerve port of entry was another durable error which lingered on despite pathological studies of Sabin and others that showed no olfactory nerve lesions in polio victims. An especially important blunder was the notion that polio virus did not enter the blood, for this implied that vaccine-induced antibodies would have little or no opportunity to counteract the virus. The few reports of *viremia*—that is, the presence of the virus in the blood-stream—were written off as examples of slovenly work.

Because many of the new findings were ignored by the orthodox, old-line virologists, the idea persisted that a safe polio vaccine could never be made since the virus would grow only in nervous tissue. And this put O'Connor and the foundation in a very tight spot. Despite the frightening increase in the number of polio cases, the "significant breakthroughs" the fund-raisers depended upon to encourage the public to give simply were not happening. Money was still being collected, but by the mid-1940s it was coming mainly from inveterate givers. These charitable souls habitually fished dimes from their pockets to fill the little containers adorned with the pathetic pictures of crippled children in heavy steel braces and wheelchairs.

But even this dribble of money, O'Connor knew, could cease if no discovery was made soon. He continued to announce "encouraging developments" to keep the contributions rolling in, ignoring strong letters of protest from indignant scientists. And he irritated many scientists even more when in 1946 he appointed Harry Weaver, a semi-retired virologist, as director of research. Most scientists believe themselves to be highly creative individuals and are loath to take directions from anybody.

Yet the appointment of Harry Weaver turned out to be one of the best moves made by the foundation. Weaver started the job with no preconceived notions about polio, and over a two-year period came to see what the old-school virologists could not or would not. Most striking, Weaver noted, was the evidence, some of it almost fifty years old, that polio was principally an intestinal infection and rarely a disease of the nervous system. In memos to Rivers and O'Connor he criticized the dogma that held polio to be a strictly neurologic illness. And in time the younger scientists were to prove Weaver correct —the first step to what O'Connor later called a "planned miracle."

Another step was soon made by three researchers at the Johns Hopkins School of Medicine—David Bodian, Isabel Morgan, and Howard Howe. Bodian and Howe had both been trained in anatomy. Isabel Morgan was the daughter of Thomas Hunt Morgan, the Nobel Prize-winning geneticist who had shown the relationship of genes to chromosomes in the fruit fly *Drosophila*. She had studied bacteriology and had worked at the Rockefeller Institute with Peter Olitsky.

Using inactivated virus suspensions, Bodian, Howe, and Morgan tried to immunize monkeys against polio. Their preparations were similar to those used by Maurice Brodie in his ill-fated 1935 effort. Some of the monkeys, they found, did develop immunity, while others did not. This work demonstrated that a killed virus vaccine might be of value—a virologic heresy at the time—and that there was apparently more than one type of polio virus. Subsequent studies suggested that there were three types, though Bodian, Howe, and Morgan could not be certain.

No one was shocked by the possible existence of more than a single type of polio virus. Other viral diseases—influenza, for example— were already known to be caused by a multiplicity of viruses. But the ineffectiveness of the Kolmer and Brodie vaccines was immediately understood; in addition to their sloppy preparation, they had contained only one type of virus. To be effective, a polio vaccine would have to immunize against all types.

But how many types of polio virus really existed? The answer to this question suddenly assumed crucial importance. Still, it was going to be difficult to obtain, since typing viruses is dull, tedious work with no particular appeal to anyone hungry for a Nobel Prize. Here Harry Weaver again proved his worth. He was certain that no older, established virologist would accept such an undignified, boring assignment. So he confined his search to young, unknown scientists. One who caught his eye was Jonas Salk, then studying flu virus at the University of Pittsburgh.

Salk, a Bronx academic prodigy, had entered the New York University Medical School in 1934, when he was only nineteen. Turned down for a Rockefeller research fellowship after graduation, he went to work for Dr. Thomas Francis at the University of Michigan, who was trying to make an influenza vaccine. The Army was financing this research, since flu epidemics were a threat to American combat troops. In 1942 Francis and Salk produced the first killed-virus vaccine effective against two types of influenza.

After a few years, however, professional jealousies began to sour the relationship between the two men. In 1947 the restless Salk, still only an assistant professor despite numerous publications, moved to the University of Pittsburgh Medical School. At the time, Pittsburgh was a decidedly second-rate institution. Salk was the only virologist, the only research worker, and the entire full-time faculty. His new job in the grimy, steel-mill-polluted city turned out to be much less attractive than his old one. Research funds were hard to come by; even a broken test tube was difficult to replace. But just as he was beginning to believe that he had reached the end of a road to nowhere, the offer from Harry Weaver came along. Salk grabbed it eagerly, although he had no experience with polio virus.

Besides his youthful lack of preconceived notions about polio, Salk presented to Weaver one other attractive aspect. At his disposal were the old contagious-disease wards of the university hospital, now emptied out by antibiotics. Large colonies of rhesus monkeys were required for the virus-typing studies, and the empty wards were an ideal place to keep them. After a minor row between the university and the foundation over who was to foot the bill for remodeling, preparation for the typing project began. In addition to Salk, Weaver recruited other typers in Kansas, Utah, and California. In 1949 the work finally got under way after more than a year of preparation.

Salk soon discovered, much to his dismay, that he was becoming little more than a glorified monkey-keeper. Much of his time was spent fussing over budgets, supply lists, and grant-renewal applications. The monkeys were expensive and difficult to maintain, but they were the only animals known to be susceptible to polio. Above all, they were vile-tempered, dangerous beasts, tricky to handle, capable of inflicting vicious bites. In 1935 a young researcher, Dr. William Brebner, was bitten by a monkey and died of a paralytic viral infection. Dr. Albert Sabin isolated the deadly organism and named it B virus after Brebner.

Even when safely caged, monkeys are still unpleasant to maintain. They are dirty animals with the annoying habit of defecating into their hands, then flinging the feces at passersby. Since most of the apes Salk received were imported from Southeast Asia, many sickened and died from respiratory disease just after arrival. Others had to be carefully nursed back to health—an expensive, time-consuming procedure.

Once the virus typing had finally begun, Salk became quickly bored. In order to expedite the process, he devised new, faster methods. This did not please Weaver or the foundation, since Salk and the other typers had been given to understand that they would stick to the prescribed methods and do precisely as they were told. Such restrictions became especially onerous when a dramatic new discovery indicated that a safe polio vaccine could be made.

In a laboratory of the Children's Hospital in Boston, three researchers—John Enders, Thomas Weller, and Frederick Robbins—succeeded in growing polio virus in cultures of nonnervous tissue. Enders' role in this stunning success was especially surprising because he had entered research much later in life than is usually the case. Born into an aristocratic Hartford family in 1897, he was the son of a banker and grandson of the president of the Aetna Insurance Company. Where Salk's early life had been marked by a desperate, intense upward struggle, Enders' was characterized by innocent dabbling in this field and that. He was a flying instructor in World War I, attended Yale, and began selling real estate after graduation. But when he learned how difficult houses were to sell, he decided to enter Harvard graduate school. He spent four leisurely years studying English literature and Celtic and Teutonic languages. He had almost finished his thesis in English literature when a roomate interested him in biology. Soon he had switched fields and obtained a Ph.D. in bacteriology.

Enders' polio discovery came as almost an accidental byproduct of his research on mumps. During World War II he had collaborated with another virologist to produce a killed-virus mumps vaccine of moderate, temporary effectiveness. Enders was troubled, however, that the virus had to be grown in the salivary glands of monkeys. In 1946 he moved to the Boston laboratory, where he was joined by Weller and Robbins. Together the three men worked to cultivate the recalcitrant mumps virus in tissue culture. By 1948 they had succeeded, first using a suspension of minced chick embryo in ox blood, then a variety of human embryonic tissues.

At the conclusion of the mumps experiments, Enders still had a few unused cultures remaining. Curious to see whether they could be used to grow polio virus, he added some "Lansing strain" virus from his freezer to preparations of human embryonic skin and muscle from a stillborn infant. The virus itself had come from an eighteen-year-old boy in Lansing, Michigan, who had died of polio. Much to everyone's surprise, it thrived in the cultures although they were not nervous tissue. The Lansing strain would even flourish in preparations of human foreskin obtained from circumcisions.

These results directly contradicted those that Sabin and Olitsky had obtained in 1935. They too had attempted to grow polio virus in human tissue culture but had been able to grow their strain in nervous tissue alone. For in an unlucky accident the two men had chosen a strain that behaved as it did only because it had been passed many times through the brains of laboratory animals. Sabin and Olitsky had not tried other types of virus because at the time no other types were known to exist.

On January 28, 1949, Enders, Weller, and Robbins published their findings in *Science*. Their article, "Cultivation of the Lansing Strain of Poliomyelitis Virus in Cultures of Various Human Embryonic Tissues," was relegated to a few obscure columns in the back pages. But five years later it was to result in the award of a Nobel Prize. Much to his credit, Enders told the Nobel Committee that he would not accept the prize unless it was shared with Weller and Robbins. Such behavior is uncommon in a scientist; it may be instructively compared with the blithe acceptance by Dr. Selman Waksman of the prize for streptomycin, which totally ignored the contributions of his two collaborators.

Now the race to produce a polio vaccine began in earnest. Each of the contenders was vying for the honor of becoming a modern Pasteur. Jonas Salk, Albert Sabin, and the group at Johns Hopkins were caught up in the excitement. So were two other virologists, Herald Cox and Hilary Koprowski; even before the announcement by Enders, these researchers in the employ of the Lederle Division of American Cyanimid were in hot pursuit of attenuated viruses for a vaccine.

The first effective polio preventive, however, did not result from the discovery of Enders, Weller, and Robbins. It was instead a by-product of the studies of blood proteins performed by another Harvard researcher, Dr. Edwin Cohn. Using special techniques to separate blood into its component fractions, Cohn was able to isolate one—gamma globulin—containing antibodies against polio and other infections. In 1951 the foundation approved a limited trial of gamma globulin prophylaxis in Provo, Utah. The results were quite encouraging but, as had been suspected, the immunity conferred was of short duration—about six weeks.

The public response was depressingly predictable. Everyone wanted gamma globulin injections for his children, and a grotesque black market could have resulted had O'Connor not immediately bought up every available drop. Anxious parents still attempted to pressure and bribe physicians to immunize their children. Emotions ran high, and many parents were terrified that because they did not have the right connections their child might contract paralytic polio.

Unfortunately, gamma globulin was costly and impossible to produce in sufficient quantity. It could only be obtained from donated human blood, and the human blood donor has never been an overabundant species. On the 1951 program alone the foundation spent more than fourteen million dollars. Figuring on the basis of six weeks' immunity from a shot, the cost came to an astounding $2.5 million per week. As rich and powerful as it was, the foundation was strained to the limit by such staggering expense. Consequently, increasing pressure was put on the scientists to come up with the long-awaited vaccine.

In 1952 a key discovery was made, strongly suggesting that an effective vaccine could be produced. While working independently, Dr. David Bodian at Johns Hopkins and Dr. Dorothy Horstman at Yale discovered polio virus in the blood of chimpanzees a few days after the animals had been fed the virus. Though the apes did not have paralytic polio at the time, many did become paralyzed later. This important finding of viremia at last brought down the hoary dogma that polio virus never entered the blood. The discovery of

Enders, Weller, and Robbins had previously shown that a safe vaccine, uncontaminated by bits of nervous tissue, was possible. Now the documentation of viremia indicated that the antibodies resulting from vaccination would have a chance to counteract the polio virus before it could do any damage. When taken with the gamma globulin trials, which demonstrated that blood antibodies could prevent paralytic polio, the new discovery eliminated any lingering doubts that a polio vaccine would work. Within days, the foundation's publicity mill had turned the studies of Bodian and Horstman into front-page news, appropriately labeled as another "encouraging development."

That the foundation finally determined to gamble on a vaccine devised by Salk was due almost solely to chance. Returning from the Second International Poliomyelitis Congress, held in Copenhagen in September 1951, Salk happened to meet Basil O'Connor aboard the *Queen Mary*. O'Connor was so impressed after this meeting that he cast the crucial vote to have the foundation sponsor a large field trial of the vaccine Salk was developing, a killed virus preparation made with formalin.

Naturally, not everyone was so favorably disposed to Salk's vaccine. Prominent among the skeptics was Enders, who believed the only way to make a vaccine was with live, attenuated virus. He was said to have referred to Salk's work as quackery.

To make his vaccine, Salk had chosen what he believed to be the most useful strains of each of the three types of polio virus. The strains had to grow well in tissue culture; additionally, they had to be virulent enough to induce antibody formation, yet be readily killed by formalin. For the type II and type III viruses, Salk had no difficulty in selecting a favorable strain. But no strain of the type I virus seemed very satisfactory. Salk finally settled on the Mahoney strain—a form of the virus with a very nasty reputation. For though the Mahoney family had survived its infection, all the children in the house next door had been paralyzed. Despite stern warnings and dire predictions of disaster from colleagues, Salk refused to relinquish the Mahoney virus. No matter how virulent a strain was in nature, he reasoned, once it was killed it was killed.

With the approval of the foundation, Salk decided to make the first human test of his vaccine on children who already had had paralytic polio. Such children would be immune to whatever type of virus had caused their illness, and this type was to be determined by blood analysis. An injection of vaccine made from the same type of virus could not do them any harm; but if the vaccine was effective, their blood antibody levels would rise. Quietly and cautiously arrangements were made to perform the study at the Watson Home for Crippled Children in Leetsdale, Pennsylvania, a Pittsburgh suburb. As Salk had predicted, his vaccine did raise the children's antibody levels. A similar effect was observed when the preparation was injected into children with no history of polio; moreover, they all stayed healthy.

No doubt Salk knew that his next step should have been the publication of these encouraging results in a professional journal. But it was January 1953, March of Dimes time again, and O'Connor could not resist telling the world about the "tremendous progress" made by the bright young man from Pittsburgh. To do this, he organized a splashy meeting at New York's Waldorf-Astoria Hotel, replete with medical dignitaries and, for some odd reason, an editor of the *Ladies' Home Journal*. Arrangements had been made to submit an article containing the contents of Salk's address to the *Journal of the American Medical Association*.

Unfortunately for Salk, the country and the press did not learn of his success from the prestigious AMA *Journal*—a proper place for a scientist to report his findings. Instead, the first announcement of the work appeared in a syndicated newspaper gossip column, "Broadway," written by Earl Wilson. Ordinarily Wilson confined himself to the activities and scandals of showfolk, and his column was the last place anyone would look to find news of a scientific breakthrough. But there it was, announced by a screaming headline, "New Polio Vaccine—Big Hopes Seen."

Now the worst possible things began to happen. Anxious parents frantically clamored for vaccine to protect their children. Virologists and other scientists denounced Salk as a publicity-seeker, a "glory hound." Salk tried to smooth things over with a national radio and television address made on the evening of March 26, 1953, but nothing could quiet the national uproar. The publicity-minded O'Connor and his flaks were squeezing every inch of fund-raising mileage out of the new hero from Pittsburgh. Fellow scientists reacted with revulsion to the spectacle that Salk seemed to be creating.

Most disturbing was Salk's uncertainty that he even had a vaccine, since it had been tested in only a small number of subjects. "Pittsburgh preparation" was the term that he used. But to everyone else it was the "Salk vaccine," and this it has remained.

Under enormous pressure, the foundation chose six companies—Cutter, Eli Lilly, Parke Davis, Pitman-Moore, Sharp & Dohme, and Wyeth—to produce the vaccine. In 1954 the first large-scale trial was held, but from the onset one crisis followed another. First a batch made by Parke Davis seemed to be contaminated with tuberculosis. Then monkeys at the National Institutes of Health Laboratory collapsed after receiving some Parke Davis vaccine. They were later found to have died from a common monkey ailment unrelated to polio, though not before the news had leaked to syndicated columnist Walter Winchell.

"Good evening, Mr. and Mrs. America, and all the ships at sea," Winchell said as he began his April 4, 1954, evening broadcast. "Attention everyone! In a few moments I will report on a new polio vaccine—it may be a killer!" After delivering a few sensational but unrelated bits of news in his dramatic staccato style, he announced that the United States Public Health Service had detected live polio virus in ten samples of the Salk vaccine. Winchell's informant was believed to be Paul de Kruif, who had been ignored by the pashas of polio since he had dredged up Maurice Brodie in 1935.

By the time of the broadcast, more than 7,500 people had received the vaccine without ill effect. The foundation answered Winchell's charges by pointing this out and adding that the finding of bad batches was a blessing, since it upheld the validity of the testing procedure. Still confident of the preparation's safety, the foundation approved an even larger trial, which began on April 26, 1954. When it was over, 441,131 children had been vaccinated. For comparison, another 201,229 children were injected with pink liquid that resembled the vaccine.

After almost a year of analysis, the results were presented on April 12, 1955. The vaccine had been found more than 90 per cent effective against types II and III polio virus, though it was not as good against type I. Most encouraging was the finding that it prevented 94 per cent of bulbar-spinal polio—the form that caused the dreaded respiratory paralysis and consigned its victims to life in an iron lung.

When the news reached the American public, the reaction was simply astounding. Men and women cried openly in the streets. "Thank you, Dr. Salk" signs appeared in store windows. Church bells rang and special prayer meetings were called. Such a massive outpouring of emotion over a medical product had never been seen before.

Salk was elevated to the status of a national hero. On the floor of Congress, one congressman proposed that a Jonas Salk dime be minted, and designs were actually submitted. Magazines hounded him for his biography. Hollywood studios wanted to make a movie of his life. President Eisenhower asked him to the White House to be awarded a presidential citation. Newspapers published editorials praising him for refusing royalties on his "discovery."

But the scientific community was far less appreciative, for Salk, in fact, had not discovered anything except how best to annoy fellow scientists. The television address, the newspaper and magazine spreads, the press conferences were too much. In 1954 the Nobel Committee totally ignored him, ostensibly because he had done no original work. He was neither the first nor the only researcher to have made a formalin inactivated vaccine. And a major disaster soon cooled the public ardor.

On April 24, 1955, a case of paralytic polio occurred in a recently vaccinated child. No one was very alarmed, since the child was assumed to have contracted the disease shortly before the injection had been given. This had occurred more than once during the field trials and was expected to occur again. But on April 26 Robert Dyer of the California State Health Department phoned the National Institutes of Health to report that six children had developed polio a week to ten days after the first shot. Dyer was especially alarmed because all the children had become paralyzed in the vaccinated arm and because in each case the vaccine had come from a batch prepared by the Cutter Company.

Cutter was immediately ordered to stop distributing its preparation. But in the meantime more cases occurred in Idaho children receiving the Cutter vaccine. Worse, the disease had spread to contacts of the vaccinated children. Public health authorities, fearing the possibility of a vaccine-induced epidemic, distributed emergency supplies of gamma globulin. In the end, there were about 250 vaccine-associated cases, 150 of which were partially or totally paralyzed. Eleven died.

Both Salk and Cutter came under intense criticism as a result of this fiasco. Virologists lambasted Salk for his use of the dangerous Mahoney strain. Congressmen delivered angry addresses about the slipshod vaccine inspections; in fact, the vaccine had not been inspected at all. Though the Mahoney strain was subsequently removed, no one was ever certain why the disaster had occurred. During the field trials and in Salk's own laboratory, an enormous amount of perfectly adequate vaccine had previously been made. "The vaccine is safe," Salk had told reporters, "and you can't get safer than safe."

Despite Salk's optimism, the Cutter disaster was one link in a chain of events that would eventually banish the Salk vaccine from the United States. For while the field trials had been going on, two rival live-virus vaccines were being perfected—one in the Lederle Pharmaceutical laboratories, the other in the laboratory of virologist Albert Sabin.

Lederle had committed itself to production of a live attenuated virus vaccine in 1946, three years before Enders had announced that the polio virus could be grown in nonnervous-tissue culture. The two scientists assigned to the project, Hilary Koprowski and Herald Cox, had an enviable virologic track record, having previously developed for Lederle a lucrative rabies vaccine that was much better than Pasteur's. It was grown in duck eggs rather than rabbit spinal cords, and so did not cause encephalitis.

By 1951, after four years' work, the Lederle researchers had produced an attenuated type II virus. Buoyed by their success, Cox and Koprowski turned to the development of an attenuated type I virus. But the previous triumph with rabies vaccine proved to be their undoing. They had been so successful growing rabies virus in eggs that they were determined to produce their attenuated type I polio virus in the same manner. Albert Sabin, their competitor, did not make this mistake.

Cox spent three disappointing years injecting one type I strain after another into hens' eggs. Finally in 1954 he had an attenuated preparation composed of the ill-behaved Mahoney strain and another, the Sickle strain. But by then Salk was inoculating thousands of children. When the Lederle vaccine was ready for mass testing of its type I and type II strains in 1956, this was no longer possible in the United States. Most of the population had already been immunized with the Salk vaccine.

After an extensive search, Koprowski was able to arrange with the government of Northern Ireland for a limited field trial there. The Irish had not yet adopted the Salk vaccine, and antibodies were believed to be low. The trials, which were a model of clinical testing, quickly revealed that the attenuated viruses reverted to virulence in the stools of immunized individuals. Both the excreted type I and type II virus were capable of producing paralysis when introduced into the brains of monkeys.

No record of the undoubtedly frenzied Lederle board meeting that resulted from this potential calamity has ever been made public. But Koprowski, the strongest company supporter of the project, resigned from Lederle shortly thereafter. He later became director of the Wistar Institute in Philadelphia. Though it had already lost several million dollars in the project, Lederle allowed Cox to continue his efforts to produce a safe live-virus vaccine. But it was Albert Sabin, with the support of the National Foundation for Infantile Paralysis, who ultimately succeeded.

Sabin had begun work on an attenuated-virus vaccine at about the same time that Salk was awarded a grant for his killed-virus vaccine. Almost immediately Sabin decided to grow the virus in kidney-tissue culture—something of an irony, since it had been he and Olitsky who in 1935 had shown, they believed, that polio virus would propagate only in nervous tissue. Despite this mistake, Sabin had risen to become one of the country's leading virologists.

Like Salk, Sabin had been born poor. His early years were spent in an impoverished Russian ghetto. In 1921, at the age of fifteen, he emigrated with his parents to the United States and went to live with relatives in Paterson, New Jersey, where he attended high school. A dentist uncle agreed to finance Sabin's education if he would study dentistry, and for two years he did so. But then, he told a *Times* reporter years later, he read de Kruif's *Microbe Hunters* and was inspired to enter medical research. The irate uncle cut off his support, and Sabin was forced to work his way through his last two years of medical school at New York University.

This formative period of hardship did nothing to help mold his personality into an especially pleasing one. "Sabin," recalled a former colleague, "couldn't say yes without antagonizing someone."

"I never did any research under anyone," Sabin once told an interviewer. "You underline that. I always developed my own ideas." Indeed, he was so successful that he was invited to join the Rockefeller Institute in 1935, only four years after his medical school graduation. His early work greatly strengthened the notion that polio is really an intestinal disease. He also showed that a widely accepted polio skin test was, in fact, worthless. In 1939 he moved to Children's Hospital in Cincinnati.

By 1956, after a few false starts, Sabin had made a vaccine containing all three types of live, attenuated polio virus. Following tradition, he and his family took the first experimental human doses. Salk, it should be mentioned, had done this also. The next subjects were two hundred convicts in federal penitentiaries. Everyone who received the vaccine developed blood antibodies to all three virus types, and no one came down with paralytic polio.

But Sabin, like Cox and Koprowski, had a problem finding a suitable location for mass testing of his vaccine. A trial in the United States would have proved nothing. Nevertheless, Sabin soon arranged for mass testing in what turned out to be an ideal spot—the Soviet Union. The powerful government control over all aspects of Russian life, he knew, was sure to make for a perfectly executed field trial.

Yet why should the Russian government submit its subjects to such an experiment?

"Well, I'll tell you," Sabin explained to an interviewer; "before 1954, they used to say in the Soviet Union, 'Under our socialist health system, we don't get polio the way they do in capitalist countries.' Then, all of a sudden, their turn came. They began to have big epidemics—18,000–20,000 paralytic cases a year—and they were frightened. I knew it, and I invited them to Cincinnati to see my experiments."

The Sabin vaccine proved to be very effective—possibly even more so than Salk's. And it had an additional advantage: It was easier and less painful to administer, being swallowed rather than injected. By 1960 it had been licensed for manufacture in the United States and quickly consigned Salk's vaccine to oblivion, both here and abroad. Salk quite naturally never accepted this situation with equanimity.

"I'm a mad dog, I'm enraged," he later fumed. "I see all this irrationality, a sea of it, an ocean of it. . . . Sabin . . . Sabin is unbelievable!"

Sabin reciprocated in kind. "Look, let's get one thing straight," he once snapped in answer to a question about his erstwhile competitor. "If you want to continue talking with me, you will never, ever mention that man's name again."

Still, despite the haggling over which vaccine was superior, both shared a frightening defect not discovered until 1960. In that year,

Dr. B. E. Eddy found that extracts of the monkey kidney-cell cultures used to grow polio virus induced malignant tumors in newborn hamsters. Two other virologists, Dr. B. H. Sweet and Dr. M. R. Hilleman, soon were able to pinpoint a virus—SV 40—as the cancer-causing agent. By this time, millions of children had received polio vaccine contaminated with SV 40 virus, and there was no way of knowing whether medical science had conquered polio at the risk of provoking a new affliction.

In a particular bind was one National Institutes of Health official, Joseph Smadel, who had played a prominent role in judging the efficacy of both vaccines. Publicly, Smadel had claimed that the preparations were as safe as grade-A pasteurized milk. But privately his sentiments were quite different, as a colleague, Dr. Anthony Morris, recalled: "Joe Smadel couldn't believe it. It was a frightening thing. It's still frightening. That information was held up for two years before it was made public, and I saw Joe Smadel fall apart under the pressure of keeping it quiet."

The contaminating virus has since been removed from polio vaccine. And the scientific consensus today is that those who were infected with it probably will not suffer any harm. Yet no one can be certain that the tumor-producing SV 40 virus will not eventually cause a cancer epidemic in the millions who received the first batches of polio vaccine. Should such an epidemic occur, it will be yet another part of the legacy of the publicity-hungry National Foundation for Infantile Paralysis and the competing scientists racing to eradicate polio.

CHAPTER NINE

Rays

In spite of the great advances made in the science of healing throughout the nineteenth century, the physician in 1895 shared one handicap with the author of the Ebers Papyrus. Both had only their sense of touch to gain information about the location of normal and diseased structures within a patient's body. But in the final decade of the century, two important discoveries—X rays and radioactivity—were to make possible for the first time the diagnosis of diseased deep structures in a living patient. In addition, the two modalities were soon found to be useful in the therapy of cancer, a disorder that had previously been successfully treated only by surgery.

X rays and radioactivity also marked another milestone in medicine, being discoveries made in the science of physics. Until the beginning of this century, physics had been used to explain many natural phenomena—gravitation, electromagnetism, light—but had had little application to medicine. Chemistry had played an infinitely greater role in understanding biologic phenomena—respiration, digestion, the composition of living tissues. Since 1900, however, physics has become increasingly more important to medicine and biology; indeed, a special branch, biophysics, now concerns itself solely with these disciplines. Biophysics may be said to have begun with X rays and radioactivity.

X Rays

On Friday, November 8, 1895, Wilhelm Conrad Roentgen, a German physicist, made the simple observation that catapulted him from semiobscurity to international fame. While experimenting with an electrical discharge tube connected to an induction coil, he noted that a nearby screen coated with barium platinocyanide was caused to fluoresce. Roentgen's famous observation was remarkable not only because of its tremendous implications but because it had been made using simple, standard equipment that was readily available to almost anyone. So easy to perform was the experiment that Roentgen said nothing about it to colleagues until he was able to publish and establish his claim to priority. He was doubtless fearful that another physicist with the same apparatus might repeat the procedure and publish first. Indeed, his fears were well grounded, for induction coils and electrical discharge tubes had been standard equipment in physics laboratories for quite some time.

The induction coil had resulted from the discovery that magnetism could be used to produce electricity, made independently in 1831 by Michael Faraday in England and Joseph Henry in the United States. Both men showed in a number of ways that an electric current is induced in a conductor when the conductor and the magnetic field are in motion with respect to each other. This fundamental discovery, basic to the science of electromagnetism, was employed in the construction of the first electric machines—the magnetoelectric generator, the electric telegraph, and the induction coil.

A presently half-forgotten device, the induction coil evolved in a relatively mature form in the short period between 1836 and 1838. Most of the basic work was performed independently by an American physician and an Irish priest. Ultimately, it played a vital part in three epoch-making discoveries: X rays, radio waves, and the electron—the first subatomic particle to be identified. It also led to the modern transformer, and before electronic devices it was one of the only sources of high-voltage current.

In its most fundamental form, the induction coil is nothing more than an iron bar wrapped with two insulated windings. A few turns of heavy wire conduct the primary current; many more turns of finer wire conduct the induced secondary current. A burst of high-voltage current is induced in the secondary winding by a collapsing magnetic field when the primary current is interrupted.

Nicholas J. Callan, a priest and physics teacher in County Kildare, Ireland, built the first simple induction coil in 1836 to study the phenomenon of secondary currents described by Faraday. Callan's coil was a horseshoe bar of iron wound with 1,300 feet of thin iron wire and 50 feet of thick copper wire. A small battery furnished the current, which was interrupted by a hand-cranked contact-breaker. Surprisingly, Faraday, who was a wizard at constructing simple but elegant gadgets to study electricity, did not invent the induction coil himself.

Over the next few months, Callan continued to make improvements in his invention. By 1837 he had published a description of "the most powerful electromagnet yet constructed" in a British technical journal, *The Annals of Electricity*. The new coil contained an iron bar more than two inches thick and thirteen feet long, wound with two insulated coils more than ten times the length of the first ones. Employing this device, Callan succeeded in generating a small arc light between carbon rods connected to the secondary terminals. Moreover, he somehow managed to survive using himself as a human voltmeter to estimate the secondary potential, though the high voltage was said to have electrocuted a chicken.

One persistent problem in Callan's coils was the need for continuous hand cranking of the contact-breaker. This tedious chore was finally obviated in the coils designed by Charles Grafton Page, a Salem physician. Before his death in 1868 Page had devised a variety of automatic contact-breakers. One of the most effective had an iron hammer that moved back and forth like the hammer in an electric doorbell. Page also built coils that worked with only a single winding —the first autotransformers.

The induction coil was quickly recognized as an excellent means of generating high voltages, both for laboratory experiments and for supposedly medicinal purposes. Daniel Davis, a Boston instrument-maker, was one of the first to manufacture and sell Page induction coils, as well as magneto machines made by Page. These devices were snapped up by academies with courses in natural philosophy, ostensibly for illustrating basic principles; more often, however, teachers liked to use the showy electrical arcs to startle bored students. Would-be healers also bought the coils for the reputed revitalizing effects of the severe electric shocks.

Throughout the mid-nineteenth century, improvements in the coil continued to be made. Heinrich Daniel Ruhmkorff, a German instrument-maker living in Paris, was one particularly successful innovator. To produce more powerful coils, Ruhmkorff used glass insulation between the primary and secondary windings. End plates to support the windings and pillars to carry the high-voltage secondary leads were also insulated with glass. Ruhmkorff coils had longer secondary windings than Page coils and also extra insulation between the layers. As a result, they could generate electrical arcs from two to three inches long. Ruhmkorff became so famous for his coils that in 1864 he was awarded a ten-thousand-dollar prize by Napoleon III for the most significant application of electrical science.

But even Ruhmkorff had not been able to overcome one major difficulty—the violent sparking between the vibrating hammer contacts that rapidly ruined the contact surfaces. This dilemma was finally solved by Armand Fizeau, the distinguished French physicist who had succeeded in accurately measuring the speed of light by means of a spinning toothed wheel. In 1853 Fizeau proposed connecting a capacitor across the hammer contacts. Made of two sheets of tinfoil interleaved with insulating layers, the capacitor was able to absorb the surges of current induced in the primary winding as the circuit was broken. In 1856 Jean Foucault, a colleague of Fizeau who demonstrated the earth's rotation by means of a pendulum, designed a sophisticated mercury contact-breaker as a substitute for the crude vibrating hammer.

Ruhmkorff coils with these two modifications were soon to be found in almost every school, college, and scientific laboratory. Besides making the snapping electric arcs, lecturers liked to awe their classes with spectacular showers of sparks produced by discharging the coil through tinfoil spangles in a glass tube. Other popular experiments: melting fine iron wire, burning wood along a track containing nitric acid as a conductor, igniting paper, setting off gunpowder, and generating a glow discharge in an evacuated tube or globe. The coils became fashionable and profitable, too, in the offices of respectable physicians, who applied the "Faradic currents" to the body with various styles of electrodes.

Showmen and traveling lecturers also became fond of the induction coil when they discovered how greatly audiences enjoyed watching shocks administered to volunteers. This dubious form of amusement was soon carried over to penny arcades in the form of an induction coil encased in a fancy box with metal handles, activated by a regulator and a coin slot.

But the induction coil was to lead to a great medical breakthrough —the discovery of X rays—as a result of serious scientific investigation into the conduction of electricity through gases. The first studies of this phenomenon were carried out by Michael Faraday and John P. Gassiot in England, and by Julius Plücker and William Hittorf in Germany. Initially, they used crude glass bowls and relied on balky friction machines—conductive leather pads rubbed on the surface of a rotating glass plate—or batteries connected in series for high voltage. Soon, however, the induction coil became the standard high-voltage source, and a much-improved tube was substituted for the glass bowl. The first of these tubes had been constructed in the mid-1850s by Heinrich Geissler, a skilled instrument-maker who worked with Plücker at the University of Bonn. Geissler's tubes had sealed-in electrodes and were connected to highly efficient mercury vacuum pumps.

Over the next two decades many properties of ionized gases and cathode rays, as they were later called, were discovered by Plücker and Hittorf, and by William Crookes in England. Crookes became internationally famous in 1879 after demonstrating the characteristics of low-pressure electrical discharges. He used a specially designed tube, soon to be named a Crookes tube, and it was this device connected to a Ruhmkorff coil that produced the X rays observed by Roentgen.

On the Friday in 1895 that he made his famous discovery, the fifty-year-old Roentgen seemed destined to remain an obscure scientist. The majority of physicists do their most innovative work in their twenties and thirties; indeed, many become quite depressed if they have done nothing outstanding by the time they are forty, because this is usually the end of the road, creatively speaking.

But then Roentgen never appeared to anybody as a man about to set the world ablaze. He had been born March 27, 1845, in the little German town of Lennep in the Ruhr valley, the son of a textile worker. His early schooling was erratic, and what little he did get was cut short by an unfortunate incident. When the prank of a schoolmate got him into trouble, he refused to name the offender and so was summarily expelled. Without the final examinations and degree necessary for admission to higher education, Roentgen's academic career appeared finished.

After a few years of study without credit, however, at the University of Utrecht, Roentgen was allowed to matriculate at the Zurich Polytechnic School, where in 1868 he was awarded a mechanical engineering degree. Ironically, though he was later to become one of the most famous physicists of his age, he never took a basic college course in physics.

Roentgen continued as a student at the Zurich Polytechnic, and in 1869 was awarded a Ph.D. with a thesis entitled *Studies on Gases*. But his early misfortune continued to plague him. When his preceptor, August Kundt, was offered a chair in physics at the University of Würzburg, he brought Roentgen along as his assistant. Here Roentgen discovered to his dismay that he could not be appointed privatdocent, the first rung in the academic ladder, because of the diploma that had been denied him when he was expelled from preparatory school. In addition to this cruel disappointment, he was forced to contend with poor laboratories and meager equipment.

The situation improved in 1872, when Kundt moved again to the Kaiser Wilhelm University at Strassburg. Roentgen came along, this time as privatdocent, and from here his career continued to progress. Over the next few years he published numerous articles, now largely forgotten, in prominent physical journals. The result was an appointment as professor of physics and director of the new physical institute at the University of Würzburg. It was at Würzburg that the famous experiment was performed and the observation made.

In fact, the first person to notice the glowing screen was not Roentgen but his laboratory assistant, or *Diener* in German. In later years this led to many humiliating jibes. Roentgen was particularly exasperated by some accounts which actually accused him of stealing his *Diener*'s discovery.

Certainly nothing could be further from the truth, since Roentgen was wholly responsible for appreciating the significance of what had occurred. The Crookes tube had been completely covered with black cardboard and the fluorescent screen was across the room. Almost immediately Roentgen realized that he was witnessing the effect of a new kind of ray, one that traveled in a straight line, penetrated opaque substances, and was not deflected by a magnetic field as were the cathode rays. He named his new rays with the mathematician's symbol for the unknown—X. On the same day he made the first medical application of his discovery—an X-ray photograph of his wife's hand.

Roentgen adamantly refused to patent any part of his discovery and indignantly rejected all commercial offers, believing that his professorial income would provide him with lifelong financial security. Alas, all his savings and even his 1901 Nobel honorarium were wiped out by the calamitous postwar German inflation. When he died in 1923, he had been reduced to a tired, despondent, lonely man and was virtually penniless.

But at least he was lucky enough not to have been maimed by his discovery. Less fortunate were many of the early radiologists. Unaware of the hazards, they continually exposed themselves to radiation while X-raying patients. Many were subsequently forced to endure a lifetime of mutilating operations to remove cancerous growths from their hands.

The safety and reliability of the early X-ray machines were greatly increased with the development of the hot cathode or Coolidge tube. The original tubes, very much like Roentgen's, contained a certain amount of gas, necessary to permit the passage of current. As the gas was gradually "used up," more gas had to be let in. Even after the introduction of automatic gas regulating devices, the X-ray output of these tubes was highly unpredictable.

The problem was solved by William David Coolidge, an engineer at the General Electric Research Laboratories in Schenectady, New York. Coolidge devised a method for producing ductile tungsten tube filaments and designed a high-vacuum tube to contain them. Both the penetrating power and the intensity of the X-ray beam from the Coolidge tube could be reliably controlled. The inauguration of this tube in 1913 ushered in what came to be called the golden age of radiology. Results could now be duplicated with an accuracy never dreamed of in the days of gas tubes.

Another significant advance came with the introduction of contrast agents. Though very dense structures, such as bones, can be distinguished from soft tissue on an ordinary X-ray film, the many soft-tissue structures—kidneys, liver, digestive tract—cannot be distinctly identified. To visualize the soft tissue structures, investigators began to administer a number of contrast agents—substances that will produce a distinct outline of the structure in which they are contained.

One of the first to employ a contrast agent was Walter Bradford Cannon, a Harvard physiologist. Recognizing that X rays could be used to study digestion, Cannon set up an apparatus in which animals could be observed. In early experiments, he watched a button pass down the esophagus of a dog and an opaque bolus slide through the neck of a goose. But soon he began to employ liquids, among them bismuth subnitrate, bismuth oxychloride, and barium sulfate. He mixed these tasteless salts of heavy metals with the animals' natural food and then would watch for hours at a time the passage of his "contrast meals" through the digestive tract, shadowed on a glowing fluoroscopic screen. Cats, he soon discovered, were especially well suited for such investigations.

During the course of his experiments, Cannon was able to observe the movements of the alimentary tract without disturbing the animal to any degree. "By use of X rays," he reported in 1898, "the rate of passage of food through the oesophagus, the speed of gastric peristalsis and rhythm, the oscillating contractions of the small intestine, the peculiar anti-peristalsis of the large intestine, the rapidity of discharge of gastric contents into the duodenum, the time required for material to be carried to the colon, and all the influences external and internal that affect these processes, can be observed continuously for as long a time as the animal remains in a state of peace and contentment. . . ."

One of Cannon's most interesting findings was the effect of changes in the emotional state on digestion. Anxiety, distress, or rage, he noted, were accompanied by complete cessation of stomach movements. Further investigation was devoted to the autonomic nervous system, which controls these movements. In 1915 he published a classic book on his work, *Bodily Changes in Pain, Hunger, Fear, and Rage.* He also coined the term *homeostasis* to designate the steady state achieved by all the co-ordinated physiologic processes.

During his many experiments, Cannon had the foresight to partially shield his X-ray apparatus with lead sheets. But, like the other early X-ray workers, he was not aware of the dangerous nature of the useful new tool. As a consequence, he suffered intensely during the last years of his life from an acute dermatitis attributed to the effects of radiation.

To the contrast agents employed by Cannon a number of others were soon added. These contained iodine and could be administered to make the gall bladder or the urinary tract visible on X-ray film. The internal architecture of the living heart, however, remained invisible to radiologists until the dramatic discovery of heart catheterization by Werner Forssmann, a German surgeon.

Until the late 1920s, inability to observe the valves and chambers of the heart frustrated any attempts at cardiac surgery. For how could mechanical disorders, such as damaged valves, be rectified if they could not be assessed before the operation? Only then would the surgeon know where to cut.

As a student, Forssmann had seen old drawings in French physiology books of a thick tube inserted through the jugular vein into the heart of a horse. He felt that the same thing might be done to a man if the tube could be put into a vein at the elbow. In the summer of 1929, shortly after graduation from medical school, he determined to try the procedure on himself.

Because his supervisor had sternly forbidden his carrying out such an apparently crazy experiment, Forssmann made his first attempt secretly one afternoon. After injecting a small amount of anesthetic into his arm, he proceeded to intubate his heart with a long tube called a catheter, ordinarily used in the urinary tract.

"When my anesthetic began to take effect," he wrote, "I quickly made an incision in my skin, inserted a Dechamps aneurysm needle under the vein, opened it and pushed the catheter about a foot inside. I packed it with gauze and laid a sterile splint over it." But as he was making an X-ray picture, a colleague named Peter Romeis burst in and became angry when he saw what was happening.

"You idiot," Romeis screamed, "what the hell are you doing?"

Romeis was so desperate, Forssmann wrote, that "he almost tried to pull the catheter out of my arm. I had to give him a few kicks on the shin to calm him down."

With a mirror placed in front of the fluoroscopic screen, Forssmann was able to see what he had accomplished: "As I'd expected, the catheter had reached the head of the humerus. Romeis wanted me to stop at this point and remove it. But I wouldn't hear of it. I pushed the catheter in further, almost to the two-foot mark. Now the mirror showed the catheter inside the heart, with its tip in the right ventricle, just as I'd envisioned it. I had some X-rays taken as documentary evidence."

When these amazing films were published in a leading medical journal, the *Klinische Wochenschrift,* in 1929, they caused an immediate sensation. A newspaper, the *Nachtausgabe,* reprinted them, and Forssmann was besieged by reporters. One magazine, the *Berliner*

Illustrierte, even offered him a thousand marks for the rights to the pictures.

But the effect on other physicians was far less favorable. Ernst Unger, an eminent surgeon, accused Forssmann of attempting to steal priority for the discovery. Unger wrote to the surgeon Ferdinand Sauerbruch, Forssmann's new supervisor, who determined to squelch the young upstart quickly.

"Very late one evening," Forssmann recalled, "I was summoned to Sauerbruch. He'd prepared himself, or been prepared, very well; on his desk lay the *Klinische Wochenschrift,* the *Nachtausgabe,* and a letter from Unger. He sat behind them and looked at me for some time in silence. Then, 'This is an absolute disgrace!' He slammed his palm down repeatedly on the *Nachtausgabe.* 'And then this!' He handed me Professor Unger's letter. 'I'm obliged to read that one of my doctors has attempted to steal priority from an eminent surgeon and disregarded the elementary rules of scientific priority. . . . As for your work, what's it all supposed to mean?'"

Patiently, Forssmann tried to explain the implications of his experiments and added that one day he hoped they would help him meet the qualifications for a lectureship.

"You might lecture in a circus about your little tricks," Sauerbruch retorted angrily, "but never in a respectable German university! What do you really want to be, an internist or a surgeon?"

"I'm afraid I can't answer that yet, Herr *Geheimrat.* I've only been qualified for nine months and I don't yet know which I'm more suited to," Forssmann answered carefully.

"There we have it! The real Forssmann who can't make up his mind about anything! *Every inch an internist!* A true surgeon thinks of only one thing: *operate! operate! operate!"*

By this time Forssmann was furious, too, and he replied with an expression that has a scatological double meaning in German: "Herr *Geheimrat* Sauerbruch, there are hunters and there are shooters."

This was too much for Sauerbruch. His eyes flashed behind his thick spectacles, and he screamed, "Get out! Leave my department immediately!"

Undaunted, Forssmann obtained another position and continued his experiments. To see whether iodine-containing contrast media were harmful in high concentrations, he injected these substances directly into the hearts of dogs through a catheter. The animals survived unscathed, though the same material was lethal for rabbits. Nonetheless, Forssmann then determined to attempt the crucial experiment: opacification of the chambers of a human heart—his own.

"People often ask me if I wasn't afraid," he recalled. ". . . I must confess that I was slightly nervous . . . and it took me a few days to make up my mind to carry out the injections. For while it was possible to remove the catheter immediately if anything went wrong, there was no way of removing the contrast media once they'd been injected."

As Forssmann had guessed, the contrast solution he prepared was indeed nontoxic. "I felt no effect when I injected it," he wrote, "only afterward a slight haziness, a disturbance of consciousness and vision which lasted only a second or two, presumably as the concentrated fluid first flowed through the brain."

Unfortunately, the X-ray films taken were not very clear because the equipment at his disposal was not powerful enough. But he had proved that contrast media could be safely injected into the human heart. A few years later two American physicians, André F. Cournand and Dickinson W. Richards, Jr., perfected Forssmann's technique, making possible the dramatic heart operations that are familiar today. In 1956 all three men were awarded the Nobel Prize in Medicine.

Within the very near future, however, X-ray pictures of the interior of the heart may be possible without contrast media and catheters. These images will be produced with the computerized axial tomographic (C.A.T.) scanner, a new device already being used to make visible previously hidden human organs, such as the pancreas.

The principle of the C.A.T. scanner was discovered by J. Radon, an Austrian mathematician, in 1917. Radon was the first to prove that a two- or three-dimensional image can be reconstructed uniquely from the infinite set of all its projections. Ordinary tomographic images or "slices" through the body have been made since 1922 by using an X-ray source which moves in one direction while a piece of X-ray film moves simultaneously in the other direction. If the patient lies in between, one thin plane slice of his body will appear on the film.

Radon's tomographic method, considerably more complex, could only be applied in practice with the arrival of the modern computer. The first C.A.T. scanners were built by a British engineer, Godfrey Hounsfield, and used in the United States at the Mayo Clinic in

1973. Though the present generation of these machines is not yet "fast" enough to stop the motion of the heart, no doubt future generations will be.

Radioactivity

Two months after Roentgen's report of X rays, Henri Becquerel, a French scientist, published the first paper describing natural radioactivity. Becquerel had noted the phenomenon after leaving some uranium salt crystals on top of a photographic plate. A few hours later, the plate had been blackened though it had not been struck by light. An Englishman, Silvanus P. Thompson, had made the same observation simultaneously, but Becquerel published first—in the *Comptes Rendus,* February 24, 1896. During the rest of the year, Becquerel wrote six more papers on the subject, and two the following year. His interest in the phenomenon then began to dwindle, but by this time a young physicist, Marie Curie, had decided to investigate natural radioactivity further as part of her doctoral thesis.

Marie Curie, née Sklodowska, had been born November 7, 1867, in a small Warsaw apartment. Her father, Jozef Sklodowska, an impecunious Polish pedagogue, had little money to spend on the education of his five children. When Marie went off to Paris to study science at the Sorbonne, she lived barely at the subsistence level. Yet she still retained a strong sense of middle-class morality and indignantly refused an offer to move in with Pierre Curie, a gifted young physicist friend. Her refusal seems to have been well considered, for shortly thereafter the free-thinking Pierre married her.

Pierre and his elder brother Jacques had already made a name for themselves while studying the generation of electric charges in heated crystals. The two soon discovered that mechanical stresses on crystals would also generate electric charges, a phenomenon later to be named *piezoelectricity,* from the Greek *piezein,* "to press." Using their discovery, they succeeded in building a highly sensitive device, the quartz piezoelectrometer, for detecting small electric currents. This electrometer proved extremely useful in the subsequent measurement of radioactivity.

Marie and Pierre Curie isolated their first new radioactive element from the ore pitchblende. On June 6, 1898, the laboratory notes, underlined with Marie's thin-nibbed pen, record that the substance was 150 times more active than uranium. "If the existence of this new metal is confirmed," the Curies wrote in their paper on the discovery, "we propose to call it polonium from the name of the country of origin of one of us."

At the time, Marie Curie believed that polonium was to be her great discovery, but she and Pierre presently identified an even more radioactive material in pitchblende. Their initial measurements revealed this substance to be an astounding nine hundred times more radioactive than uranium. In mid-December 1898 they decided to name the element radium; yet they needed a much larger quantity than they had on hand in order to characterize it fully.

The principal European source of pitchblende was the St. Joachimsthal mine in Bohemia, a part of the Austrian Empire. The Austrian government worked this mine with considerable profit, as the uranium it contained was quite valuable. The Curies knew, however, that once the recoverable uranium had been extracted, the residual material was discarded as waste. Through the Vienna Academy of Science, they succeeded in persuading the Austrian government to intercede with the Joachimsthal mine authorities on their behalf. The aim of their research, Marie emphasized, was purely scientific and would benefit the Joachimsthal factory, since it could sell or otherwise exploit the valueless residues. With their own funds, the Curies were quickly able to obtain several tons of dirt-cheap residue, which the Bohemians were doubtless overjoyed to see removed from their dumping ground at a small profit. Little did anyone suspect how precious the radium extract would eventually prove to be.

In the early months of 1899 the first heavy sacks of extracted pitchblende were dumped in the yard of the School of Physics and Chemistry near the Curies' laboratory. To the eye, the mixture appeared to be composed of nothing more than brown dust and pine needles. But tests for radioactivity revealed that the material was "hotter" than the unrefined pitchblende from which it had come.

By March 28, 1902, according to Marie Curie's laboratory notes, one-tenth gram of radium chloride had been isolated from the yardful of sacks. On that day Marie had recorded the estimation of molecular weight that had required over two years' work—Ra = 225.93. The element was so radioactive that it was beyond the range of the delicate charged electrometer. Even today, three quarters of a century since they were first contaminated by the fingers of Marie and Pierre, the laboratory notebooks are still considered dangerous to handle.

Like the early X-ray workers, the Curies had no notion of the hazards they were facing. So beneficial to mankind did Marie believe radium to be that as the end of her life approached she refused to accept the fact that the element was harmful as well. Yet the warnings were certainly dramatic. Shortly after they had begun working with radium, the Curies had noticed the early signs of what was later recognized as radiation sickness—weakness, severe fatigue, rheumatic pains. Pierre's fingers became so sore that he could scarcely hold a pen; permanent scars were left on his skin.

Pierre continued to sicken, and his severe malaise may have been indirectly responsible for his untimely death. On April 19, 1906, the forty-seven-year-old physicist was struck by a large cart while crossing a street.

"He was walking quickly, his umbrella was up in his hand and he literally threw himself on my left side horse," the driver told reporters. Pierre's head was smashed into fifteen or sixteen pieces by the rear wheel, and a large crowd gathered to watch the blood mix with the rain in the gutter.

Marie's life entered a long period of decline after her husband's death. When she had recovered from her grief, she entered into an affair with a young physicist, Paul Langevin. A married man with four children, Langevin maintained a small *pied-à-terre* in Paris, and here the trysts took place. On November 4, 1911, *Le Journal* learned of the situation, and it became a sensation.

"A Story of Love. Mme. Curie and Professor Langevin," blared the headlines. Under a striking photograph of *"pécheuse"* Marie, the titillating story began, "The fire of radium had lit a flame in the heart of a scientist, and the scientist's wife and children were now in tears."

By the next day, every newspaper in Paris carried the story, and news of the scandal had passed by wireless to tabloids in London, Berlin, New York, and San Francisco. There was even speculation that Pierre had been driven to suicide when he learned that his wife was carrying on with a former pupil. White with rage, Langevin challenged the newspaperman who had broken the story to a duel. The event, complete with pistols and seconds, took place at the Parc-des-Princes bicycle stadium. Fortunately, at the count of *trois,* neither man would fire at the other. Greatly relieved, the seconds removed their hats, wiped their brows, and cautiously took the pistols from the contestants. The weapons were discharged into the air, the doctors closed their bags, and the reporters put away their notebooks. The farce had come to an end; Langevin's marriage and the well-publicized affair soon ended also.

The situation had been too much for Marie. On December 29, 1911, she was carried off by stretcher to a sanatorium. Sympathetic with her plight, the Nobel Committee awarded her the prize in chemistry; she had previously shared the 1903 physics prize with her husband and Henri Becquerel.

In the years following her recovery, Marie worked for increased application of her discovery. The usefulness of radium in the treatment of cancer, especially of the cervix and uterus, was ascertained, and a Curie Institute in Paris was founded. During the First World War, Marie and her daughter Irène instructed the Allied soldiers in radiology. Marie suffered greatly during her last years from radiation burns to her hands. In 1934 she died of leukemia, another sequela of radiation exposure.

CHAPTER TEN

Diabetes Mellitus and Insulin

One day, many millions of years ago, one of the numerous individual living cells floating in the waters of our primitive earth decided—for better or worse—to stop going its own separate way and join together with another cell. Thus were the multicellular organisms first formed.

From the beginning, advantages accrued to this merger of talents. A single cell no longer had to serve as a jack of all trades. Digestion, defense, respiration, locomotion, and other functions could be taken over by specialists; single-cell general practitioners were relegated to the evolutionary backwaters. But as more complex organisms began to develop, one big problem had to be overcome.

Cells had to tell each other what was going on and what to do. If this could not be accomplished, activities in various parts of the organism could not be co-ordinated, and existence would be constantly threatened. In animals, the evolution of the nervous system filled the need for some forms of co-ordination, especially in movement.

Equally as important as physical co-ordination was molecular co-ordination, the synchronization and control of metabolic activities of the many distinct forms of cells. Nerves, however, were not chosen by nature for this task; instead, a swift and unique messenger was selected—a chemical messenger.

As far back as the time of Hippocrates, physicians suspected that chemicals within the body were important for proper function. The venerable theory of the four humors (blood, phlegm, yellow bile, and black bile) formed the basis of a medical doctrine lasting for centuries, eventually falling into disrepute only after a mound of scientific evidence had proved it to be worthless. In the mid-nineteenth century Claude Bernard, a French physiologist, demonstrated that the liver releases glucose into the blood, which in turn carries this common form of sugar to the tissues of the body. Once again the idea that the blood carries important substances from one part of the body to another became widespread, based this time on solid scientific evidence. Bernard referred to his discovery as an internal secretion.

By the late 1800s certain glandular structures without secretory ducts were seen as having some type of secretory function. In 1849 a substance made in the testis was demonstrated to cause a cock's comb to grow. This observation was not widely recognized, however, and another fifty years passed before such glandular structures as the thyroid were accepted as releasing into the blood chemical messengers which have specific effects on distant tissues.

In June 1905 the term *hormone* was first used by E. H. Starling, a British physiologist. Starling found that substances secreted by the stomach incited the production of pancreatic digestive enzymes and hydrochloric acid. These first-known hormones were named after a Greek word meaning "I excite," and were seen to have the following properties:

a) secreted by living cells in trace amounts from within the organism
b) transported by the blood to a specific site of action
c) not used as a source of energy
d) act to regulate and not initiate chemical reactions

Hormones quickly became familiar to scientists after Starling's work. By 1915 Dr. E. C. Kendall had investigated thyroxine, the thyroid hormone. But world attention was not caught by the search for hormones until 1921. On July 30 one of the great medical discoveries of the twentieth century was made.

That night was a hot, humid, and uncomfortable one in Toronto, the Canadian metropolis that spreads northward from the shores of Lake Ontario. In a laboratory under the eaves of the medical building on the campus of the University of Toronto two young investigators, Dr. Frederick Banting, a twenty-nine-year-old surgeon, and Charles Best, a twenty-one-year-old medical student, fought off drowsiness in the stifling air. At 12:15 A.M. they aroused their patient—a diabetic dog. Blood and urine samples were taken, and five cubic centimeters of a pancreatic extract from a vial floating in a bowl of ice was injected.

When the routine tests were done, Banting and Best realized they had made a momentous find. There was no sugar in the dog's urine, and the animal's blood sugar had been lowered by half. The two men looked at one another incredulously for a moment, then shouted with triumph and danced about for joy. They had isolated the hormone which had eluded generations of scientists: insulin.

The discovery of insulin revolutionized the treatment of diabetes—a medical problem for more than two thousand years. The most prominent symptom of the disease, excessive urination (polyuria), was recorded in the Ebers Papyrus from ancient Egypt before the year 30 B.C.; the accompanying emaciation and lack of pain were also definitely noted by Egyptian physicians.

In the first century A.D. Aretaeus the Cappadocian coined the name *diabetes* from the Greek word for "passing through." Aretaeus left this vivid description: "Diabetes is a wonderful affection, not very frequent among men, being a melting down of the flesh and limbs into urine. Its cause is of a cold and humid nature, as in dropsy. The course is the common one, namely the kidneys and bladder; for the patients never stop making water, but the flow is incessant, as if from the opening of aqueducts. The nature of the disease, then, is chronic, and it takes a long period to form; but the patient is short-lived, if the constitution of the disease be completely established; for the melting is rapid, the death speedy. Moreover, life is disgusting and painful; thirst unquenchable; excessive drinking, which, however, is disproportionate to the large quantity of urine, for more urine is passed; and one cannot stop them either from drinking or making water. Or if for a time they abstain from drinking, their mouths become parched and their bodies dry; the viscera seem as if scorched up; they are affected with nausea, restlessness, and a burning thirst; and at no distant term they expire."

Diabetes was also known in the Far East. The Chinese physician Tchang Tchong-king described the disorder in A.D. 200 as the disease of thirst; another writer of A.D. 600 identified excessive hunger, excessive thirst, and excessive urination as a triad of symptoms that almost certainly indicated diabetes. In the sixth century Aetius of Amida left his imprint on treatment by recommending bleeding, narcotics, and agents that produced vomiting; these methods continued to be used for many years to come. Narcotics in diabetes, though, were probably not a new development. Another physician, Archigenes, had recorded their use in the second century.

In A.D. 1000 Avicenna, an Arab physician, first described diabetic gangrene. Some translations also credit Avicenna with the first hypothesis of a nervous origin for diabetes and the first theory of the role of the liver. But Avicenna does not appear to have influenced later thinking to any extent. Any beneficial results from his prescribed treatment of fenugreek, lupin, and wormseed were probably due to the nauseating effects of these compounds.

The association between sugar and diabetes was initially recognized in the sixth century A.D. An Indian physician, Susruta, wrote of diabetes as the honey urine disease. In addition, Susruta noted the high frequency of skin infections and tuberculosis as complications of diabetes.

Unfortunately, Susruta's writings were unknown to early European doctors. In the sixteenth century Paracelsus evaporated urine from diabetic patients, recovering what he called a salt. A hundred years later Dr. Thomas Willis added the tasting of urine to the time-honored practice of "urine gazing." Discovering diabetic urine to be "wonderfully sweet, as if imbued with honey or sugar," Willis wondered why salt should have such a flavor.

The answer to Willis's question came in 1775 with the beginnings of modern chemistry. In that year Matthew Dobson recognized that the sweet material in diabetic urine was indeed sugar, and by 1815 Michel Chevreul had identified the sugar as glucose, the same as that in grapes. Doctors were finally spared taste-testing urine for glucose in 1841, when Karl Trommer, a German chemist, developed a qualitative test for sugar. A quantitative test—still used in elementary chemistry classes—was perfected nine years later by another German, Hermann von Fehling.

The discovery of chemical tests for glucose led to the first understanding of the ways in which the body uses this form of sugar. In 1848 Claude Bernard demonstrated glucose in the liver veins of dogs fed either sugar or protein. His isolation of the starch glycogen from the liver led Bernard to postulate that the body can synthesize its own chemicals and that the elevated blood sugar of diabetics results from overproduction of sugar by the liver. By puncturing a chamber of the brain, Bernard was able to cause an elevation in blood sugar, thus exhibiting a cerebral role in glucose metabolism. Bernard also showed that there was a kidney threshold for glucose; only when blood sugar rose above this level would sugar begin to "spill" into the urine. The recognition of this threshold allowed Bernard to postulate that patients had glycosuria—sugar in the urine—when the blood sugar was too high or the kidney threshold too low. The latter condition, called renal glycosuria, was later identified in humans by a German physician, Georg Klemperer. Dr. Bernard Naunyn, another German physician, was the first to recognize that glycosuria caused by high blood sugar is diagnostic of diabetes.

When abnormal glucose metabolism was recognized as the primary abnormality in diabetes, the disease was given its last name, *mellitus,* from a Greek word meaning "honeyed" or "sweet." And this sweetness brought about the first rational approach to treatment —diet.

The first dietary regimen for diabetes was devised by Thomas Willis in the seventeenth century, and the practice of undernutrition set was to be followed in diabetic diets for the next two hundred years. Willis believed that salts were being lost in the urine and advised lime water replacement. Antimony and opium concoctions were also prescribed, remaining in vogue for over a hundred years after Willis's death in 1675.

One famous modification of the Willis diet was made by Dr. John Rollo. Rollo restricted his patients to animal foods—unappetizing, nauseating old meats, fat, and milk—to which lime water, laxatives, and opium were added. Erroneously believing diabetes to be a primary and peculiar affliction of the stomach, Rollo aimed to upset digestion—a feat his regimen accomplished admirably.

A much more rational diet was devised by the nineteenth-century French physician Apollinaire Bouchardat. Using the newly devised Trommer's test for urinary sugar, Bouchardat required that each diabetic patient analyze his urine daily. Discriminating application of exercise was introduced for the first time and was shown to increase carbohydrate tolerance. "You shall earn your bread by the sweat of your brow," was the famous admonition to each new case. Bouchardat was responsible for the introduction of gluten bread, and he often eliminated bread and milk from the diet entirely to reduce carbohydrate, substituting fat and alcohol. Starch in vegetables was diminished by discarding the water in which they were cooked. "Eat the least possible," Bouchardat advised.

Modifications of the Bouchardat diet and a pioneering observation were made by Arnoldo Cantani, a nineteenth-century Italian physician. Unlike Bouchardat, Cantani customarily allowed his patients the maximum number of calories that would not produce urinary sugar. But the importance of preventing the appearance of sugar in the urine was paramount, and Draconian measures were taken to enforce this goal. Patients would be locked in their rooms if need be to implement dietary restrictions. Cantani's greatest contribution to the knowledge of diabetes came from his research interest. Performing microscopic studies of various organs from thousands of cases, Cantani noted that fatty changes and shrinking were more frequently found in the pancreas of a diabetic than of a nondiabetic. But nineteenth-century researchers seem to have disregarded this important finding until an experimental case of diabetes in an animal was accidentally produced a few years later.

In 1898 Dr. Bernard Naunyn published the authoritative nineteenth-century study of the disease, *Der Diabetes Mellitus*. In this monumental work Naunyn described the studies of diabetic coma made by him and his close associates. The urine of comatose patients was found to contain, after distillation, large quantities of the compound diacetic acid. The blood was filled with high concentrations of a group of chemical compounds called ketones and markedly changed in one physical characteristic, carbon dioxide combining power.

Normal blood can be induced to combine with large quantities of the gas carbon dioxide, a byproduct of cellular metabolism. Naunyn and his associates observed that the carbon dioxide combining power of blood from patients in diabetic coma was quite low; the body was overproducing acid, exhausting its normal alkaline reserves. Coma and death were the end results. To describe this condition, Naunyn introduced the term *acidosis*.

Throughout his long life Naunyn continued to study diabetes and remained the dominant figure in this field until after the turn of the century. Recognizing that all foods contributed ultimately to the sugar in the blood, this researcher emphasized that the total caloric intake of the diabetic's diet should be closely regulated—not just the carbohydrate intake, as earlier physicians had believed.

The experimentally documented observation that severe undernutrition could prolong the life of a diabetic was made by an American physician, Dr. Frederick M. Allen. Until insulin, this dietary restriction was the best hope a diabetic had for a longer life.

Allen showed that weight loss due to caloric restriction was beneficial to overweight diabetics, whereas an uncontrolled diet accompanied by weight loss and urinary sugar was detrimental. Continued appearance of sugar in the urine indicated progression of the diabetes. Even some very severe diabetics could be kept alive, Allen found, if a normal blood sugar could be maintained with rigid dietary control. Allen's principles of control were adopted by Dr. Elliott P. Joslin, founder of the famed Joslin Diabetes Foundation and Joslin Clinic in Boston. Yet the great breakthrough in diabetes treatment was to come not from the refinements in diet but from the basic physiological studies of glucose metabolism begun in the latter half of the nineteenth century.

In 1867 a German pathologist, Dr. Paul Langerhans, reported his results of an exhaustive microscopic study of the anatomy of the pancreas. Langerhans observed that most of the pancreatic tissue was made up of groups of cells, called acinar cells, centered around a duct; Dr. Claude Bernard had already shown that these cells produce the enzymes capable of digesting food. Langerhans also noted that scattered throughout the pancreas were small, distinct clusters of totally different cells bunched in formations that he called islets.

The significance of this now-celebrated discovery was not appreciated by Langerhans, who went to his grave not realizing what he had found. Then in 1893 Dr. Gustave E. Laguesse, a French physiologist, made the remarkable guess that these structures were endocrine glands. In honor of their discoverer, Laguesse named them the islets of Langerhans.

Laguesse's striking conjecture was based on evidence obtained from a new experimental procedure—pancreatectomy, or the removal of the pancreas. In 1889, after performing a pancreatectomy on a dog, two German physiologists, Dr. Joseph von Mering and Dr. Oskar Minkowski, discovered that they had produced a diabetic animal. Other scientists might not have noticed such a finding, but this famous accident, like many others throughout the history of science, was observed by a prepared mind. For Minkowski, it seems, had previously made extensive studies of the physiology of diabetes and had only lately begun to work on the pancreas. Grasping the significance of what had occurred, the two men immediately confirmed their work and reported it.

Now attention was riveted on the pancreas—particularly the islets of Langerhans—as the most likely source of some internal secretion vital to normal glucose metabolism. Shortly after the turn of the century the observed pancreatic changes in diabetes led Dr. E. L. Opie and Dr. L. V. Sobolev to advance independently the theory that diabetes resulted from diseased changes within the islet tissue, and that the islets were needed for the control of carbohydrate metabolism, while the digestive-enzyme-producing acinar cells were not. Dr. Robert Bensley made further microscopic studies of the fine structure of the islet cells, and in 1907 M. L. Lane, one of Bensley's students, described the distinguishing microscopic features of the two types of human islet cells, alpha and beta. Today we know that only the beta cells are capable of insulin production.

Yet in spite of these rapid advances in knowledge and prodigious efforts by numerous scientists, no one was able to extract the mysterious substance insulin from a pancreas, and no one knew why. For thirty years failure was piled upon failure. Sobolev had suggested in 1900 that tying off the pancreatic duct might isolate the islets of Langerhans anatomically so that their chemical properties could be studied; in this way a rational form of therapy for diabetes would be possible. Had Sobolev acted upon his own suggestion, he might have changed the history of medicine by making himself the discoverer of insulin.

By 1921 most of the world's foremost authorities on carbohydrate metabolism were certain that no internal pancreatic secretion controlled the utilization of glucose. A few researchers, however, continued to entertain the notion that such a substance did, indeed, exist. One of these was Dr. Moses Barron of the University of Minnesota. In the October 1920 issue of *Surgery, Gynecology, and Obstetrics,* Dr. Barron published an article commenting on the work of Minkowski and Mering. Had their experiments been carried further, Barron suggested, a substance secreted by the pancreas might have been found; and, perhaps, such a substance might alleviate diabetes. This article inspired the discovery of insulin by Frederick Banting and Charles Best.

Dr. Banting was born November 14, 1891, near the small country town of Alliston, some sixty miles north of Toronto. He grew up on his father's farm, received a local education, and sought to oblige his parents by studying for the ministry. This proved the wrong choice, however, and he switched to the study of medicine at the University of Toronto. After a medical education hurried by the advent of World War I, Banting, fresh from medical school, was shipped overseas as an officer of the Fifteenth General Hospital Unit of the Canadian Army Medical Corps. In France the young physician had abundant opportunities to gain the surgical experience later used in his research. He was wounded only six weeks before the end of the war.

Banting returned to Canada following his recuperation and joined the orthopedic department of the Toronto Hospital for Sick Children. After completion of his surgical training he accepted an instructorship in orthopedic surgery at the University of Western Ontario, in London. In addition, he opened a modest office as an orthopedic surgeon and awaited patients. Few came. In his considerable free time, Banting began to frequent the medical library, reading one journal after another. While preparing a lecture on the functions of the pancreas, he came across Dr. Barron's article in *Surgery, Gynecology, and Obstetrics*.

That night Banting reviewed the article in his mind, and thought back to his childhood when he had watched a bright, active girl playmate wither and die of diabetes. After many tosses and turns, the sleepless physician found a notebook and scribbled the following: "Ligate the pancreatic ducts of dogs. Wait six to eight weeks for degeneration. Remove the residue and extract."

During the next few days, Banting discussed his nocturnal inspiration with faculty associates and received some encouragement. Everyone knew, however, that the facilities of the University of Western Ontario were inadequate for carrying out the proposed experimental work. Knowledgeable colleagues suggested consultation with Professor John James Rickard Macleod, chairman of the physiology department of the University of Toronto, regarded by many as the world's outstanding authority on carbohydrate metabolism.

Two trips to Toronto in a battered car netted Banting only a polite but firm turndown by Professor Macleod. The erudite physiologist cited literature on the pancreas over the centuries—and volunteered his own formidable opinion—that the organ secreted no such chemical as Banting hoped to find. And, Macleod pointed out none too tactfully, predecessors in pancreatic investigation, such as Minkowski and Mering, had the advantage of extensive research training, of which Banting had none.

Perhaps Macleod cannot really be faulted for his lack of confidence in Banting's idea. Under the best of circumstances, medical research is an uncertain endeavor. For every investigator who makes a significant discovery, a thousand more equally competent scientists wander down promising paths leading nowhere and waste precious, scarce research funds in the process.

But Banting was persistent; and when, on his third visit, he came armed with pleas for consideration voiced by a number of Professor Macleod's own associates, Macleod gave ground and agreed that Banting might have some test animals and take over a temporarily unused laboratory for eight weeks during the summer. Recognizing that Banting had little knowledge of the chemical aspects of the problem, Macleod inquired of his final-year class in physiology and biochemistry whether a student would like to help a young surgeon with some experiments relative to diabetes. Charles Best, who was about to graduate and had no fixed plans for the summer, volunteered. Macleod then left on vacation for his native Scotland.

Best was born of Canadian parents in 1899, in the village of West Pembroke, a small settlement on the United States side of the Maine–New Brunswick border. As soon as he was old enough to accompany his physician father, Charles Best was assisting at surgical operations frequently performed on kitchen tables in northern Maine and in New Brunswick. Like Banting, the young Best had already seen death from diabetes close up. A favorite aunt, Anna Best, trained as a nurse at the Massachusetts General Hospital in Boston, had died of the disease while under the care of Elliott Joslin, the Boston diabetes specialist.

His education at the University of Toronto interrupted by World War I, Best returned after the armistice to physiology and biochemistry courses, writing his final examinations only the day before he and Banting began work. Banting had hardly enough money to support himself and was unable to pay anything to his new assistant.

On the morning of May 17, 1921, the young men began their project. After a study of the discouraging literature on the subject, they put the assigned laboratory in order. It was a small, dirty room under the eaves of the medical building that had not been used for some time; the walls and floor had to be thoroughly scrubbed, and since there were no assistants, Banting and Best had to do the job themselves.

After the test dogs had been situated in the animal room next door, Banting, with Best assisting, began the surgical procedures. The pancreatic ducts of several of the animals were tied off. Then Best, with Banting assisting, carried out numerous chemical tests on blood and urine.

Banting's theory was that other investigators had failed because the pancreatic enzymes capable of digesting food had destroyed the extracted glucose-lowering substance. If no attempt were made at extraction until the pancreas was tied off and given six weeks to degenerate, the islets of Langerhans containing the substance would remain free and clear.

When six weeks of the eight weeks allotted by Professor Macleod had passed, the abdomens of the test animals were reopened. To the dismay of the two investigators, the catgut sutures used to tie off the pancreatic ducts had broken. All the pancreatic tissue was still healthy.

With six weeks' time lost, Banting and Best repeated the tying off of the ducts with a more stable suture material. The allotted research time passed, but fortunately Macleod remained in Scotland. Toward the end of July another experimental dog was made diabetic by removal of its pancreas. Again the test dogs were examined.

Now the results were more favorable. The cells that produce digestive enzymes had deteriorated, while the islets of Langerhans remained intact. The altered pancreatic tissue was removed from the animals and ground up with sand in a chilled mortar. This material was suspended in a saline-containing liquid called Ringer's solution and filtered to remove loose sand and ground tissue. The temperatures were kept as low as possible to prevent any digestive activity by remaining enzymes. This was the material which, when injected, successfully lowered the blood sugar of the diabetic dog on the night of July 30, 1921.

Now Banting and Best began work day and night to confirm their results. Test animals became infected; there was no measure of the strength of their pancreatic extract; yet the substance was undeniably effective, since diabetic animals died when it was withdrawn. By September the two researchers had repeated their work sufficiently to be certain that the extract would prevent the death of diabetic dogs. They named it *isletin* after the islets of Langerhans from which it was extracted. Later, Banting was persuaded to adopt *insulin,* a more easily pronounced term.

When Macleod returned from Scotland and was first presented

with the experimental data, he was unconvinced. How could two young, inexperienced workers discover anything that had been over-looked by the best European physiologists for thirty years? The professor asked for repetition of the experiments, and these repetitions produced a wide rift and bitterness between Macleod and Banting.

By late 1921 Macleod was convinced that a diabetes-controlling substance had been isolated. Between Christmas 1921 and February 1922 newspapers picked up the story, making the discovery front-page news throughout the world. Appeals flooded into the University of Toronto for insulin to save the lives of countless diabetics, though only very small quantities of unstandardized hormone were available. And insulin had not yet been tried on a human being.

Banting and Best first injected themselves with their extract to test for safety. Then in February 1922 word came that a twelve-year-old boy in the Toronto General Hospital, Leonard Thompson, was near death from diabetes. Insulin made from beef pancreas was adminis-tered to the child by his physician, Dr. Walter Campbell, with as-tounding results: The boy made steady recovery and was able to live with the aid of insulin for several years until his death in a motorcy-cle accident.

Early in 1922 manufacture and sale of insulin was begun by Eli Lilly & Company. Banting and Best refused to profit directly from their discovery. Only after repeated requests did they apply for pat-ents on insulin, with the understanding that these would be accepted and administered by the University of Toronto.

Throughout his lifetime Banting remained bitter at Macleod, who, he felt, had tried to take credit for the discovery from him and Best. As Best later remarked, there soon developed considerable pressure "exerted by senior and more experienced investigators, who had not invested an hour's work before the discovery, but who were now more than anxious to appropriate a share of it." Ironically, the 1923 Nobel Prize in Medicine was awarded jointly to Banting and Mac-leod. When Banting announced that he would split his share of the prize money with Best, Macleod, not to be outdone, immediately de-clared that he would share his with Dr. J. B. Collip, whom he had appointed after the discovery to assist with chemical procedures.

Unfortunately, the work of one other diabetes researcher, Nicolas Constantin Paulesco, was completely ignored during this un-gentlemanly fracas. A Rumanian physiologist, Paulesco had first be-come interested in diabetes while working as a student with Mering and Minkowski. In 1916 he discovered that an aqueous pancreatic extract injected into a diabetic dog gave immediate, though temporary, relief of symptoms. His research was interrupted by the First World War, but he was able to resume in 1920. In August 1921 he published his results, which proved convincingly that he had isolated insulin and had used it to lower the blood sugar in both normal and diabetic dogs. Yet by a regrettable oversight the Nobel Committee overlooked Paulesco, as it had Best, when making its 1923 award—engendering considerable resentment in Rumania. Years later, Professor Tiselius, head of the Nobel Institute, acknowledged that Paulesco was as deserving of a share of the prize as were Macleod and Banting.

The epoch-making insulin extraction was Banting's first and only piece of research; perhaps any subsequent project would have been anticlimactic. He opened a surgical office in Toronto, while Best was appointed director of insulin production at Connaught Laboratories. In 1941 Banting's life was cut tragically short: After re-entering the army, he was killed in a military plane crash during a storm over Newfoundland.

The first insulin used on a human being was known in its purified form as "regular insulin." Initially, the unmodified extract was employed, but chemists soon discovered that the compound could be crystallized by adding zinc, thus making purification easier. Injection of regular insulin leads to a rapid lowering of blood sugar. When given one-half hour to two hours before a meal, the action will parallel the absorption of glucose from food. So regular insulin is valuable for the treatment of diabetic patients in coma, since rapid action is essential.

The drawback to regular insulin in the routine management of diabetics is obvious: The quick, unsustained effect requires multiple injections throughout the day. As early as 1923 attempts were made to prolong the blood-sugar-lowering activity of regular insulin. Relatively insoluble in an acid solution, regular insulin is most easily dissolved and taken up in the slightly alkaline body fluids. Researchers recognized this phenomenon and began searching for an insulin preparation that would dissolve slowly in the body. They found that the compound protamine, when mixed with insulin, was only poorly soluble in body fluids and therefore was absorbed slowly. Injection of this preparation beneath the skin makes available a depot supply from which insulin can gradually be withdrawn. In fasting diabetics, a single injection of protamine zinc insulin has maintained low-blood-sugar levels for as long as forty-eight to seventy-two hours.

Assessing and increasing the strength of insulin preparations was another task confronting researchers. A reference standard was initially established by measuring the blood-glucose-lowering effect of individual insulin solutions on rabbits. This crude biological method was later supplanted by an exact measurement when chemists were able to prepare solid insulin in a dry, stable crystalline form. The first commercially available insulin solutions contained only three insulin units per cubic centimeter. Today, five hundred units of insulin have been compressed into the same volume of fluid, allowing more convenient administration to diabetic patients.

Shortly after its discovery, insulin was recognized as a polypeptide (small protein). In 1955 Dr. F. Sanger and his colleagues were able to determine the exact chemical structure of insulin, and in 1963 three groups of researchers simultaneously achieved a total chemical synthesis of material with insulin activity. Unfortunately, synthetic insulin cannot be prepared in sufficient quantity to treat the diabetic population. Perhaps in the future, scientists may be able to transplant the human insulin gene into bacteria in laboratory cultures, permitting the bacteria to produce large amounts of pure human insulin.

Epilogue

What next?

The possibilities are endless. For example, Dr. Robert White of the Brain Research Laboratory in Cleveland's Metropolitan General Hospital is now successfully transplanting the brains of rhesus monkeys—a feat believed impossible only a few years ago.

Other researchers are using drugs to extend the mammalian life span. Dr. George Cotzias of New York's Sloan-Kettering Institute has found that the lives of both humans and rats can be significantly prolonged by administration of the drug L-dopa. Such an agent may eventually prove to be the long-sought fountain of youth.

But there are also potential dangers ahead. While smallpox now appears to have been totally eradicated from the earth, samples of the virus have been stored at the federal government's Center for Disease Control in Atlanta, and in a few other laboratories as well. What if a terrorist should get hold of one of these samples? He could threaten to wipe out most of the world's population with an epidemic if his demands were not met.

Another equally frightening prospect: the destruction of antibiotic effectiveness. Animal raisers routinely add antibiotics to animal feeds, since these drugs have been found to be powerful growth stimulants. But the U. S. Food and Drug Administration and many scientists fear that this practice will eventually produce medicine-resistant bacteria capable of causing untreatable diseases in humans. Yet the animal-raisers refuse to stop, since their concern is only profit, not potential dangers to humanity.

These and other applications of the science of healing give pause for thought. The great discoveries have in the past been applied almost solely for the benefit of mankind. We can only hope that the future will bring more of the same.

Bibliography

Chapter One

Bender, George A. *Great Moments in Medicine.* Detroit: Northwood Institute Press, 1971.

Bronowski, Jacob. *The Ascent of Man.* Boston: Little, Brown & Company, 1973.

Duveen, Dennis. "Lavoisier." *Scientific American,* May 1956.

Foster, M. *Lectures on the History of Physiology.* Cambridge: Cambridge University Press, 1901.

Fulton, John F. "The Place of William Withering in Scientific Medicine." *Journal of the History of Medicine and Allied Sciences,* 8:1–15 (1953).

Goodman, Louis, and Alfred Gilman. *The Pharmacological Basis of Therapeutics,* 3rd ed. New York: Macmillan Company, 1965.

Hall, Marie Boas. "Robert Boyle." *Scientific American,* August 1967.

Keynes, Geoffrey. "William Harvey." *Encyclopaedia Britannica.* Chicago, 1974.

Kilgour, Frederick. "William Harvey." *Scientific American,* June 1952.

Leake, Chauncey D. "The Development of Knowledge About the Cardiovascular System." In *The Historical Development of Physiological Thought,* ed. C. Brooks. New York: Hafner Publishing Company, 1959.

Majno, Guido. *The Healing Hand.* Cambridge, Mass.: Harvard University Press, 1975.

Marks, Geoffrey, and William K. Beatty. *The Medical Garden*. New York: Charles Scribner's Sons, 1971.

Mettler, Cecilia C. *History of Medicine*. Philadelphia: The Blakiston Company, 1947.

Palmer, R. R., and Joel Colton. *A History of the Modern World*. New York: Alfred A. Knopf, 1965.

Robinson, Victor. *The Story of Medicine*. New York: Medical Life Press, 1931.

Talbott, John H. *A Biographical History of Medicine*. New York: Grune & Stratton, 1970.

Wilson, Mitchell. "Priestley." *Scientific American*, October 1954.

Chapter Two

Asimov, Isaac. *A Short History of Biology*. New York: American Museum Science Books, 1964.

Bragg, W. L. "X-ray Crystallography." *Scientific American*, July 1968.

Bronowski, Jacob. *The Ascent of Man*. Boston: Little, Brown & Company, 1973.

Mirsky, Alfred E. "The Discovery of DNA." *Scientific American*, June 1968.

Posner, E. "The Enigmatic Mendel." *Bulletin of the History of Medicine*, 40:430–40 (1966).

Sayre, Anne. *Rosalind Franklin and DNA*. New York: W. W. Norton, 1975.

Sturtevant, A. H. *A History of Genetics*. New York: Harper & Row, 1965.

Sullivan, Navin. *The Message of the Genes*. New York: Basic Books, 1967.

"Tinkering with Life." *Time*, April 18, 1977, pp. 32–45.

Watson, James D. *The Double Helix*. New York: Atheneum Publishers, 1968.

Chapter Three

Atkinson, D. T. *Magic, Myth and Medicine*. New York: World Publishing Company, 1956.

Burlingham, Bo. "Politics Under the Palms." *Esquire,* February 1977, pp. 47–125.

Fülöp-Miller, René. *Triumph over Pain.* Trans. Eden and Cedar Paul. New York: The Literary Guild of America, Inc., 1938.

Goodman, Louis, and Alfred Gilman. *The Pharmacological Basis of Therapeutics,* 3rd ed. New York: Macmillan Company, 1965.

Karen, Robert. "Dr. LaVerne's Magic Gas." *New York,* July 4, 1977, pp. 43–49.

MacQuitty, Betty. *Victory over Pain.* New York: Taplinger Publishing Company, Inc., 1971.

Robinson, Victor. *Victory over Pain.* London: Sigma Books, Ltd., 1947.

Talbott, John H. *A Biographical History of Medicine.* New York: Grune & Stratton, Inc., 1970.

Wyckoff, James. *Franz Anton Mesmer.* Englewood Cliffs, N.J.: Prentice-Hall, 1975.

Young, Hugh Hampton. *A Surgeon's Autobiography.* New York: Harcourt, Brace and Company, 1940.

Chapter Four

Bender, George A. *Great Moments in Medicine.* Detroit: Northwood Institute Press, 1966.

Burget, G. E. "Lazzaro Spallanzani." *Annals of Medical History,* 6:177–84 (1924).

Dawson, Percy M. "Semmelweis, An Interpretation." *Annals of Medical History,* 6:258–79 (1924).

de Kruif, Paul. *Microbe Hunters.* New York: Harcourt, Brace and Company, 1926.

Edgar, Irving I. "Ignatz Philipp Semmelweis." *Annals of Medical History,* 1:74–96 (1939).

"Found: The Philly Killer, Perhaps." *Time,* January 31, 1977, p. 47.

Haden, Russell L. "The Origins of the Microscope." *Annals of Medical History* 1:30–44 (1939).

Majno, Guido. *The Healing Hand.* Cambridge, Mass.: Harvard University Press, 1975.

Nicolle, Jacques. *Louis Pasteur.* New York: Basic Books, 1961.

Reid, Robert. *Microbes and Men.* New York: E. P. Dutton & Company, Saturday Review Press, 1975.

Robinson, Victor. *Pathfinders in Medicine.* New York: Medical Life Press, 1929.

"The Microscope." *Encyclopaedia Britannica*. Chicago, 1975.

"The 30th Fatality." *Time,* November 29, 1976, p. 67.

Weise, E. Robert. "Semmelweis." *Annals of Medical History,* 2:80–88 (1930).

Young, Hugh Hampton. *A Surgeon's Autobiography.* New York: Harcourt, Brace and Company, 1940.

Chapter Five

Bender, George A. *Great Moments in Medicine*. Detroit: Northwood Institute Press, 1966.

Finney, J. M. T. *A Surgeon's Life*. New York: G. P. Putnam's Sons, 1940.

Franz, Caroline Jones. "Johns Hopkins." *American Heritage,* February 1976, pp. 31 ff.

Fulton, John F. *Harvey Cushing*. Springfield, Ill.: Charles C. Thomas, 1946.

Garraty, John A. *The American Nation*. New York: Harper & Row, 1966.

Graham, Harvey. *The Story of Surgery*. New York: Doubleday, Doran & Company, 1939.

Harvey, A. McGhee. *Adventures in Medical Research*. Baltimore: Johns Hopkins University Press, 1976.

———. "Harvey Williams Cushing: The Baltimore Period, 1896–1912." *The Johns Hopkins Medical Journal,* 138:196–216 (1976).

McCullough, David. "Steam Road to El Dorado." *American Heritage,* June 1976, pp. 54 ff.

Majno, Guido. *The Healing Hand*. Cambridge, Mass.: Harvard University Press, 1975.

Metz, Robert. "The Biggest Man in Broadcasting." *New York,* July 1975, p. 44.

Penfield, Wilder. "Halsted of Johns Hopkins." *Journal of the American Medical Association,* 210:2214–18 (1969).

Richardson, Robert G. *Surgery: Old and New Frontiers*. New York: Charles Scribner's Sons, 1968.

Sharpe, William. *Brain Surgeon*. New York: The Viking Press, 1952.

Young, Agatha. *Scalpel*. New York: Random House, 1956.

Young, Hugh Hampton. *A Surgeon's Autobiography.* New York: Harcourt, Brace and Company, 1940.

Chapter Six

Bettman, Otto. *A Pictorial History of Medicine.* Springfield, Ill.: Charles C. Thomas, 1956.

Bradbury, Saville. *The Evolution of the Microscope.* Oxford: Pergamon Press, 1967.

de Kruif, Paul. *Microbe Hunters.* New York: Harcourt, Brace and Company, 1926.

Krebs, Albin. "Dr. Paul de Kruif, Popularizer of Medical Exploits, Is Dead." New York *Times,* March 2, 1971.

McNeill, William. *Plagues and Peoples.* Garden City, N.Y.: Doubleday & Company, Inc., 1976.

"Malaria." In *The Merck Manual,* 12th ed. Rahway, N.J.: Merck & Company, 1972.

Marks, Geoffrey, and William K. Beatty. *The Medical Garden.* New York: Charles Scribner's Sons, 1971.

Nicolle, Jacques. *Louis Pasteur.* New York: Basic Books, 1961.

Pappenheimer, A. M. "The Diphtheria Bacilli and the Diphtheroid." In René Dubos and J. Hirsch, eds., *Bacterial and Mycotic Infections of Man,* 4th ed. Philadelphia: J. B. Lippincott, 1966.

Reid, Robert. *Microbes and Men.* New York: E. P. Dutton & Company, Saturday Review Press, 1975.

Robinson, Victor. *Pathfinders in Medicine.* New York: Medical Life Press, 1929.

Schorer, Mark. "Afterword." In Sinclair Lewis, *Arrowsmith.* New York: New American Library, 1961.

——. *Sinclair Lewis: An American Life.* New York: McGraw-Hill Book Company, 1961.

Talbott, John H. *A Biographical History of Medicine.* New York: Grune & Stratton, 1970.

Tobey, James A. *Riders of the Plagues.* New York: Charles Scribner's Sons, 1930.

Warshaw, Leon J. *Malaria: The Biography of a Killer.* New York: Rinehart & Company, Inc., 1949.

Chapter Seven

Bender, George A. *Great Moments in Medicine*. Detroit: Northwood Institute Press, 1975.

Bickel, Lennard. *Rise Up to Life*. New York: Charles Scribner's Sons, 1972.

Cartwright, Frederick F. *Disease and History*. New York: T. Y. Crowell & Company, 1972.

de Kruif, Paul. *Microbe Hunters*. New York: Harcourt, Brace and Company, 1926.

"Dr. Schatz Wins 3% of Royalty; Named Co-finder of Streptomycin." New York *Times*, December 30, 1950.

Epstein, Samuel, and Beryl Williams. *Miracles from Microbes*. New Brunswick, N.J.: Rutgers University Press, 1946.

Majno, Guido. *The Healing Hand*. Cambridge, Mass.: Harvard University Press, 1975.

Marx, Rudolph. *The Health of the Presidents*. New York: G. P. Putnam's Sons, 1960.

Reid, Robert. *Microbes and Men*. New York: E. P. Dutton & Co., 1975.

Robinson, Donald. *The Miracle Finders*. New York: David McKay Company, Inc., 1976.

Rosebury, Theodor. *Microbes and Morals*. New York: The Viking Press, 1971.

Schatz, A., E. Bugie, and S. Waksman. "Streptomycin, Substance Exhibiting Antibiotic Activity Against Gram Positive and Gram Negative Bacteria." *Proceedings of the Society for Experimental Biology and Medicine*, 55:66–69 (January 1944).

Schickel, Richard. *The Disney Version*. New York: Simon & Schuster, 1968.

"Streptomycin Profit Asked by Ex-student." New York *Times*, March 11, 1950.

"Streptomycin Suit Is Labeled 'Baseless.'" New York *Times*, March 13, 1950.

"Streptosettlement." *Time*, January 8, 1951, p. 32.

"Waksman Royalty Is Put at $350,000." New York *Times*, April 29, 1950.

Wilson, David. *In Search of Penicillin*. New York: Alfred A. Knopf, 1976.

Chapter Eight

Bean, William B. "Walter Reed and the Ordeal of Human Experiments." *Bulletin of the History of Medicine,* 51:75–92 (1977).

Beecher, Henry K. "Ethics and Clinical Research." *The New England Journal of Medicine,* 274:1354–60 (1966).

Cartwright, Frederick F. *Disease and History.* New York: T. Y. Crowell, 1972.

Dudar, Helen. "The Price of Blowing the Whistle." New York *Times Magazine,* October 30, 1977.

Gross, Ludwik. *Oncogenic Viruses,* 2nd ed. Oxford: Pergamon Press, 1970.

Harmetz, Aljean. *The Making of the Wizard of Oz.* New York: Alfred A. Knopf, 1977.

Henderson, Donald A. "The Eradication of Smallpox." *Scientific American,* October 1976.

Johnson, H. N. "Rabies Virus." In F. Horsfall and I. Tamm, eds., *Viral and Rickettsial Infections of Man,* 4th ed. Philadelphia: J. B. Lippincott, 1965, pp. 814–15.

Klein, Aaron E. *Trial by Fury.* New York: Charles Scribner's Sons, 1972.

Langer, William L. "Immunization Against Smallpox Before Jenner." *Scientific American,* January 1976.

McCullough, David. *The Path Between the Seas.* New York: Simon & Schuster, 1977.

McNeill, William H. *Plagues and Peoples.* Garden City, N.Y.: Doubleday & Company, Anchor Press, 1976.

Rapoport, Roger. *The Superdoctors.* Chicago: Playboy Press, 1975.

Robinson, Donald. *The Miracle Finders.* New York: David McKay Company, 1976.

Williams, Greer. *Virus Hunters.* New York: Alfred A. Knopf, 1959.

———. *The Plague Killers.* New York: Charles Scribner's Sons, 1969.

Chapter Nine

Bender, George A. *Great Moments in Medicine.* Detroit: Northwood Institute Press, 1974.

Forssmann, Werner. *Experiments on Myself.* New York: St. Martin's Press, 1974.

Gordon, Richard, et al. "Image Reconstructions From Projections." *Scientific American,* October 1975, pp. 56–58.

Grigg, E. R. N. *The Trail of the Invisible Light.* Springfield, Ill.: Charles C. Thomas, 1965.

Reid, Robert. *Marie Curie.* New York: E. P. Dutton, 1974.

Shiers, George. "The Induction Coil." *Scientific American,* May 1971, pp. 80–87.

Chapter Ten

Bender, George A. *Great Moments in Medicine.* Detroit: Northwood Institute Press, 1974.

Diabetes. Kalamazoo: Upjohn Laboratories, 1965.

Diabetes Mellitus, 7th ed. Indianapolis: Eli Lilly Research Laboratories, 1967.

Murray, Ian. "Paulesco and the Isolation of Insulin." *Journal of the History of Medicine and Allied Sciences,* 26:150–57 (1971).

Swan, Clark T. *The Hormones.* Boston: Little, Brown & Company, 1969.

Index